Instant Clinical Diagnosis in Ophthalmology

Lens Diseases

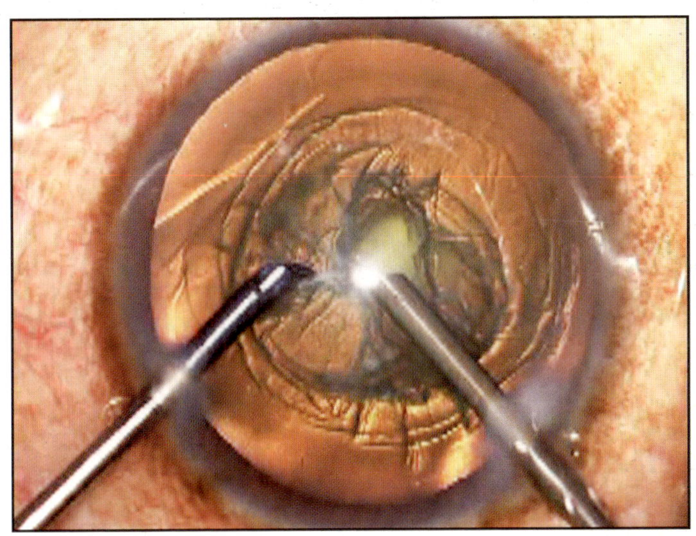

INSTANT CLINICAL DIAGNOSIS IN OPHTHALMOLOGY

LENS DISEASES

Series Editors

Ashok Garg MS PhD FIAO(Bel)
FRSM FAIMS ADM FICA
International and National Gold Medalist
Chairman and Medical Director
Garg Eye Institute and Research Centre
235-Model Town, Dabra Chowk
Hisar-125 005 (India)

Emanuel Rosen MD
Medical Director
Rosen Eye Associates
Harbour City
Salford Quays
M50 3 BH, UK

Editors

Gian Maria Cavallini MD
Director
Institute of Ophthalmology,
University of Modena and Reggio Emilia
via del Pozzo 71-41100, Modena
Italy

Arturo Perez Arteaga MD
Medical Director
Centro Oftalmologico Tlalnepantla
Dr Perez-Arteaga Vallarta No 42
Tlalnepantla, Centro,
Estado de, Mexico, 54000, Mexico

Boris Malyugin MD PhD
Chief of Department of Cataract and
Implant Surgery
Deputy Director General
S Fyodorov Eye Microsurgery
Complex State Institution
Beskundnikovsky blvd 59A
127486 Moscow, Russia

Bojan Pajic MD
Chief Corneal and
Refractive Surgery
Department Vision Care
Klinik Pallas
Louis Giroud
Str.20, 4600 Olten
Switzerland

Foreword
Robert J Weinstock

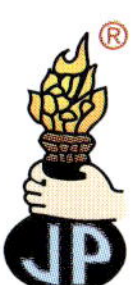

JAYPEE BROTHERS MEDICAL PUBLISHERS (P) LTD

New Delhi • Ahmedabad • Bengaluru • Chennai • Hyderabad
Kochi • Kolkata • Lucknow • Mumbai • Nagpur • St Louis (USA)

Published by

Jitendar P Vij
Jaypee Brothers Medical Publishers (P) Ltd

Corporate Office
4838/24 Ansari Road, Daryaganj, **New Delhi** 110 002, India, +91-11-43574357

Registered Office
B-3 EMCA House, 23/23B Ansari Road, Daryaganj, **New Delhi** 110 002, India
Phones: +91-11-23272143, +91-11-23272703, +91-11-23282021,
+91-11-23245672, Rel: +91-11-32558559 Fax: +91-11-23276490, +91-11-23245683
e-mail: jaypee@jaypeebrothers.com, Visit our website: www.jaypeebrothers.com

Branches

- 2/B, Akruti Society, Jodhpur Gam Road Satellite
  Ahmedabad 380 015 Phones: +91-79-26926233, Rel: +91-79-32988717
  Fax: +91-79-26927094 e-mail: ahmedabad@jaypeebrothers.com
- 202 Batavia Chambers, 8 Kumara Krupa Road, Kumara Park East
  Bengaluru 560 001 Phones: +91-80-22285971, +91-80-22382956,
  +91-80-22372664, Rel: +91-80-32714073
  Fax: +91-80-22281761 e-mail: bangalore@jaypeebrothers.com
- 282 IIIrd Floor, Khaleel Shirazi Estate, Fountain Plaza, Pantheon Road
  Chennai 600 008 Phones: +91-44-28193265, +91-44-28194897,
  Rel: +91-44-32972089 Fax: +91-44-28193231 e-mail: chennai@jaypeebrothers.com
- 4-2-1067/1-3, 1st Floor, Balaji Building, Ramkote Cross Road
  Hyderabad 500 095 Phones: +91-40-66610020,
  +91-40-24758498, Rel:+91-40-32940929
  Fax:+91-40-24758499, e-mail: hyderabad@jaypeebrothers.com
- No. 41/3098, B & B1, Kuruvi Building, St. Vincent Road
  Kochi 682 018, Kerala Phones: +91-484-4036109, +91-484-2395739,
  +91-484-2395740 e-mail: kochi@jaypeebrothers.com
- 1-A Indian Mirror Street, Wellington Square
  Kolkata 700 013 Phones: +91-33-22651926, +91-33-22276404,
  +91-33-22276415, Rel: +91-33-32901926
  Fax: +91-33-22656075, e-mail: kolkata@jaypeebrothers.com
- Lekhraj Market III, B-2, Sector-4, Faizabad Road, Indira Nagar
  Lucknow 226 016 Phones: +91-522-3040553, +91-522-3040554
  e-mail: lucknow@jaypeebrothers.com
- 106 Amit Industrial Estate, 61 Dr SS Rao Road, Near MGM Hospital, Parel
  Mumbai 400012 Phones: +91-22-24124863, +91-22-24104532,
  Rel: +91-22-32926896 Fax: +91-22-24160828, e-mail: mumbai@jaypeebrothers.com
- "KAMALPUSHPA" 38, Reshimbag, Opp. Mohota Science College, Umred Road
  Nagpur 440 009 (MS) Phone: Rel: +91-712-3245220,
  Fax: +91-712-2704275 e-mail: nagpur@jaypeebrothers.com

USA Office
1745, Pheasant Run Drive, Maryland Heights (Missouri), MO 63043, USA,
Ph: 001-636-6279734
e-mail: jaypee@jaypeebrothers.com, anjulav@jaypeebrothers.com

Instant Clinical Diagnosis in Ophthalmology (Lens Diseases)

First Edition: **2009**

ISBN: 978-81-8448-482-3

Typeset at JPBMP typesetting unit
Printed at Ajanta Offset & Packagings Ltd., New Delhi

Dedicated to

— My Respected Param Pujya Guru Sant Gurmeet Ram Rahim Singh Ji for his blessings and motivation
— My Respected parents, teachers, my wife Dr Aruna Garg, son Abhishek and daughter Anshul for their constant support and patience during all these days of hard work
— My dear friend Dr Amar Agarwal, a renowned International Ophthalmologist for his constant support, guidance and expertise

— Ashok Garg

The memory of my step daughter Nicola Ross who enjoyed benefits from refractive surgery, were cut short by a tragic fatal illness

— Emanuel Rosen

I dedicate my work to all the people in the world with ophthalmic diseases, with the best wish to improve our quality of care with this kind of material. I also dedicate this opus to Prof Ashok Garg, because he has trusted me a lot

— Arturo Perez Arteaga

To my father Edvard Malyugin for everything and to my wife Natalia for her continuous support and love

— Boris Malyugin

To my son Valentin Aleksandar

— Bojan Pajic

Contributors

A Dhivya MS
Dr. Agarwal's Eye Hospital
19, Cathedral Road
Chennai 600 086, India

AK Grover MD FRCS
Chairman
Department of Ophthalmology,
Sir Gangaram Hospital
Rajinder Nagar
New Delhi
India

Alejandro Tello MD
Centro Oftalmologico Virgilio Galvis
Bucaramanga, Santander
Colombia

Amar Agarwal MS, FRCS, FRC Ophth
Consultant
Dr Agarwal's Eye Hospital
19, Cathedral Road
Chennai 600 086, India

Armando Capote MD
Vice Chairman Microsurgery Center
Cuban Institute of Ophthalmology
Ramon Pando Ferrer
Havana
Cuba

Arturo Perez Arteaga MD
Medical Director
Centro Oftalmologico Tlalnepantla
Dr. Perez Arteaga Vallarta no. 42
Tlalnepantla, Centro, Estado de Mexico
54000, Mexico

Ashok Garg MS PhD FRSM
Chairman and Medical Director
Garg Eye Institute and Research Centre
235-Model Town, Dabra Chowk
Hisar 125 005 (India)

Athiya Agarwal MD, DO, FRSH
Consultant
Dr. Agarwal's Eye Hospital
19, Cathedral Road
Chennai 600 086, India

Bassam El Kady MD
Faculty of Medicine
Ain Shams University and
Clinical Research Fellow
Vissum-Instituto Oftalmologico de Alicante
Department of Research and Development
Alicante, Spain

Bojan Pajic MD
Department of Ophthalmology
Vedis, Klinik Pallas
4600 Olten
Switzerland

Boris Malyugin MD PhD
Chief of Department of Cataract and Implant Surgery
Dy Director General
S. Fyodorov Eye Microsurgery
complex State Institution
127486 Moscow
Beskudnikovsky blvd 59A
Russia

Brigitte Pajic Eggspuehler MD
AugenZentrumPajic (AZP) Research Institute
Titlisstrasse 44, 5734
Reinach, Switzerland

C Cheisi MD
Institute of Ophthalmology
University of Modena and Reggio Emilia
via del Pozzo 71-41100, Modena
Italy

Chandresh Baid MS
Dr Agarwal's Eye Hospital
19, Cathedral Road
Chennai 600 086, India

Cristina Masini MD
Institute of Ophthalmology
University of Modena and Reggio Emilia
via del Pozzo 71-41100, Modena
Italy

Cyres K Mehta MS FSVH FAGE
Director and Consultant
Mehta International Eye Institute
Seaside, 147, Colaba Road
Mumbai 400 005, India

Elizabeth A Davis MD
Minnesota Eye Consultants
9117, Lyndale Aves, Bloomington
MN 55420, USA

Emanuel Rosen MD
Medical Director
Rosen Eye Associates
Harbour Cty
Salford Quays
M50 - 3 BH, UK

Eneida de la C Perez MD
Cuban Institute of Ophthalmology
Ramon Pando Ferrer
Havana, Cuba

Forrest Fleming MD
Cataract and Refractive Surgeon
The Eye Institute of West Florida
148, 12th Street SW
Largo, Florida 33770, USA

Frederic Hehn MD
Centre de La Vision
Nations Vision
23, Boulevard de l'europe
54500 Vandoeuvre, France

Gauri Nagpal MD
Senior Resident
Department of Ophthalmology
Sir Gangaram Hospital
Rajinder Nagar, New Delhi
India

Gian Maria Cavallini MD
Director
Institute of Ophthalmology
University of Modena and Reggio Emilia
via del Pozzo 71-41100, Modena
Italy

Hiroshi Tsuneoka MD
Associate Professor
Deptt of Ophthalmology
Jikei University Daisan Hospital
4-11-1, Izumihoncho, Komae
Tokyo 201-8601, Japan

Jasna Ljubic MD
General Hospital
Department of Physical Medicine and
Rehabilitation, 16000, Leskovac
Serbia, Switzerland

Jorge L Alio MD PhD
Instituto Oftalmologico De Alicante
Avda. Denia 111, 03015
Alicante, Spain

Jose L Rodriguez Prats MD PhD
Consultant Ophthalmologist
Instituto Oftalmologico De Alicante
Alicante, Spain

P Kaushik MBBS
Doctor Eye Institute
Spenta Mansion, Ist floor,
SV Road, Andher (W), Mumbai

Kayo Nishi MD
Nishi Eye Hospital
Osaka, Japan

Keiki Mehta MS DO FIOS
Chairman and Medical Director
Mehta International Eye Institute
147, Shahid Bhagat Singh Road
Colaba Road
Mumbai 400 005, India

Kumar J Doctor MD
MS (Ophth), DNB (Ophth)
Doctor Eye Institute
Spenta Mansion, Ist floor,
SV Road, Andher (W)
Mumbai

Luca Campi MD
Institute of Ophthalmology
University of Modena and Reggio Emilia, via del Pozzo 71-41100, Modena, Italy

Luis Felipe Vejarano MD
Medico Oftalmologo
Fundacion Oftalmologica Vejarano
Nacional Bascom Palmer Eye Institute
Carrera 3, No. 5-54
Popayan, Cauca-Colombia
South America
572-8241926

Marcelino Rio MD
Cuban Institute of Ophthalmology
Ramon Pando Ferrer
Havana, Cuba

Okihiro Nishi MD
Director
Nishi Eye Hospital
Osaka, Japan

Pawel Klonowski MD PhD
Vissum-Instituto Oftalmologico de Alicante, Department of Research and Development, Alicante, Spain

Peter W Reick MD
Director der Augenklinik
Charite-Universitatsmedizine
Berlin
Campus Virchow Klinikum
Augustenburger Platz 1
13353, Berlin
Germany

Richard L Lindstrom MD
Minnesota Eye Consultants, PA
710 East, 24th Street, Suite 106,
Minneapolis, MN 55404
USA

Roberto Bellucci MD
Chief of Ophthalmic Unit
Hospital of Verona
University of Verona
Italy

Robert J Weinstock MD
Director
Cataract and Refractive Surgeon
The Eye Institute of West Florida
148, 12th Street SW
Largo, Florida 33770
USA

Roberto Pinelli MD
Director
Istituto Laser Microchirurgia Oculare
Crystal Palace
Via Cefalonia, 70
25124 Brescia
Italy

Rohit Om Parkash MS
Director
Dr. Om Parkash Eye Institute
117-A, The Mall
Amritsar
India

Rupesh V Agrawal MD
Consultant
Comprehensive Ophthalmology
Uveitis and Ocular Trauma
LV Prasad Eye Institute
Kallam Anjil Reddy Campus
Banjara Hills
Hyderabad 500 034
India

Satish Desai MD
Comprehensive Ophthalmology
Uveitis and Ocular Trauma
LV Prasad Eye Institute
Kallam Anjil Reddy Campus
Banjara Hills
Hyderabad 500 034
India

Shaloo Bageja MS
Consultant
Ophthalmologist
Department of Ophthalmology
Sir Gangaram Hospital
Rajinder Nagar
New Delhi
India

Shiao Chang MD
Nishi Eye Hospital
Osaka, Japan

Shilpa Kodkany MS
Asst Professor of Ophthalmology
JN Medical College, Belgaum

Simonetta Morselli MD
Director
Anterior Segment Surgery
Ophthalmic Unit
Hospital of Verona
University of Verona, Italy

Simone Pelloni MD
Institute of Ophthalmology
University of Modena and Reggio Emilia
via del Pozzo 71-41100,
Modena, Italy

SK Gibran MD
Consultant
St Paul's Eye Unit
Royal Liverpool University Hospital
Prescot Street
Liverpoor - L 78 XP, UK

Soosan Jacob MS
Dr Agarwal's Eye Hospital
19, Cathedral Road
Chennai 600 086
India

Stephen M Weinstock MD
Cataract and Refractive Surgeon
The Eye Institute of West Florida
148, 12th Street SW
Largo, Florida 33770
USA

Sunita Agarwal MS DO PSVH
Dr Agarwal's Eye Hospital
19, Cathedral Road,
Chennai 600 086
India

Yutaro Nishi MD
Nishi Eye Hospital
Osaka
Japan

Foreword

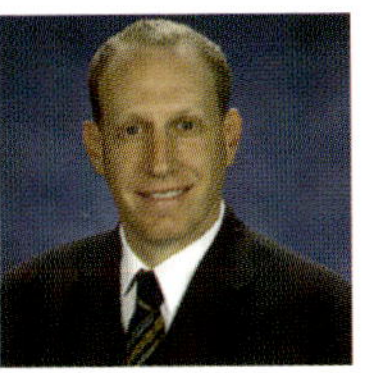

As Ophthalmologists and Cataract Surgeons, we are all fascinated by the human lens. When I was a young medical school student, I vaguely remember one small section in the anatomy and physiology textbook discussing the human lens. Then there was embryology, which maybe, gave a little more attention to this tiny part of the body and two pages was devoted to the topic.

Now, many of us find that our daily life revolves around this complex delicate tissue that is so vital to the visual system. We look at the lens many times a day under high magnification at the slit lamp. We spend countless hours in the operating room carefully trying to remove cataracts without damaging other parts of the delicate eye. And of course, the ophthalmic industry and surgeons are continuously trying to replicate the crystalline lens and reproduce artificial lens for implantation in the human eye that functions like the natural lens.

Regarding lenticular surgery, it is hard to imagine that there is another subspecialty in medicine that has improved and evolved so rapidly. Within a few decades, cataract removal in developed countries has gone from a high risk and high morbidity procedure to possibly the safest and most efficient surgery available with such a dramatic effect on quality of life.

We are extremely grateful to Dr Ashok Garg and his co-editors for assembling this thorough and definitive textbook on the human lens and lenticular surgery. Seldom do you find a reference so complete, starting with the basics of clinical lenticular disease and finishing with state-of-the-art advanced surgical techniques for lens removal.

His panel of international experts have dissected every facet of the human lens and presented highly detailed and informative chapters. By tapping into resources and perspectives from around the globe, Dr Garg and his co-editors have provided the most comprehensive and encompassing lens textbook available.

Whether you are a novice Ophthalmologist who is just beginning to explore the depths of cataract surgery, or a well-seasoned Cataract Surgeon who is looking to add new techniques and improve your results, you will find this reference to be a valuable companion. Through the efforts of leading surgeons from around the world, we are able to benefit from their experience and allow patients to receive better care.

Dr Robert J Weinstock MD
Cataract and Refractive Surgeon
The Eye Institute of West Florida
148 13th Street SW Largo, Florida 33770, USA
Tel. : 001-727- 585-6644, E-mail : RJWeinstock@yahoo.com

Preface

The modern day busy and fast life Ophthalmologists are glued to their clinical and surgical practice and have little time to read large volume books. The need of hour is to have a pocket size ready reckoner enriched with complete and up-to-date information of diseases in a most comprehensive manner. At present, very few Quality Ready Reference Books are available at an International level.

After a detailed research and according to the need of Ophthalmologists, we have developed a series of 10 Volume Ready Reference Books termed as Instant Clinical Diagnosis in Ophthalmology. This series covers Oculoplastic and Reconstructive Surgery, Retina, Lens, Glaucoma, Refractive Surgery, Pediatric Ophthalmology, Strabismus, Anterior Segment Diseases, Cornea and Neuro-ophthalmology. The present series has been designed to provide up-to-date information of concerned diseases in a comprehensive and lucid manner along with high quality clinical photographs in an easy to read format. International Masters of concerned subject have contributed chapters in this series covering pathophysiology, clinical signs and symptoms, investigations, differential diagnosis, treatment and prognosis in a simplified manner.

This volume deals with Lens Diseases. Section 1 deals with clinical aspects of various types of lens diseases. Congenital and developmental anomalies, various senile cataracts, traumatic cataracts, complicated and dismetabolic cataracts are covered nicely in this section. Section 2 deals with special surgical aspects of lens diseases available today. International experts have covered microphaco, micro coaxial, biaxial, torsional phaco and 3-D cataract surgery comprehensively for the benefit of the readers. The unique concept of combining clinical and surgical aspects of lens diseases is to have an edit attraction of this volume.

We are highly thankful to our publisher M/s Jaypee Brothers Medical Publishers (P) Ltd. specially Sh. Jitendar P Vij (CEO), Mr. Tarun Duneja (Director, Publishing) and all staff members for their dedication and hard efforts put in the preparation of High Quality Series of Instant Clinical Books.

We hope this 10 volume set of ready reference pocket size books shall provide complete and useful clinical information to Ophthalmologists all around the world and shall help them accurately and precisely diagnose, treat and manage their clinical case confidently to the satisfaction and expectations of their valued patients. We also hope this Ready Reckoner shall serve as a useful companion onto every clinician desk.

Editors

Contents

SECTION 1
LENS DISEASES (CLINICAL)

SECTION 2
LENS DISEASES (SURGICAL)

Lens Diseases (Clinical)

Section **1**

1

Congenital Lens Anomalies

- **Congenital Lens Anomalies**
  Bojan Pajic, Brigitte Pajic-Eggspuehler
  Jasna Ljubic (Switzerland)
- **Congenital Cataract**
  Arturo Perez Arteaga (Mexico)

Congenital Lens Anomalies

Bojan Pajic, Brigitte Pajic-Eggspuehler, Jasna Ljubic
(Switzerland)

Lenticonus Posterior

KEY FACTS

- Can be associated with persistent hyperplastic primary vitreous (PHPV)
- Ectasia of the posterior lens surface
- Commonly bilateral, not always symmetric
- Frequently associate with cataract

CLINICAL FINDINGS

- Myopia and astigmatism, frequently progressive in power and axis
- Monocular diplopia and anisometropia
- Visual acuity decreasing
- Cataract
- Amplyopia

ANCILLARY TESTING

- Biomicroscopy with the slitlamp
- Topographic
- Wavefront analysis

DIFFERENTIAL DIAGNOSIS

- Keratoconus
- Cataract without ectasia
- Myopia magna with retinal astigmatism
- Megalocornea
- Megalophthalmus anterior
- Microspherophakie
- Ectopia lentis

TREATMENT

- **Mild expression**
- Prescribe best optical correction
- May tolerated contact lenses for ever in cases of an isometropia and advanced myopia and astigmatism
- Amblyopia treatment

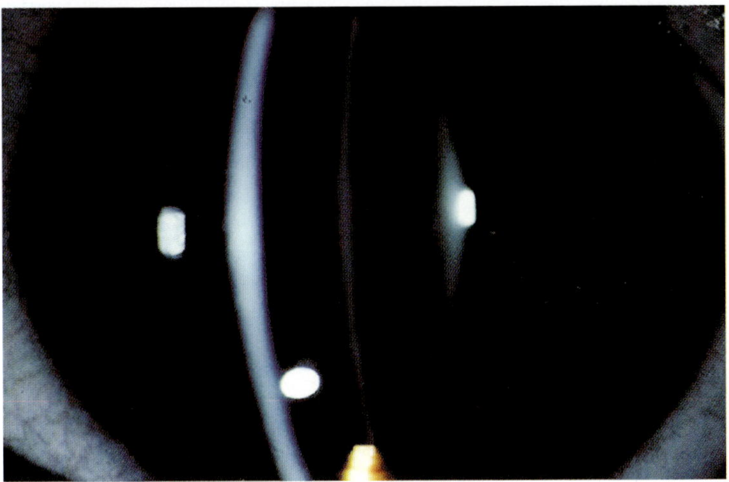

Fig. 1: Lenticonus posterior

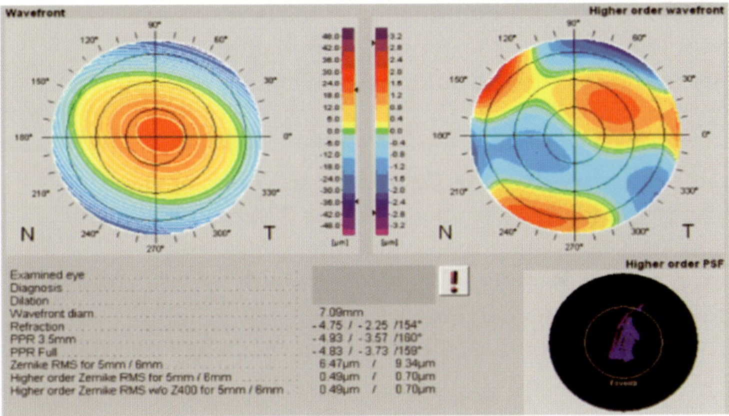

Fig. 2: Wavefront analysis of a lenticonus posterior. The PSF prove a higher order aberration. Topography analysis of the same patient is regular (here not shown)

- **Advanced expression**
- Cataract surgery with implantation of an intraocular lens depending of the patient age
- Amblyopia treatment
- Options for rehabilitation are best optical correction with classes, contact lens correction, intraocular lens implantation

PROGNOSIS

- Significant visual impairment is unusual
- If not treated early in the childhood an amblyopia may lead to a significant visual acuity decrease

Lentiglobus

KEY FACTS

- Lentiglobus is a spheric deformation of the lens surface
- Posterior lentiglobus (90%), typically a unilateral condition
- Usually involves only the outermost layers of the adult nucleus and the cortex
- A hyaloid remnant is often, but not always, seen adherent to the globus
- The rarer anterior lenticonus (lentiglobus) is often bilateral
- An opacity is usually associated with the defect
- Lentiglobus is associated with congenital glaucoma
- Anterior polar cataracts, posterior lentiglobus, and unilateral PHPV generally are not associated with a systemic disorder
- In a child who is otherwise healthy, approximately one-third of cataract cases are idiopathic

CLINICAL FINDINGS

- Associated with opacities in the region of the bulge of the posterior lentiglobus
- Visual acuity decrease
- Binocular visual function decrease
- Strabismus
- Amplyopia
- Pendular nystagmus

ANCILLARY TESTING

- Biomicroscopy investigation with the slitlamp
- Skiascopy
- Stereo Test Lang, Hirschberg-Test, Brueckner-Test
- Best visual acuity measurement, Moiré measurement

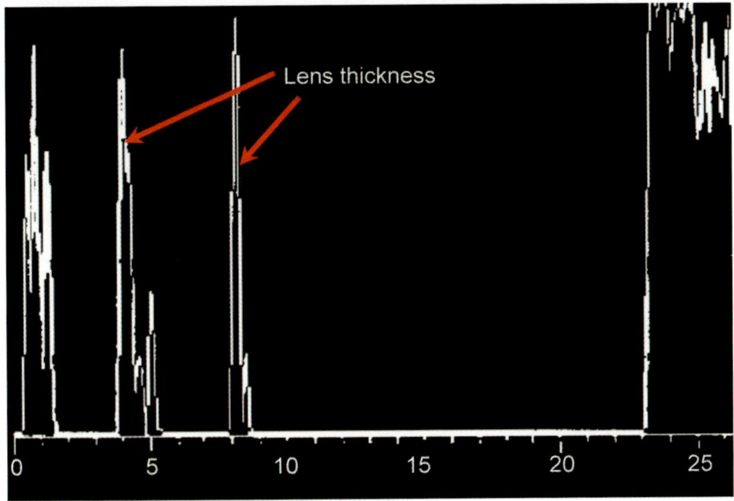

Fig. 3: Ultrasound biometry shows a very lens thickness in the case of lentiglobus

- Systemic metabolic investigation
- Glaucoma exclusion
- Ultrasound examination
- In the case of a congenital cataract in an otherwise healthy child, galactokinase deficiency must be excluded
- Fifty percent of all hereditary cataracts are new mutations
- Between 8.3% and 23% of cataracts are familial, with autosomal dominant heredity being the most frequent mode of inheritance

DIFFERENTIAL DIAGNOSIS

- Leukokorie
- Any opacity in the anterior segment
- Lenticonus anterior and posterior

TREATMENT

- Pediatric consultation for treatment the basis desease, i.e. galactosemia
- Treatment of a associated eye desease, i.e. congenital glaucoma
- Amblyopia treatment for child younger than 10 years old
- In cases with a central lens opacity, a trial of a long-acting cycloplegic agent may be used to improve visual acuity
- Cataract surgery with implantation of an intraocular lens depending of the patient age with days or weeks after diagnosis if the opacity is clinical relevant
- Importance of capsulorhexis posterior with vitrectomy anterior performance during cataract surgery of juvenile cataract
- Options for rehabilitation are best optical correction with classes, contact lens correction, intraocular lens implantation

PROGNOSIS

- Significant visual impairment is unusual
- If not treated early in the childhood an amblyopia may lead to a significant visual acuity decrease

Lens Coloboma

KEY FACTS

- Lens has a natural tendency to assume a more spherical shape
- This phenomenon accounts for accommodation, when the circular muscle of the ciliary body contracts, allowing the zonules to relax
- This tendency probably also explains lens coloboma, in which the lens zonules are missing in the area of a ciliary body coloboma and the lens appears notched in that area

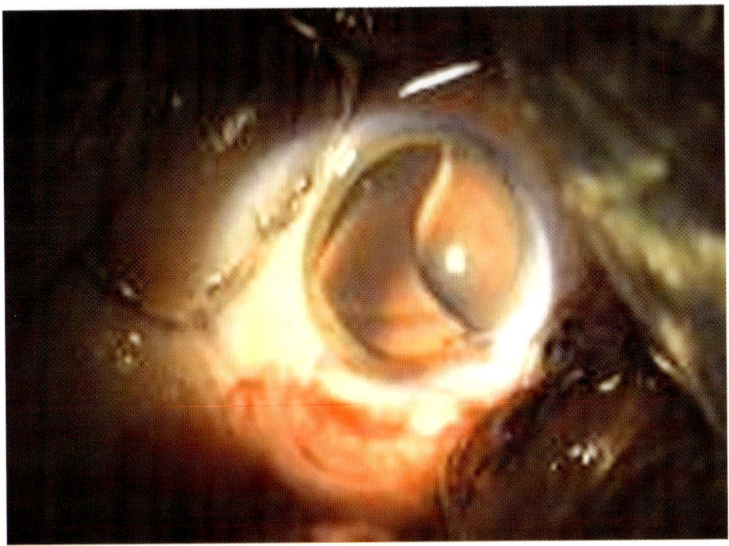

Fig. 4: Lens coloboma

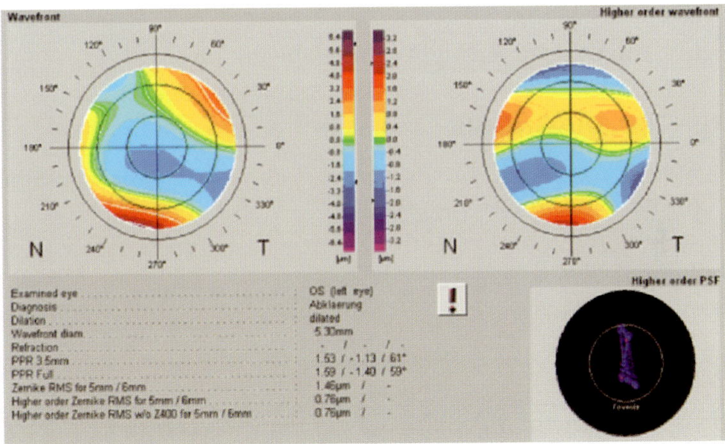

Fig. 5: Higher order aberration analysis of lens coloboma

- Because there are no zonules in the area of the coloboma, the lens takes on its more natural spherical shape, forming a notch in this area.

CLINICAL FINDINGS

- Spherical shape
- Refraction may get more myope
- Decrease of accomodation
- Visual acuity decrease
- Binocular visual function decrease
- Amblyopia may occur
- Diplopia

ANCILLARY TESTING

- Biomicroscopy investigation with the slitlamp
- Looking for lentodonesis
- Skiascopy
- Best visual acuity measurement, Moiré measurement
- Ultrasound examination inclusively with measurement of the lens thickness
- Wavefront analysis of the higher order aberration

DIFFERENTIAL DIAGNOSIS

- Leukokorie
- Any opacity in the anterior segment
- Lenticonus anterior and posterior
- Lentiglobus
- Primary lentodonesis

TREATMENT

- Amblyopia treatment for child younger than 10 years old
- Best possible correction with glasses or contact lenses before surgery. If the visual acuity is not satisfying than cataract surgery is suggest.
- In cases with a central lens opacity, a trial of a long-acting cycloplegic agent may be used to improve visual acuity.
- Cataract surgery with implantation of an intraocular lens depending of the patient age with days or weeks after diagnosis if the opacity is clinical relevant
- Importance of capuslorhexis posterior with vitrectomy anterior performance during cataract surgery of juvenile cataract
- Options for rehabilitation are best optical correction with classes, contact lens correction, intraocular lens implantation

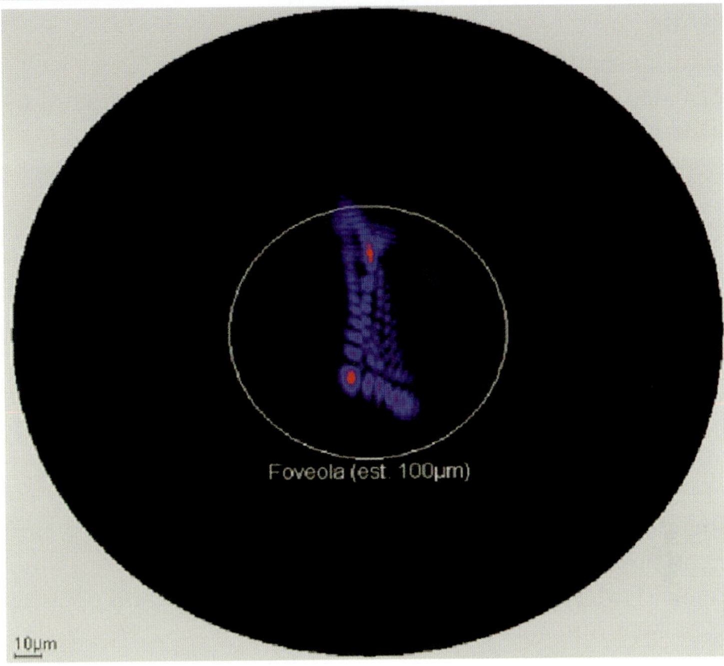

Fig. 6: PSF HOA analysis which shows two focal points with consecutive diplopia

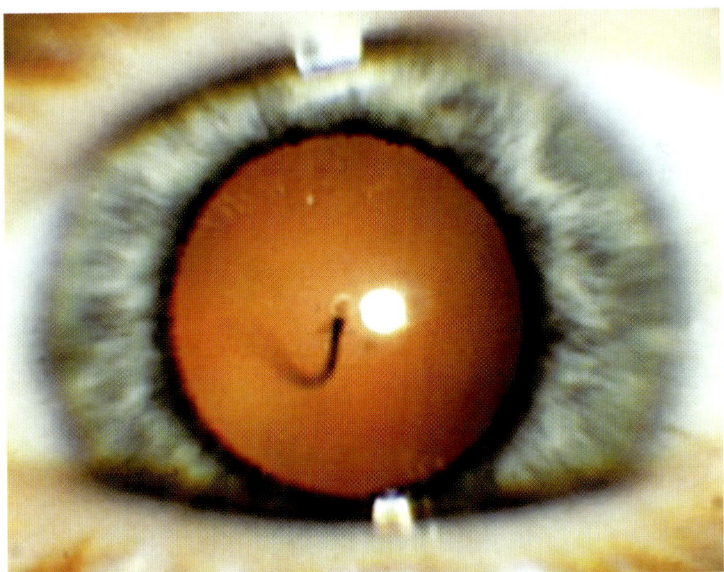

Fig. 7: Mittendorf dot

PROGNOSIS

- Significant visual impairment is unusual
- If not treated early in the childhood an amblyopia may lead to a significant visual acuity decrease

Mittendorf Dot

KEY FACTS

- A failure to retract the anterior portion of the hyaloid artery completely may result in the formation on the posterior capsule of the lens
- Evidence of remnants of the hyaloid artery can be found in most patients
- In about 10% of all children, the attachment of the hyaloid artery can be seen on the posterior lens capsule inferior and slightly nasal to the posterior pole
- A Mittendorf dot, also called spurious posterior polar cataract, can be fairly large and appear as a round, dense capsular opacity.
- The hyaloid artery can be seen in premature infants, and occasionally the vessel persists into adult life

CLINICAL FINDINGS

- A ophthalmoscopically, a persistent hyaloid artery appears as a single vessel extending from the optic disk anteriorly through Cloquet's canal.
- It may be filled with blood but usually is bloodless after birth and can extend as far anteriorly as the posterior capsule of the lens
- Usually, the insertion on the posterior capsule is located inferonasal to the visual axis
- Occasionally, after the vessel has regressed, only the circular point of insertion remains
- A remnant of the posterior primary vitreous can occasionally be identified on the optic disk.
- This remnant, representing the embryonic point of exit of the hyaloid vascular system from the optic nerve head, is known as Bergmeister's papilla
- Visual acuity decrease can be seen in dependency of the position of the hyaloid artery at the posterior lens membrane
- An amplyopia can occur

ANCILLARY TESTING

- Biomicroscopy investigation with the slitlamp
- Skiascopy
- Best visual acuity measurement, Moiré measurement

DIFFERENTIAL DIAGNOSIS

- Any opacity in the anterior segment
- Lenticonus posterior

TREATMENT

- Best possible correction with glasses or contact lenses
- Amblyopia treatment for child younger than 10 years old

PROGNOSIS

The condition rarely interferes with vision.

Congenital Cataract

Arturo Perez Arteaga (Mexico)

Introduction

A congenital cataract is an opacification of the lens present at birth. Not all cataracts are visually significant, but if a lenticular opacity is located in the visual axis, it is considered visually significant and because may lead to blindness, should require treatment. If the cataract is small, in the anterior portion of the lens, or in the periphery, no visual loss may be present; a close monitoring long-life is mandatory.

Investigation

The lens forms during the invagination of surface ectoderm overlying the optic vesicle. The embryonic nucleus develops by the sixth week of gestation. Surrounding the embryonic nucleus is the fetal nucleus. At birth, the embryonic and fetal nuclei make up most of the lens. In the postnatal period, cortical lens fibers are laid down from the conversion of anterior lens epithelium into cortical lens fibers. Unilateral cataracts are usually isolated sporadic incidents. They can be associated with ocular abnormalities (e.g. posterior lenticonus, persistent hyperplasic primary vitreous, anterior segment digenesis, and posterior pole tumors), trauma, or intrauterine infection, particularly rubella. Bilateral cataracts are often inherited and associated with other diseases. They require a full metabolic, infectious, systemic, and genetic investigation. The common causes are hypoglycemia, trisomy (e.g. Down's, Edwards' and Patau's syndromes), myotonic dystrophy, infectious diseases (e.g. toxoplasmosis, rubella, cytomegalovirus, and herpes simplex), and prematurity.

Differential Diagnosis

All close family members should be examined. Infectious causes of cataracts should be investigate and include rubella (the most common), chickenpox, cytomegalovirus, herpes simplex, herpes zoster, poliomyelitis, influenza, Epstein-Barr virus, syphilis, and toxoplasmosis. In unilateral cataracts, prenatal and family history should be taken; slitlamp examination in both eyes (dilated pupil); dilated fundus examination; laboratory studies include TORCH titers and VDRL test, are mandatory. In bilateral cataracts, prenatal and family history, slitlamp examination in both eyes (dilated pupil), dilated fundus examination, genetics evaluation and laboratory studies include CBC, BUN, TORCH titers, VDRL, urine for reducing substances, red cell galactokinase, urine for amino acids, calcium, and phosphorus.

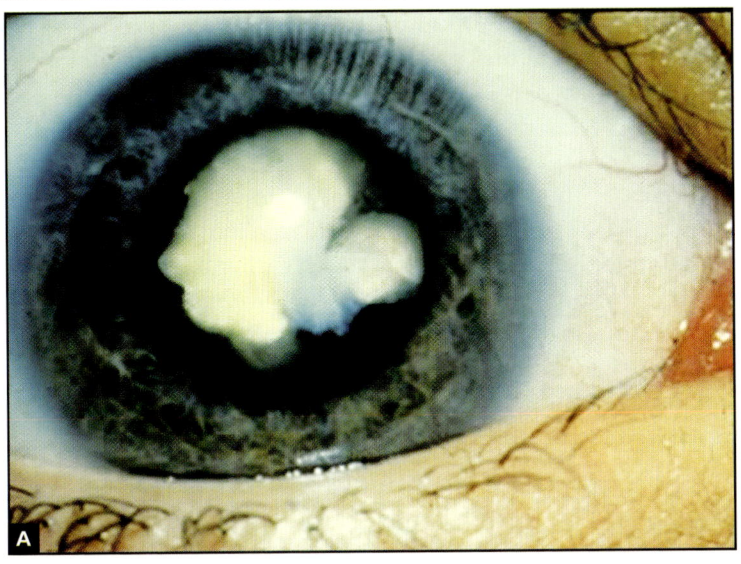

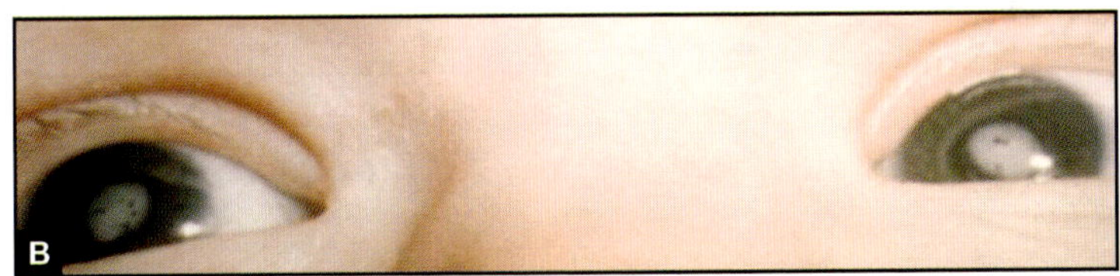

Figs 1A and B: Congenital cataract

Some other causes of leukokoria should be excluded like persistent hyperplasic primary vitreous, prematurity retinopathy and retinoblastoma.

Treatment

Cataract surgery is the treatment of choice and should be performed when patients are younger than 17 weeks to ensure minimal or no visual deprivation. Most ophthalmologists opt for surgery much earlier, ideally when patients are younger than 2 months, to prevent irreversible amblyopia and sensory nystagmus in the case of bilateral congenital cataracts. The delay in surgery is because of fear to glaucoma, since glaucoma occurs in 10% of congenital cataract surgery. A link to long-term visual rehabilitation is mandatory; the patient must be followed up, during the entire life.

Prognosis

Congenital cataracts usually are diagnosed at birth. If a cataract goes undetected in an infant, permanent visual loss may ensue. Of persons with unilateral cataracts, 40% develop vision of 20/60 or better. Of persons with bilateral congenital cataracts, 70% develop vision of 20/60 or better. Prognosis is poorer in persons with other ocular or systemic involvement.

2

Developmental Lens Abnormalities

- **Developmental Lens Abnormalities**
  Arturo Perez Arteaga (Mexico)
- **Management of Ectopia Lentis**
  SK Gibran (UK)

Developmental Lens Abnormalities

Arturo Perez Arteaga (Mexico)

Introduction

Developmental cataract is a type of small cataract in youth, resulting from heredity, malnutrition, toxicity, or inflammation, seldom affecting vision. Types are as follows:

1. Punctate
   a. Blue dot
   b. Sutural
   c. Central pulvurental
2. Zonular
3. Fusiform
4. Nuclear
5. Coronary
6. Anterior capsular (Polar)
7. Posterior capsular (Polar)

INVESTIGATIONS

Etiology can include maternal (and infantile) malnutrition, maternal viral infection (e.g. Rubella), placental hemorrhage causing deficient fetal oxygenation, hypocalcemia, chromosomal abnormality (e.g. Down's syndrome) and metabolic disorders (e.g. galactosemia). In some cases the cause can remain unknown.

CLINICAL SIGNS AND SYMPTOMS

Symptoms

The informant, usually parents talk about a history of white spot at the pupillary area. The child is usually brought with history of diminution of vision referring that is unable to follow or recognize objects and parents. Some other symptoms can be unsteady and deviated eyes. Associated symptoms of systemic disease, if present, are usually recognized.

Signs

Decreased visual acuity, many times difficult to establish in very young children, lenticular opacity (leukokoria), nystagmus, deviation of eye, usually convergent strabismus. There may be other ocular and systemic abnormalities in cases of rubella nuclear cataract or other systemic conditions.

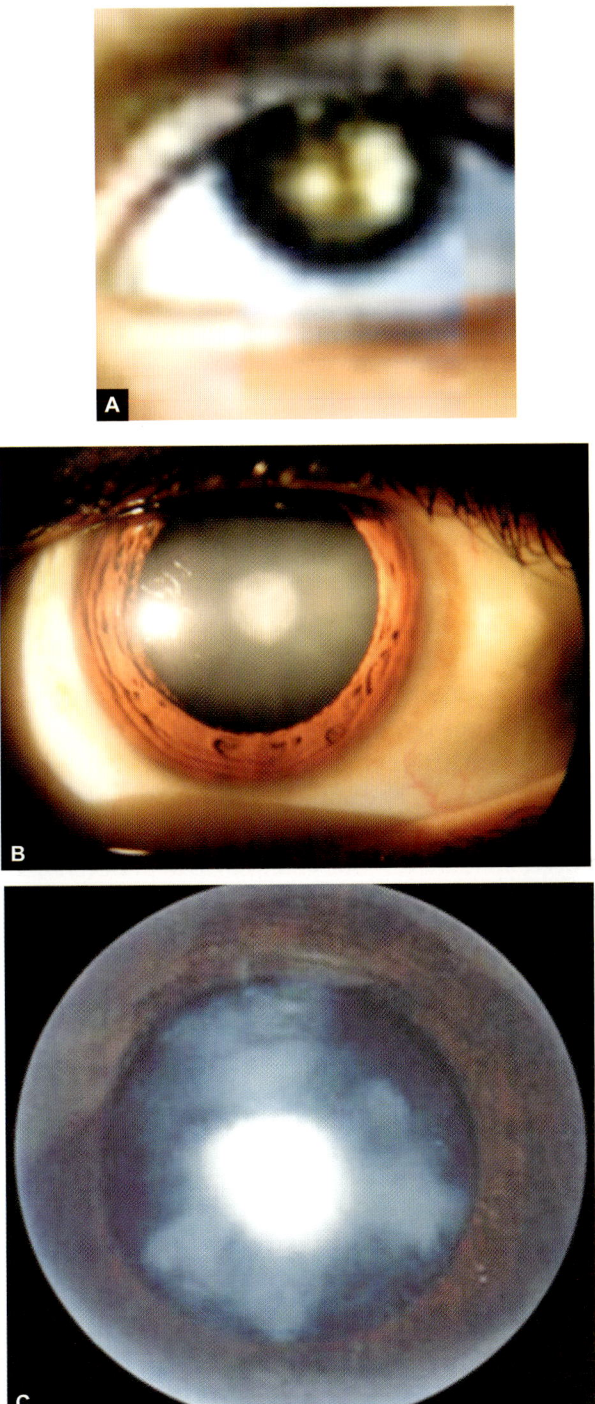

Figs 1A to C: Developmental cataract

DIAGNOSIS

1. *Detailed clinical history:* Because many times developmental cataracts can be part of a systemic disorder, clinical history is of vital importance.
2. *Detailed clinical examination:* It should include visual status, intraocular pressure, fundus examination (when possible), B-scan ultrasonography to exclude posterior segment abnormality like a retinoblastoma or other causes of leukokoria, A-scan to determine axial length of the eye, retinoscopy and cover test.
3. *Laboratory investigations:* Blood test including blood glucose, calcium and phosphorus, RBC transferase and galactokinase levels, TORCH test and hepatitis B virus. Urine analysis includes reducing substance for galactosemia and for amino acids (to exclude Lowe's syndrome in suspected cases).

TREATMENT

It can include different options according the case, described as follows:

a. *No treatment at all:* No treatment is an option if vision is not affected significantly. Sometimes use of mydriatics if opacity is central and vision improves with pupil dilation.

b. *Surgery:* Timing of surgery is of particular importance. In case of a bilateral dense cataract the time is 6 weeks. In case of bilateral partial, if vision is not significantly affected, surgery may be delayed up to the age of 2 years or up to puberty. Uniocular dense cataract, oblige to urgent surgery within days. In partial uniocular cataract, when vision is not significantly affected, surgery may be delayed up to the age of 2 years or up to puberty. In cases in Rubella cataract, operation can be delayed till 1-2 years of age. But early surgery may be indicated if cataract is total, or if eye deviation and/or nystagmus are present.

c *Surgical technique:* Operative procedures available are aspiration and irrigation (ECCE), lensectomy (Pars plana or anterior route), aspiration and irrigation (ECCE) with primary posterior capsulotomy with partial anterior vitrectomy; it all depending the particular case.

d. *Rehabilitation:* Posterior chamber IOL, contact lens, aphakic spectacles, occlusion therapy for treatment and prevention of amblyopia. Long life-term follow-up is mandatory.

PROGNOSIS

It depends upon the particular case, the associated damage and the systemic disease.

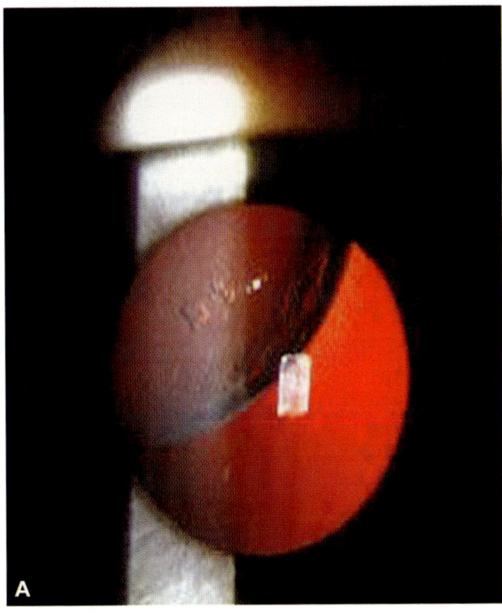

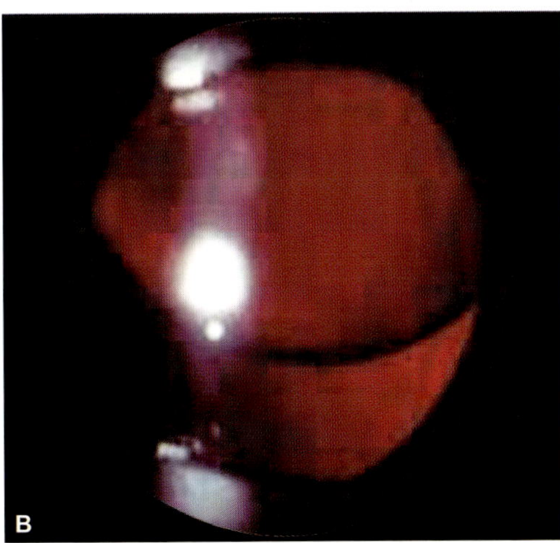

Figs 2A and B: Marfan's syndrome

Marfan's Syndrome

INTRODUCTION

Marfan's syndrome is inherited as a dominant trait. It is carried by a gene called FBN1, which encodes a connective protein called fibrillin-1. Parents have a 50/50 chance of passing on the gene to their children. People with Marfan's are typically tall, with long limbs and long thin fingers. The most serious complication is defects of the heart valves and aorta artery but it also affects the lungs, eyes, dural sac and hard palate. In addition to being a connective protein that forms the structural support for tissues outside the cell, fibrillin-1 binds to another protein. Researchers now believe that the inflammatory effects of transforming growth factor beta (TGF-β), at the lungs, heart valves, and aorta, weaken the tissues and cause the features of Marfan's syndrome.

CLINICAL SIGNS AND SYMPTOMS

Although there are no unique signs or symptoms of Marfan's syndrome, the characteristics of long limbs, dislocated crystalline lenses, and aortic root dilation is sufficient to make the diagnosis with confidence. There are more than thirty other clinical features that are variably associated with the syndrome most of them involving the locations of connective tissue like skeleton, skin, and joints. There is a great deal of clinical variability even within families that carry the identical mutation.

Marfan's syndrome affects the eyes and vision in many characteristic ways. Myopia (particularly high myopia) and astigmatism are common, but hyperopia can be present in some patients. Subluxation (dislocation) of the crystalline lens in one or both eyes can occur in 80% of the patients. In Marfan's the dislocation is typically superotemporal whereas in the similar condition called homocystinuria the dislocation is inferonasal. Retinal detachment and early onset glaucoma can decrease the visual prognosis in these patients.

INVESTIGATIONS

Marfan's syndrome is caused by mutations in the *FBN1* gene on chromosome 15, which encodes a glycoprotein called fibrillin-1, a very important component of the extracellular matrix. The Fibrillin 1 protein is essential for the proper formation of the extracellular matrix including the biogenesis and maintenance of the elastic fibers. The extracellular matrix is critical for both the structural integrity of connective tissue and recently has been involved as a reservoir for growth factors. Elastin fibers are found throughout the body but are particularly abundant in the aorta artery, ligaments and in particular at the zonular ligament; so, as a consequence these areas are among the more affected.

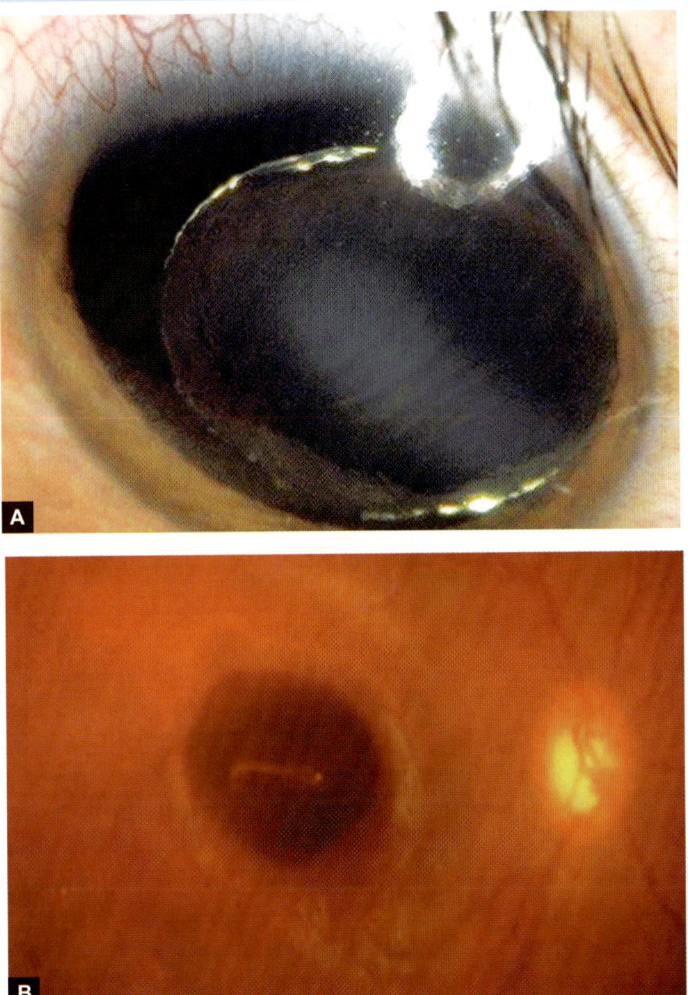

Figs 3A and B: Homocystinuria

DIAGNOSIS

The following conditions may result from Marfan's syndrome but may also occur in people without any known underlying disorder. A diagnosis of Marfan's syndrome is based on family history and a combination of major and minor indicators of the disorder, rare in the general population, that occur in one individual. For example, four skeletal signs with one or more signs in another body system such as ocular and cardiovascular in one individual. Aortic aneurysm, arachnodactyly, bicuspid aortic valve, dural ectasia, crystalline lens subluxation, flat feet, gigantism, glaucoma, hernia, mitral valve prolapse, myopia, obstructive lung disease, pneumothorax, retinal detachment, scoliosis and stretch marks.

The differential diagnosis must take in count the following disorders that have similar signs and symptoms of Marfan's syndrome: congenital contractural arachnodactyly, Ehlers-Danlos syndrome, homocystinuria, Loeys-Dietz syndrome, MASS phenotype, Stickler syndrome and multiple endocrine neoplasias.

TREATMENT

There is no cure for Marfan's syndrome, but life expectancy has increased significantly over the last few decades, and clinical trials are underway for promising new treatments. The syndrome is treated by addressing each issue as it becomes clinically significant, and, in particular, considering preventive medication, even for young children, to slow progression of aortic dilation.

In ophthalmology the surgical treatment of ectopia lentis must be consider. If vision is unaffected no surgery is indicated, only refractive correction is used. When an important subluxation is present, surgery can be useful. Many approaches can be done according the surgeon: intracapsular extraction with anterior chamber IOL, or a posterior chamber IOL fixated to sulcus or to iris; phacoemulsification with endocapsular rings and sometimes sutures, to preserve the capsular bag and "in the bag" IOL implantation; pars plana vitrectomy with lensectomy. In every case, a particular care of the retina is mandatory. Retinal detachment is treated as usual; nevertheless the prognosis is not good. Glaucoma is treated with medication as usual.

PROGNOSIS

It may have variations from patient to patient according the severity of the case, the time of diagnosis and the onset of the particular treatment. A long-life term of follow-up must be carried by many physicians.

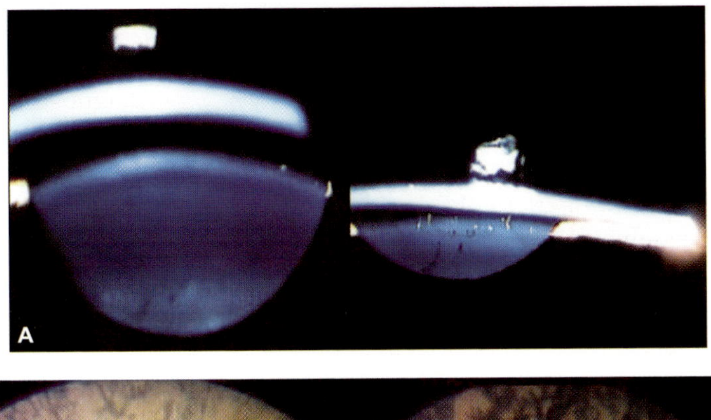

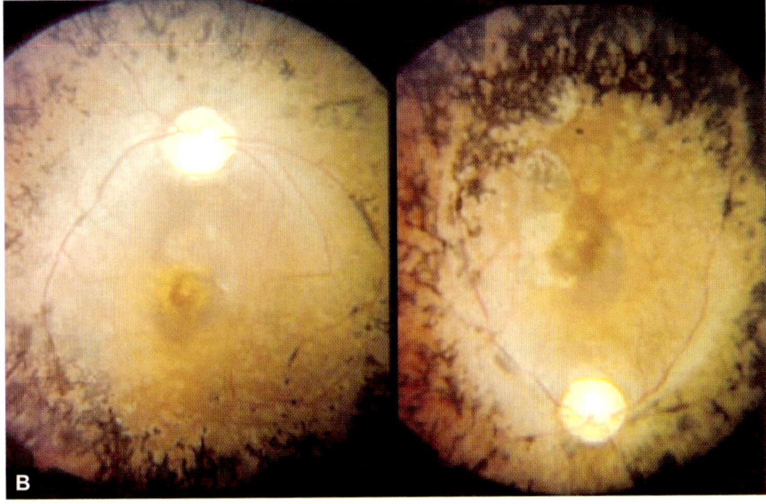

Figs 4A and B: Weill-Marchesani syndrome

Homocystinuria

INTRODUCTION

Homocystinuria is an inherited autosomal recessive defect in methionine metabolism that is caused by a deficiency in the enzyme cystathionine synthase that leads to a multisystem disorder of the connective tissue, muscles, central nervous system, and cardiovascular system. These groups of hereditary metabolic disorders are characterized by an accumulation of homocysteine in the serum and an increased excretion of homocysteine in the urine.

CLINICAL SIGNS AND SYMPTOMS

Even that an infant with homocystinuria is usually healthy when newborn, three important systems involved, representing the landmark of the disease (neurological, vascular and ophthalmic). The neurologic features include thromboembolic complications of the central nervous system and psychomotor delay occurring during the first year of life. A developmental delay is noted when patients are aged 2-3 years. Psychiatric symptoms are present in approximately one-half of patients with homocystinuria. Pyramidal symptoms are occasionally observed in areas like as the legs. In the skeletal and muscular apparatus the characteristic long and thin extremities with arachnodactyly may not appear until late in childhood or until adolescence. Sometimes, osteoporosis is already present for sometime before. Vascular occlusive disease is an important and serious feature. Thromboembolic events, such as cerebrovascular occlusions or pulmonary emboli, usually do not occur until adulthood but are reported sometimes in childhood and infancy.

The ophthalmologic features include severe myopia and the characteristic sign of ectopia lentis that may precede lens dislocation. Once established, ectopia lentis progresses, even when good biochemical control of the disease is performed. The ophthalmologic findings are similar to those in patients with Marfan's syndrome. Ectopia lentis is an almost universal feature in patients older than 10 years (the dislocation of the ocular lenses usually occurs in patients aged 4-10 years) and it can even be present in newborns. Other findings can include myopia, iridopathy (atrophy), cataracts, secondary glaucoma, and retinal degeneration. Atrophy of the optic nerve, strabismus, nystagmus, or diminished convergence is less frequent findings.

INVESTIGATIONS

On the basis of the type of homocystinuria, the following 3 nosologic units are distinguished as follows: Homocystinuria can be caused by the deficiency of cystathionine synthase; can be caused by insufficient vitamin B_{12} synthesis resulting from a defect in the remethylation of homocysteine to methionine; can

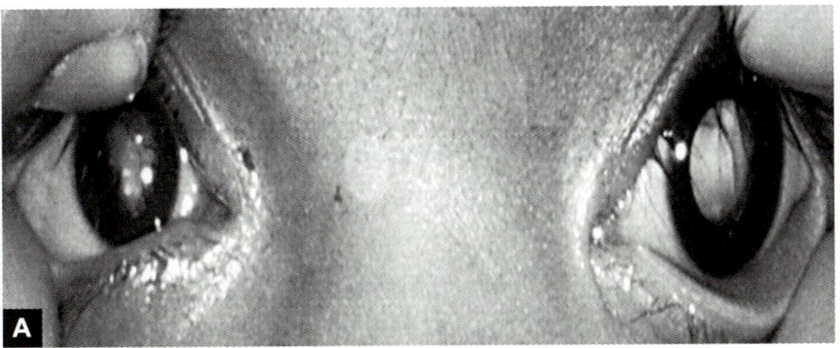

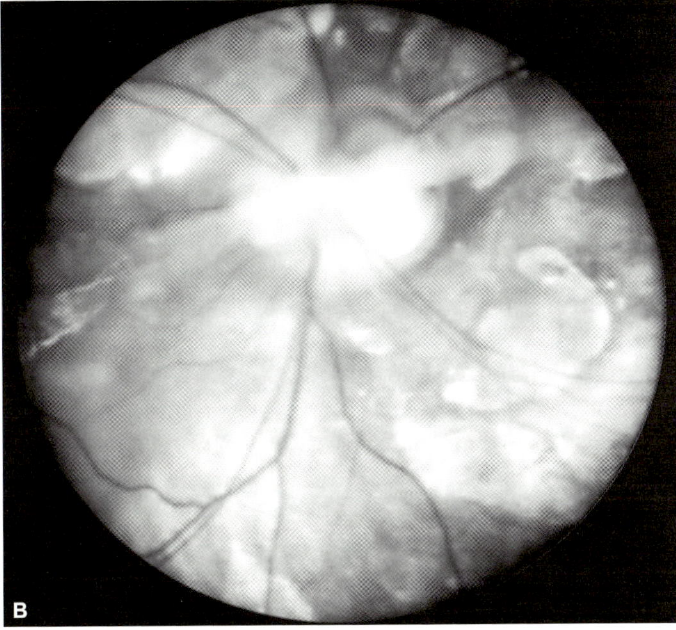

Figs 5A and B: Persistent fetal vasculature

be caused by a deficiency in methylenetetrahydrofolate reductase. The methionine level is within the reference range. In all cases the basis of the disease is a defect of the gene coding for L-serine dehydratase cystathionine synthase, which converts homocysteine and serine into cystathionine. Deficient activity of this enzyme has been demonstrated in liver extracts, in brain tissue, and in cultured skin fibroblasts and lymphocytes. The deficiency leads to an accumulation of homocysteine and methionine and to its conversion into homocysteine, which is excreted in the urine. The accumulation of homocysteine leads to damage of the collagen and elastic fibers. The binding of homocysteine to lysine residues results in the formation of thiazine bonds.

DIFFERENTIAL DIAGNOSIS

The diagnosis is based on the clinical picture and the results of laboratory analysis. The cyanide nitroprusside reaction in the urine is used as the Brand reaction. The reference range methionine level is less than 1 mg/dL (30 µM). Homocysteine levels of up to 0.2 µmol/mL and methionine levels of up to 2 µmol/mL characterize cystathionine synthetase deficiency.

Marfan's syndrome is the primary differential diagnosis. Clinical features of homocystinuria, such as ectopia lentis, dolichocephalia, and chest and spinal deformities, are similar to the features found in patients with Marfan's syndrome, although the cerebral symptoms, the changes in the hair, and the disorders of mental development are absent in patients with Marfan's syndrome. Generalized osteoporosis, arterial and venous thrombosis, and mental retardation, which are features of homocystinuria, do not occur in patients with Marfan's syndrome. In addition, and as a final feature, homocysteine is not detectable in the urine of patients with Marfan's syndrome.

TREATMENT

Neonates in whom homocystinuria is diagnosed have had a benign course when they are fed on methionine-restricted cysteine-supplemented diets. Homocysteine Reduction Formula, a special nutritional supplement created by Brimhall, can also lower homocysteine levels. Cysteine can be supplemented to a maximum of 500 mg per day. The administration of pyridoxine in high doses (300-600 mg/d) has demonstrated to be effective in some patients. Other possible treatments include the use of folic acid.

Surgical treatment should be considered, especially in patients with pupillary-block glaucoma or in those with recurrent lens dislocation into the anterior chamber. Other ophthalmologic or orthopedic disorders should be corrected.

PROGNOSIS

The diagnosis should be established as early as possible. The prognosis is favorable if patients use adequate diet alimentation; even so, nearly 25% of patients die before age 30 years.

Weill-Marchesani Syndrome

INTRODUCTION

In 1932, Georges Weill reported eight patients with dislocation of the lens and other dysmorphic features. Several of these persons had arachnodactyly and were regarded as having the Marfan's syndrome, but two were of stunted stature with short, stiff digits.

Some years after, in 1939, Marchesani documented a boy aged eight years and three siblings in another family, all of whom had ectopia lentis. He recognized that although ectopia lentis was a feature of the Marfan's syndrome, the patients whom he had studied had short fingers rather than arachnodactyly. He emphasized this point by including comparative photographs in his article, in which he termed the disorder "brachydactyly and congenital spherophakia". The condition was first named for Marchesani, but when Weill's earlier report was recognized, the conjoined eponym came into general use.

INVESTIGATIONS

The precise mode of inheritance of Weill-Marchesani syndrome is still uncertain. Most of the reports support an autosomal recessive pattern of inheritance. The heterozygous patients may have short stature or brachydactyly and may suffer from refractive errors (mostly myopia) but not ectopia lentis. The consanguinity among parents suggests autosomal recessive inheritance. However, a high degree of inbreeding in some family pedigrees makes it difficult to decide the type of inheritance.

CLINICAL SIGNS AND SYMPTOMS

Typically, these patients have small shallow orbits, mild maxillary hypoplasia, narrow palate, small spherical crystalline lenses, and myopia with or without glaucoma, frequent ectopia lentis, occasional blindness, malformed and misaligned teeth, and cardiac defect. Late ossification of the epiphyses is a constant feature. The typical clinical findings are enough to establish the diagnosis.

DIAGNOSIS

Diagnosis is made when several characteristic clinical signs are observed. There is no single test to confirm the presence of Weill-Marchesani syndrome.

Exploring family history or examining other family members may prove helpful in confirming this diagnosis. Even so, a variety of manifestations of Weill-Marchesani syndrome can present a diagnostic problem. A diagnosis should be based only on the combination of specific ocular and skeletal abnormalities. The physician should take in count that isolated ocular or skeletal features can occur as isolated familial anomaly or as a part of some other diseases.

The main differential diagnosis is with Marfan's syndrome, because both present similar features but also sharp contrast. A typical Marfan's patient is tall, lean, with high arm span, arachnodactyly and hyper-extensible joints, while Weill-Marchesani individuals are short in stature, with brachymelia, brachydactyly, stubby spade-like hands and feet, and limitation of mobility of joints.

TREATMENT

Physical therapy and orthopedic treatments are generally prescribed for problems stemming from mobility from this connective tissue disorder. However, this disorder has no cure, and generally, treatments are given to improve quality of life.

Despite the systemic features ophthalmic surgery has been documented to help those with ocular diseases, such as some forms of glaucoma; however, long-term medical management of glaucoma associated with this disease has not proven to be successful. To maintain vision, an early diagnosis is necessary. Peripheral iridectomy, lens extraction and recently laser iridotomy are used in the treatment.

PROGNOSIS

It may have variations from patient to patient according the severity of the case, the time of diagnosis and the onset of the particular treatment. A long-life term of follow-up must be carried by many physicians.

Persistent Fetal Vasculature

INTRODUCTION

Persistent fetal vasculature syndrome (PFVS) is a new term that has replaced the older name of persistent hyperplastic primary vitreous. This new name is better than older because it recognizes that two parts of the fetal vasculature can persist leaving the eye with an opaque lens and vascular stalk of tissue. One of the changes that the name does not imply is that the retina may also be altered (retinal dysplasia) either in larger or microscopic amounts.

CLINICAL SIGNS AND SYMPTOMS

Usually, PFVS is found in one eye that is somewhat smaller than the better eye (dominant) and has a white pupil reflex (leukokoria) and elongated ciliary processes. This set of findings does not assure whether retinal dysplasia is present or not. In some eyes the stalk of persistent fetal vessels may not opacify the visual axis of the lens (some part of the light rays may pass through the lens allowing vision). This stalk can pull on the retina and disturb it as well as pull on the lens causing it to be poorly shaped (posterior lenticonus). This child that usually does not have the white pupil, is often diagnosed at a later age, decreasing this way the visual prognosis.

INVESTIGATIONS

Ultrasound studies, visual evoked potential response or electroretinography testing are helpful in evaluation but finally the clinical evaluation should be performed. At this time there are no other known systemic problems associated. At this time no genetic mutations have been associated with the typical unilateral PFVS. About 10% of infants affected by PFVS have both eyes involved. These children more frequently have retinal dysplasia. Bilateral PFVS is also not associated with systemic changes.

DIFFERENTIAL DIAGNOSIS

The disease that can be indistinguishable from bilateral PFVS with extensive retinal dysplasia is called Norrie's disease. In this process the child may be affected with hearing loss or other central nervous system problems. Genetic testing is available for Norrie's disease. As with many diseases known to be under genetic control, there may be several mutations. Norrie's disease testing will confirm the diagnosis in 80% of the cases, leaving 20% of children where a mutation cannot be found, but clinical examination confirms the diagnosis of Norrie's disease.

TREATMENT

Treatment for PFVS is surgical, usually with removal of the lens and persistent vascular stalk tissue. It can accomplish several things. It may reduce the risk of glaucoma and usually clears the opaque tissue out of the eye allowing light to reach the retina. It also can relieve pulling or distortion of the retina because of tractions. When the media are clear the physician can form an opinion as to the amount or absence of retinal dysplasia. The flourescein angiography and OCT testing in infants under anesthesia can be much more accurate about microscopic retinal dysplasia; it can be done during the same surgical procedure.

PROGNOSIS

If the eye has no retinal dysplasia the visual prognosis improves; even so there still is a great challenge to overcome occlusive amblyopia. This can often be helped by contact lenses and occlusive therapy.

Management of Ectopia Lentis

SK Gibran (UK)

Introduction

Normally, the crystalline lens is suspended in its anatomical place behind the iris diaphragm by the zonular fibers of the ciliary body. Abnormalities of the suspensory system resulting from a developmental defect, disease, or trauma may result in instability or displacement of the lens.

Etiology

Table 1 summarizes the causes and associations of ectopia lentis.

TABLE 1: Associations of ectopia lentis

- Trauma
  - Isolated subluxation
  - Frenkel's syndrome (Ocular contusion syndrome)
- Heritable
  - Simple Ectopia Lentis
  - Ectopia Lentis et Pupillae
- Ocular Conditions
  - Uveitis
  - Intraocular tumor
  - Congenital glaucoma
  - High myopia
  - Aniridea
  - Megalocornea
  - Cataract
  - Coloboma of iris and choroid
- Systemic Associations
  - Marfan's syndrome
  - Homocystinuria
  - Weill-Marchesani syndrome
  - Hyperlysinemia
  - Syphilis
  - Scleroderma
  - Porphyria
  - Reiger's syndrome
  - Sulfite oxidase deficiency
  - Ehler-Danlos syndrome
  - Sturge-Weber syndrome
  - Crouzon's syndrome
  - Klippel-Feil syndrome
  - Oxycephly
  - Mandibulofacial dysostosis

A syndrome of dominantly inherited blepharoptosis, high myopia, and ectopia lentis has also been described.

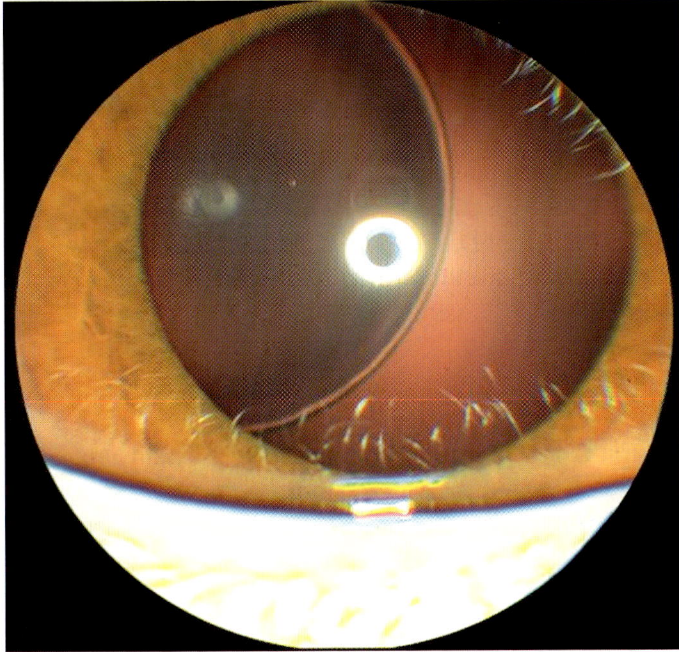

Fig. 1: Lens subluxation as a result of Simple Ectopia Lentis in a 6-year Caucasian male. Note >180 degree zonular dehiscence

A major cause of lens displacement is trauma. It can cause isolated subluxation of the lens or a manifestation of Frenkel's syndrome.

Frenkel's syndrome (Ocular contusion syndrome), a syndrome studied by French Henri Frenkel in 1931. It comprises mydriasis, a tear of the iris and a subluxation of the crystalline lens.

There are heritable forms of ectopia lentis and those associated with systemic disease. Displacement of the lens occurring as a heritable ocular condition unassociated with systemic abnormalities is referred to as simple ectopia lentis. Simple ectopia lentis is usually transmitted as an autosomal dominant condition. The lens is generally displaced upwards and temporally. The onset may be congenital or may occur between 20 and 65 years of age.

Another form of heritable dislocation is *ectopia lentis et pupillae*. In this condition, both the lens and pupil are displaced, usually in opposite directions. This condition is generally bilateral, with one eye being the mirror image of the other. Ectopia lentis et pupillae is a recessive condition, although variable expression with some intermingling with simple ectopia lentis has been reported.

Ectopia lentis occurs in approximately 80% of patients of Marfan's syndrome, and in about 50% of patients the ectopia is evident by the age of 5 years. In most cases, the lens is displaced superiorly and temporally; it is almost bilateral and relatively symmetric. In *homocystinuria*, the lens is displaced inferiorly and somewhat nasally. It occurs early in life and is often evident by 5 years of age. In Weill-Marchesani syndrome the displacement of the lens is often downwards and forwards, and the lens tends to be small and round.

Clinical Symptoms and Signs

Displacement of the lens is classified as *luxation* (dislocation-complete displacement of the lens) or as *subluxation* (partial displacement-shifting or tilting of the lens). Symptoms include blurring of vision, which is often the result of refractive change such as myopia, astigmatism, or aphakic hyperopia. Some patients develop diplopia and photophobia.

An important sign of displacement is iridodenesis, a tremulousness of the iris caused by the loss of its usual support. Also, the anterior chamber may appear deeper than normal.

Sometimes, the equatorial region (edge) of the displaced lens may be visible in the pupillary aperture.

On retroillumination, this may appear as a black crescent. Also, the difference between the phakic and aphakic portion can be appreciated when focusing on the fundus.

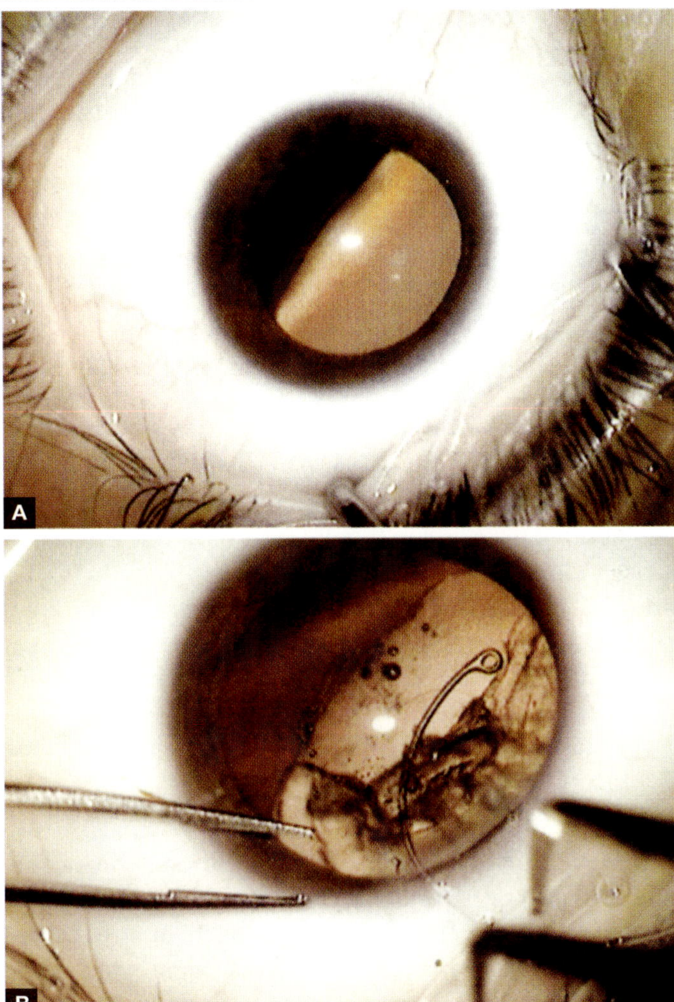

Figs 2A and B: (A) Lens subluxation in Marfan's syndrome. Note <180 degree zonular dehiscence. (B) After partial removal of lens capsule tension ring (OPHTEC BV) is being introduced

Management

The management of ectopia lentis can be challenging for an ophthalmologist. The greatest obstacle to obtaining good visual acuity in ectopia lentis patients is form-deprivation amblyopia. Displacement of the lens often results only in optical problems; in others, however more serious complications may develop, such as glaucoma, uveitis, retinal detachment, or cataract. Management must be individualized according to the type of displacement, its etiology, and the presence of any complicating ocular or systemic conditions. Patients with lens abnormalities may benefit from evaluation by a pediatrician or a geneticist.

CONSERVATIVE MANAGEMENT

For many patients, optical correction by spectacles or contact lenses can be provided, depending upon the compliance of the patient.

Manipulation of the pupil with mydriatic or miotic drops may sometimes help improve vision.

In many children, treatment of any associated amblyopia must be instituted early.

In addition, for children with ectopia lentis, safety precautions should be taken to prevent injury to the eye.

In selected cases, the best treatment is surgical removal of the lens.

SURGICAL MANAGEMENT

Surgical intervention needs to be a combined team approach of the ophthalmologist, orthoptist and parents. It is indicated for associated cataract, lens induced glaucoma, uveitis, endothelial touch, or if the other methods are inappropriate. Any conservatively untreatable visual obstacle is amblyogenic, in order to obtain good visual acuity results, surgery must be completed in the first few months of life and the visual axis kept clear postoperatively.

In children up to the age of two years of age, in whom spectacles contact lenses are the preferred means of aphakic optical correction, lensectomy is performed through a small limbal or parsplana incision with dry (non-irrigating) or wet (irrigating) vitreous cutter. If dry cutter is used, infusion can be provided by separate cannula.

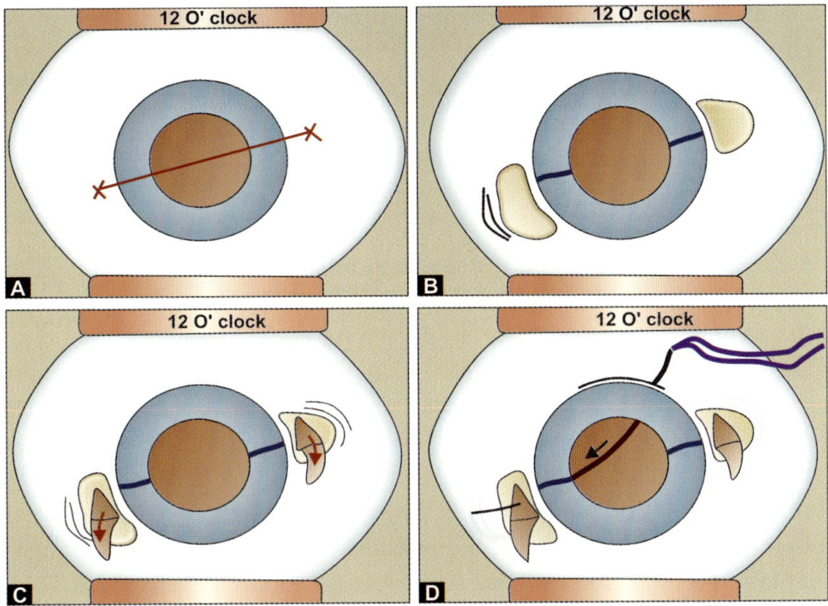

Figs 3A to D: (A) Marking the site for scleral flaps. (B) Conjunctival periotomy and cauterizing the sclera. (C) Triangular partial thickness scleral flaps with apex towards 12 O' clock and base inferiorly. (D) Ab interno approach, i.e. direct insertion of the needle through the corneal incision to the scleral flap site

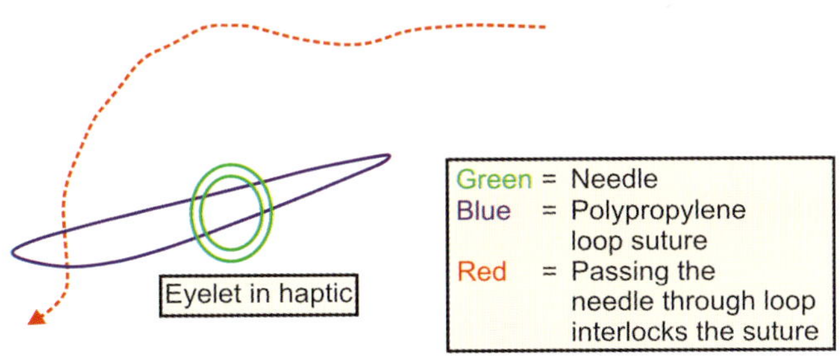

Fig. 4: Interlocking of 10/0 polypropylene loop suture on eyelet in the haptic of scleral sutured IOL

In monocular cases, immediate optical correction and patching therapy needs to be instituted in postoperative period. Part-time patching (50-70% of waking hours) is usually utilized in order to avoid risk of occlusion amblyopia in fixing eye (rare) and, more importantly the induction of nystagmus in the fixing eye. Periodic re-evaluation of the refractive error with refitting of the appropriate contact lens is mandatory. Secondary intraocular lens (IOL) is considered at later date.

In binocular cases, if surgery and visual rehabilitation is completed before nystagmus appears, often little or no significant binocular form-deprivation amblyopia will be apparent. Once amblyopia supervenes, however, visual acuity levels are significantly reduced even with aggressive therapy. In many cases of binocular form deprivation, monocular deprivation is also seen and patching of the preferred fixing eye needs to be undertaken if visual acuity results are to be equalized. Even so, a significant percentage of patients treated in this manner will not develop good visual acuity. Binocular cases will do better, but never obtain normal visual acuity levels. For children older than 2 years of age IOL implantation is preferred by some surgeons. Although long-term risks of IOLs are unknown, accumulating evidence of IOLs in children to date has been promising.

In my experience, children older than 5 years are good candidates to consider IOL implantation.

Further in this chapter, option of secondary implant at the time of lensectomy in older children is discussed in detail.

PREOPERATIVE EVALUATION

A detailed family history, pediatric physical, ocular examination and biometric studies should be performed. It is important to rule out posterior segment pathology and any systemic association or abnormality. If cooperation is the issue, examination under anesthesia is performed.

Parents should be explained in detail and counselled appropriately. Surgical options should be discussed in layman terms with the parents and mutual decision is made. A detailed consent is obtained.

The surgical options of implanting IOL, depending upon degree of dislocation include following:

- Lensectomy and anterior stabilization of capsular bag with IOL implant
- Vitreolensectomy and sulcus scleral sutured IOL/Iris clipped lens.

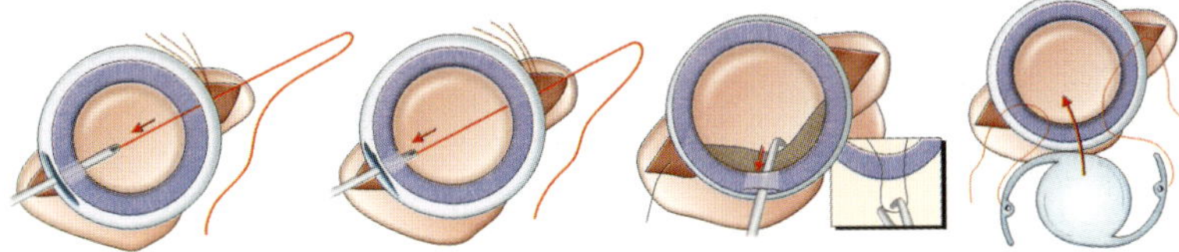

Fig. 5: Ab externo technique of scleral fixation sutures (surgical steps; from top to bottom)

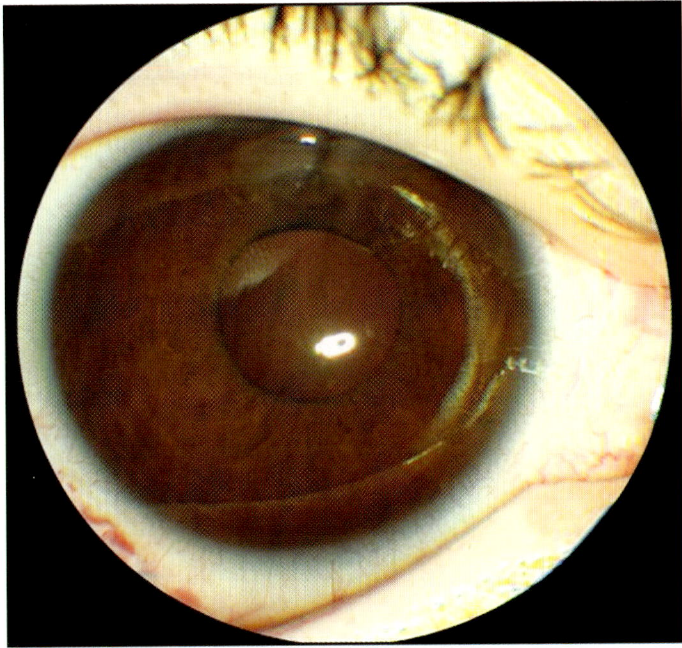

Fig. 6: Same patient in Fig. 1, after vitreolensectomy and scleral sutured IOL (Alcon.CZ70BD)

SURGICAL TECHNIQUE

Lensectomy and Anterior Stabilization of Capsular Bag with Intraocular Lens (IOL) Implant

This approach is appropriate in cases of 90-180 degree subluxation and healthy condition of remaining zonules. After stepped corneal section, low cohesive viscoelastic is injected in anterior chamber and small continuous capsulorhexis (CCC) is performed. Hydrodissection and aspiration of the lens is carried out. Low irrigation and aspiration setting are used to avoid vitreous aspiration. Once the lens is partially removed, a small amount of viscoelastic is injected in the bag to inflate it and capsule tension ring is inserted. Aspiration of the lens is completed and the IOL is inserted in the bag. Viscoelastic is removed and Miochol is used to constrict the pupil. If any vitreous (rarely) is identified, anterior vitrector is used to remove it. Completion of surgery is achieved in usual manner.

Patient is given an intensive course of postoperative topical (usually sufficient) antibiotics and steroids.

Vitreolensectomy and Sulcus Scleral Sutured IOL/Iris Clipped Lens

Sulcus scleral sutured IOL

The conjunctiva is retracted superiorly at the 2 and 8 O' clock positions. Scleral surface is cauterized in wet field. Two triangular partial thickness scleral flaps measuring 2 mm at the base are raised with apices pointing superiorly. I prefer the dissection of triangular scleral flaps with apices pointing toward 12 O'clock because it is much easier and simpler as compared to traditional limbal based rectangular flaps. At 2 and 8 O' clock positions the curvature of the eye slants away and the scleral dissection often results in button holes, dehiscence or free flaps. The flaps are centred at the site where the needle with the suture is expected to exit the eye, 1.5 mm from the limbus. A partial thickness shelved peripheral corneal limbal incision measuring 7 mm was prepared for the IOL at 12 O'clock.

Lensectomy is performed either by anterior or posterior approach depending upon surgeon's choice. Some commonly used models of scleral sutured IOLs include the CZ70BD (Alcon Laboratories, Inc., Fort Worth, TX) and the C540MC (CIBA Vision, Duluth, GA). A scleral sutured IOL is prepared by passing a loop of 10/0 polypropylene suture (ALCON: 307901 on PC 9 needle) through the eyelets in the haptics and interlocking it. Viscoelastic is injected in anterior chamber to protect corneal endothelium and stabilize the anterior chamber. The scleral fixation sutures, using 10/0 polypropylene, can be inserted using an *ab externo* technique or an *ab interno* technique.

I prefer *ab interno* technique as it avoids the complications of multiple puncture holes. It also simplifies and expedites the surgical technique. Gentle

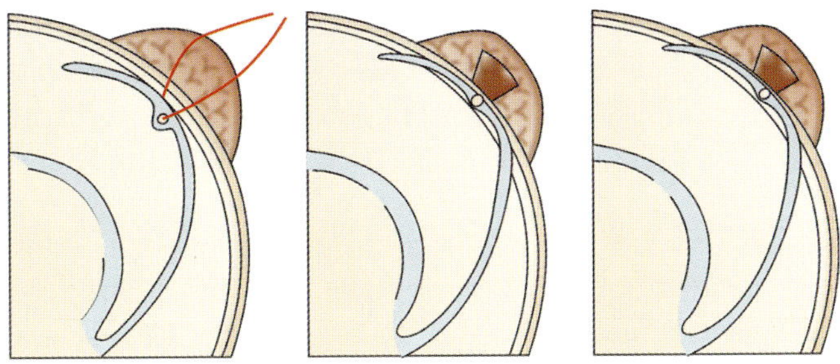

Fig. 7: Note proper fixation of IOL in ciliary sulcus by double 10/0 polypropylene suture

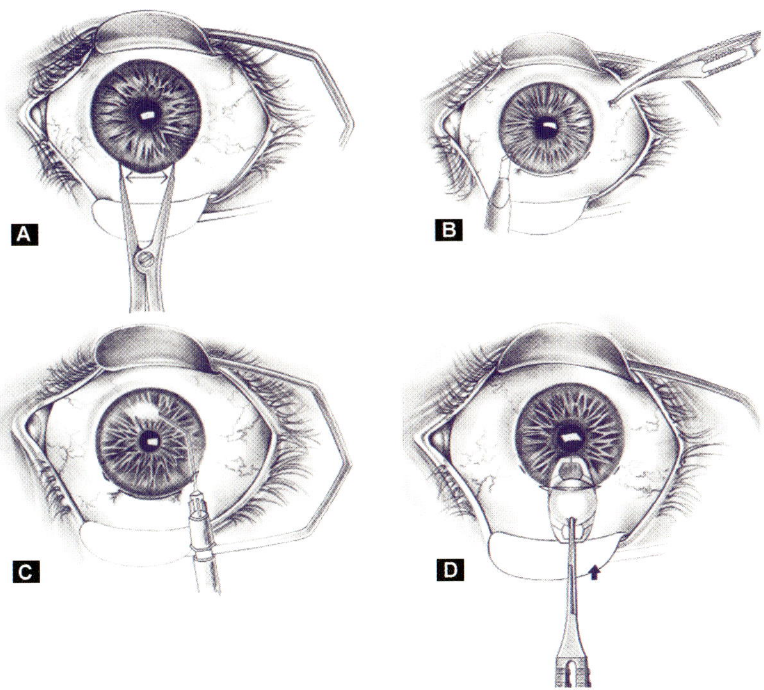

Figs 8A to D: (A) Calipers are used to indicate the proper incision size. (B) Making paracentheses for introduction of the enclavation needles. Watch the direction in which the knife is orientated. (C) The injection needle is passed through one of the paracenteses and Miochol is injected. (D) Introduction of IOL in a vertical position at 12 O'clock

cautery is applied at the bed of scleral flaps as it minimizes the chances of choroidal and scleral bleed. The suture needle is passed *ab interno* (inside out) through the center of the bed of scleral flaps avoiding the iris capture. The IOL is inserted in ciliary sulcus (CS) and sutures are pulled simultaneously. Once IOL is in CS, one suture of the loop is cut and a partial thickness scleral bite is taken in the scleral bed by the needle and tied with the cut end of the suture. Viscoelastic is washed out from anterior chamber, miochol is injected and any vitreous presence is cautiously observed and cleared. The scleral flaps were closed with 8/0 vicryl and interrupted 10/0 nylon was applied to the corneal wound. Conjunctival continuity was achieved with 10/0 vicryl and knots are buried to minimise the postoperative irritation.

I prefer one piece solid poly-methyl methacrylate (PMMA) IOL (ALCON: CZ70BD; optic 7.0 mm, length 12.5 mm) with a larger optic in order to reduce the incidence of pupillary and centration problems.

This technique can be employed to suture a foldable IOL but to date, no foldable IOL is available, which is designed to place in CS and have haptic modifications to secure the scleral fixation suture.

Complications of sutured IOLs

Complications like *IOL subluxation* due to suture breakage have been described. I use a 10/0 polypropylene loop suture on a long curved needle (ALCON: 307901 on PC 9 needle) to lock one haptic of the IOL. After suturing it to the sclera with multiple knots each haptic is secured by two 10/0 polypropylene sutures, which act in a complementary mechanical fashion. The careful closure of the superficial scleral flaps is aimed at preventing the external exposure and erosion of the suture ends and subsequent risk of postoperative *endophthalmitis*.

Retinal detachment (RD) remains a concern. The incidence of RD has been quoted as 1.1 to 4.9%. Simple ectopia lentis has less incidence of retinal detachment than ectopia lentis associated with Marfan syndrome, homocystinuria and ocular trauma. Careful attention to the needle passage helps to avoid retinal perforation and minimizes the risk of retinal detachment. In cases of suspected retinal touch, peroperative cryotherapy/indirect diode laser posterior to the scleral flaps may be carried out but this is controversial.

The surgical technique of "Scleral sutured posterior chamber IOL" is an alternative approach in solving the challenge of selected cases of ectopia lentis with satisfactory postoperative visual rehabilitation.

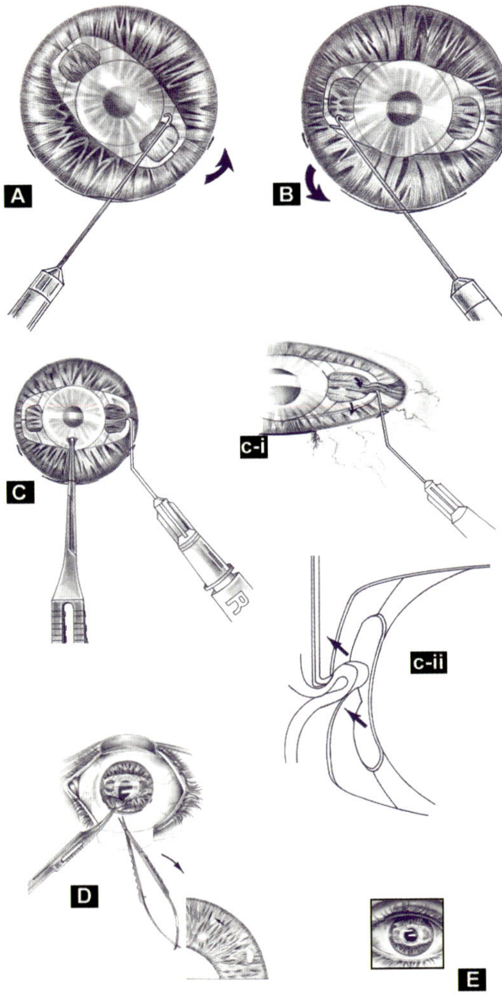

Figs 9A to E: (A,B) Rotation of the artisan IOL in the horizontal position. (C) Firmly grasping the artisan IOL with the Implantation Forceps, the Enclavation Needle creates a "fold" of iris tissue "Snowploughing movement" (ci and cii; magnified views). (D) Peripheral iridectomy. (E) Final position of IOL. Note centeration and round pupil

Iris clipped IOLs

The new generation of iris clipped IOLs (Artisan: OPHTEC BV) is promising and proves to be satisfactory alternative with relative ease of surgery. This option needs to be evaluated for the long term safety and efficacy. The technique is as follows:

After vitreolensectomy, use calipers to mark the 5.2 or 6.2 mm incision width, depending on the size of the optic (5 or 6 mm). Create a non-perforating initial section of the central corneal incision. Make 2 paracenteses of 1.2 mm, one beginning at 2 O'clock and one beginning at 10 O'clock. The tip of the knife should be pointed downwards, oriented towards the enclavation sites for introduction of the enclavation needles. Inject miochol into the anterior chamber to constrict the pupil. The pupil has to be very small to facilitate the centration of the IOL around the pupil. Filling the AC with a high viscosity viscoelastic substance greatly facilitates the visibility of the various manoeuvres, creates space and protects the corneal endothelium. The IOL is introduced in a vertical position with the artisan implantation forceps. Insert the lens through the incision and gently apply some viscoelastic on top of the lens to prevent movement of the lens during the enclavation procedure. Rotate the lens into the desired position (usually haptics at 3 and 9 O'clock) with the artisan lens manipulator to make sure that the lens is centered over the pupil, not on the cornea. Care must be taken to avoid contact with the corneal endothelium. Insert the enclavation needle (left or right) through one of the paracenteses to fixate the lens to the iris, while securely holding the lens body with the implantation forceps use the enclavation needle to create a small "knuckle" of iris tissue. Make a "snow-ploughing" movement at the desired fixation site. Hold the "knuckle" of iris with the needle while gently pressing the slotted center of the lens haptic over the knuckle, thus grasping the iris tissue. A significant fold of iris tissue must be delivered through the haptic slot to ensure adequate lens stability. If the fold of the lens is too small, the IOL can luxate into the AC and cause damage to the endothelium. Carefully retract the enclavation needle to avoid damage to the iris surface. Transfer the instruments to the opposite hands and repeat the enclavation for the second haptic while ensuring that the lens is well-centered and pupil stays round. It is recommended to perform a small superior iridotomy. Carefully remove all of the viscoelastic by making a semi-circular movement from 6 O'clock towards the main incision with manual/automated irrigation and aspiration using BSS. Incomplete removal of the viscoelastic may cause high intraocular pressure. Close the corneal incision with 10/0 nylon. At the end of implantation pupil should be round and centered on the optic of artisan IOL.

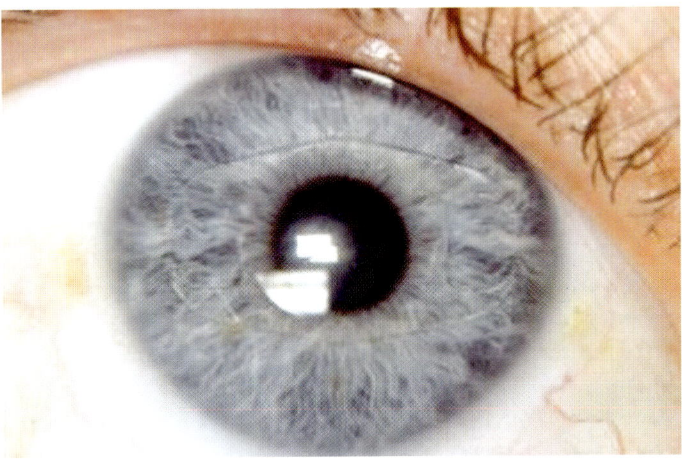

Fig. 10: After vitreolensectomy and artisan implantation in a 9-year old Caucasian female

Complications

Most postoperative complication of iris clipped IOLs can be avoided at the time of surgery. Judicious use of viscoelastic prevents *corneal endothelium damage*. Ensuring sufficient iris tissue is clipped in the haptics avoids future *unclipping* (if it happens it can be re-clipped with ease). *Centration* on the pupil can be gauged during the surgery. One concern is *uveitis* by the continuous irritation of iris tissue trapped in haptics. Fluorescein angiographic studies have shown a non leakage from the iris vessels and preservation of blood-ocular barrier.

The surgical intervention for ectopia lentis provides rapid visual improvement in younger patients. Without surgery, amblyoia may have occurred in one or both eyes.

In these cases, it is frequently difficult to provide adequate visual rehabilitation with contact lenses or aphakic glasses. Several surgical options for the centration for capsular bag and IOL insertion have been discussed.

In my opinion, one should master a technique that is safe in their hands and carries minimal chances of complications.

3

Senile Cataract

- Nuclear Cataract
- Cortical Cataract
- Posterior Subcapsular Cataract
- Posterior Polar Cataract

Arturo Perez Arteaga (Mexico)

Introduction

Senile cataract is a vision-impairing disease characterized by gradual, progressive thickening of the lens. It is one of the leading causes of blindness in the world today. Considering that the visual morbidity brought about by age-related cataract is reversible, to know that this is a cause of blindness is unfortunate. Early detection, close monitoring, and timely surgical intervention must be observed in the management of senile cataracts.

Senile cataract can be classified into 3 main types: nuclear cataract, cortical cataract, and posterior subcapsular cataract.

Nuclear Cataract

INTRODUCTION

Nuclear cataracts result from excessive nuclear sclerosis and yellowing of the crystalline lens, with consequent formation of a central lenticular opacity; this can be very hard and dense, of particular importance for surgery purposes. In some instances, with the time, the nucleus can become very opaque and brown, termed a brunescent nuclear cataract, sometimes very difficult to operate by conventional phacoemulsification.

CLINICAL SIGNS AND SYMPTOMS

Patients with nuclear sclerotic cataracts present to the consultation with decreased vision, not many times with decreased distance acuity and good near vision. Myopic shift and second sight are also very common and are not seen in cortical and posterior subcapsular cataracts; the patient refers that "has recovery his near vision".

At the clinical examination the cataract is seen, and before pupil dilation the surgeon must remember that the visual significance of oil droplet nuclear cataracts is evaluated best with a normal-sized pupil to determine if the visual axis is affected. Then with pupil dilation, the nuclear size and the brunescence should be determined prior to phacoemulsification surgery as indicators of cataract density. The lens position and integrity of the zonular fibers also should be checked because of possible lens subluxation. Direct and indirect ophthalmoscopy (when possible) for evaluation of the integrity of the posterior pole are very important for the prognosis of visual recovery.

INVESTIGATIONS

Nuclear cataracts have been studied by many investigators regarding its particular features, and some have concluded that they appear to have a correlation with smoking, calcitonin and milk intake. In histological studies

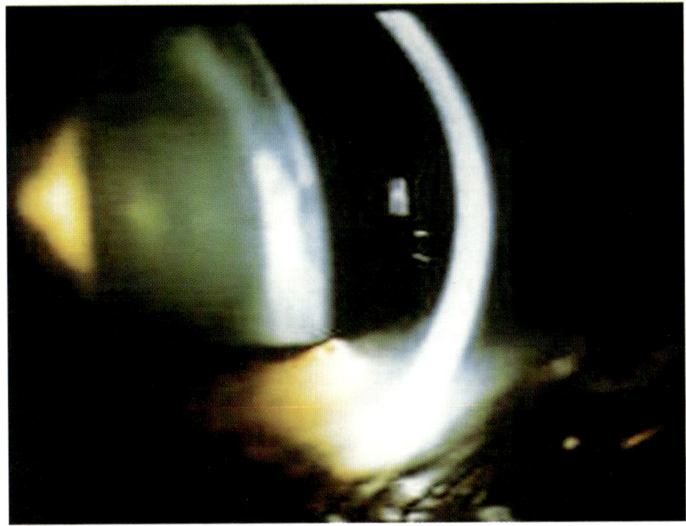

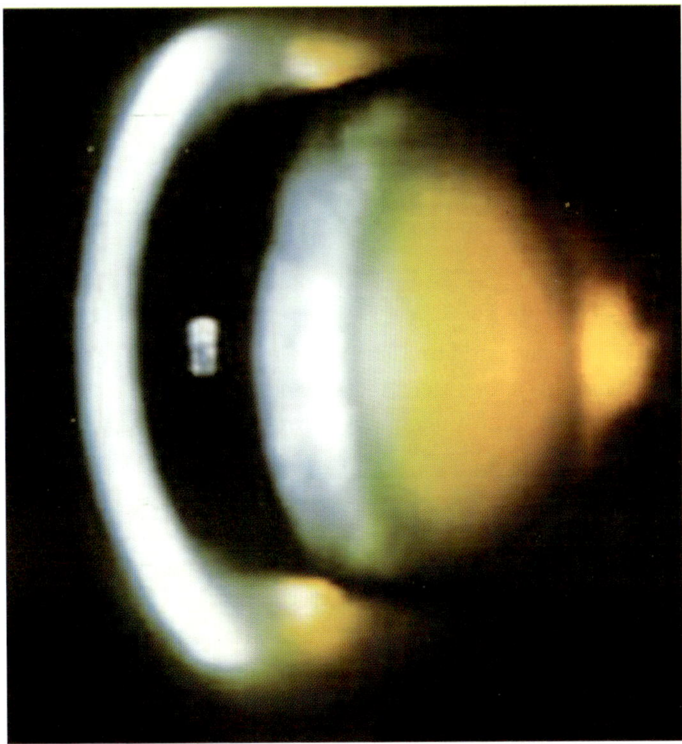

Figs 1 and 2: Nuclear cataract

nuclear cataracts are characterized by homogeneity of the lens nucleus with loss of cellular laminations.

DIAGNOSIS

Ocular imaging studies are requested when posterior pole pathology is suspected and an adequate view of the back of the eye is obscured by the dense cataract; of particular helpful is the Mode-B echography that can be accompanied by an accurate biometry to calculate the IOL power to be used. Corneal integrity, specifically the endothelial layer, should be studied in some particular cases of suspected endothelial cells damage (specular microscopy).

TREATMENT

Conventional phacoemulsification can be very difficult in some cases of nuclear cataracts, in particular in the brunescent types; new techniques for hard nucleus management should be taken in count, either, coaxial or biaxial. For some instances a planned extracapsular technique (Conventional or Small Incision Cataract Surgery), can be a better option, in particular in cases with low endothelial cells count, avoiding this way the exposure to ultrasonic force.

PROGNOSIS

Frequently good if proper preoperative evaluation and surgical technique are performed.

Cortical Cataract

INTRODUCTION

Cortical cataract corresponds to the opacity of the cortical material of the lens, with less involvement of the nucleus. Some changes in the ionic composition of the lens cortex and the eventual change in hydration of the lens fibers produce a cortical cataract.

CLINICAL SIGNS AND SYMPTOMS

A cortical cataract is generally asymptomatic until late in its progression when cortical spokes compromise the visual axis. However, instances exist when a solitary cortical spoke occasionally involves the visual axis. After dilation, cortical spikes and cataract density can be evaluated prior to phaco-emulsification surgery. The lens position and integrity of the zonular fibers also should be checked because lens subluxation. The direct and indirect ophthalmoscopy to evaluate the integrity of the posterior pole if frequently easy because the transparency of the nucleus.

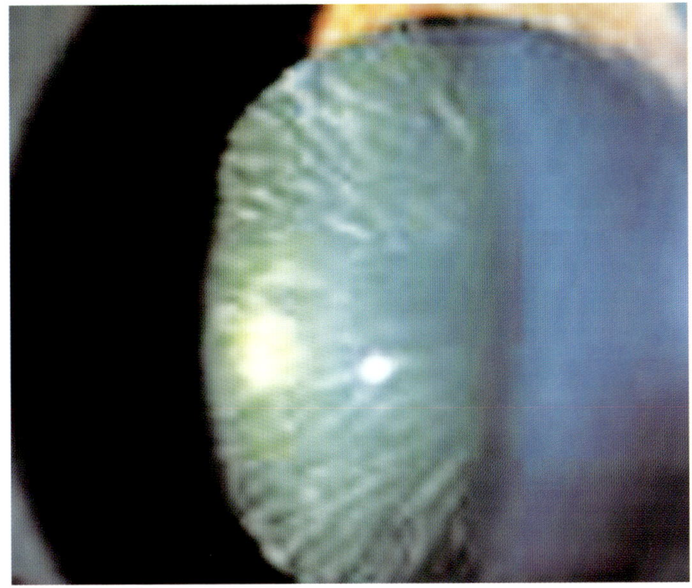

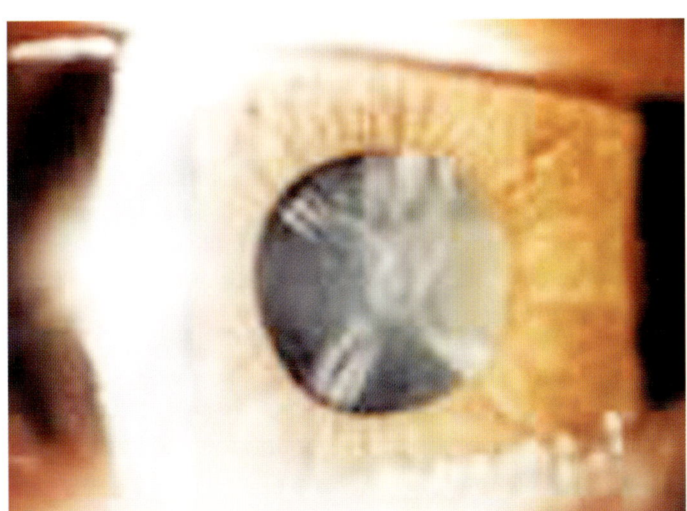

Figs 3 and 4: Cortical cataract

INVESTIGATIONS

Some investigators have demonstrated that cortical and posterior subcapsular cataracts are related closely to environmental stresses, such as ultraviolet (UV) exposure and drug ingestion; the association of UV light and development of senile cataract has generated much interest; some cortical cataracts are associated with the presence of diabetes for more than 5 years and increased serum potassium and sodium levels. One hypothesis implies that senile cataracts, particularly cortical opacities, may be the result of thermal damage to the lens. Histological studies demonstrated that cortical cataracts typically manifest with hydropic swelling of the lens fibers with globules of eosinophilic material (morgagnian globules) seen in slit like spaces between lens fibers.

DIAGNOSIS

Ocular imaging studies, like Mode-B echography are requested when posterior pole pathology is suspected and an adequate view of the back of the eye is obscured by the dense cataract; for some authors it is also helpful even when the posterior pole is visible. An accurate biometry also should be performed to calculate for the IOL power to be used. Corneal integrity, specifically the endothelial layer should be studied in some particular cases of suspected endothelial cells damage (specular microscopy).

TREATMENT

Conventional or microincisional phacoemulsification are the treatments of choice for cortical cataracts; because many times the nucleus remains unaffected, they are very soft cataracts very easy to emulsificate; also capsulorhexis performance is very easy because there is almost every time a nice red reflex. Rarely extracapsular procedures are needed.

PROGNOSIS

Frequently good if proper preoperative evaluation and surgical technique are performed.

Posterior Subcapsular Cataract

INTRODUCTION

This is a type of senile cataract where there is a formation of granular and plaque like opacities in the posterior subcapsular cortex; sometimes can cover by complete the subcapsular space and some other times only the center, compromising so the visual acuity. Small opacities seen in the lens at presbiopic age, often heralds the formation of posterior subcapsular cataracts.

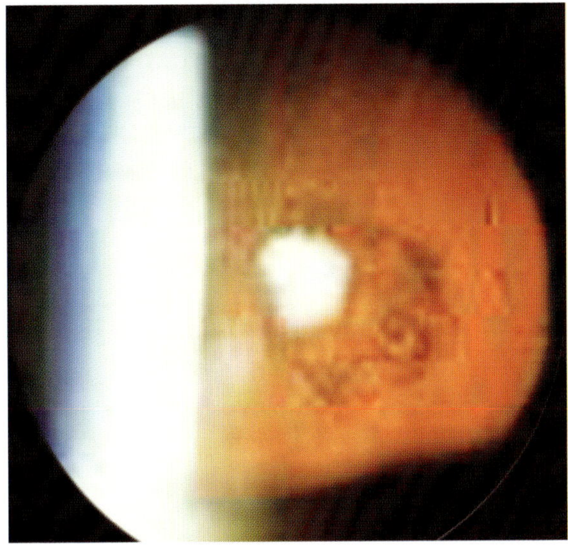

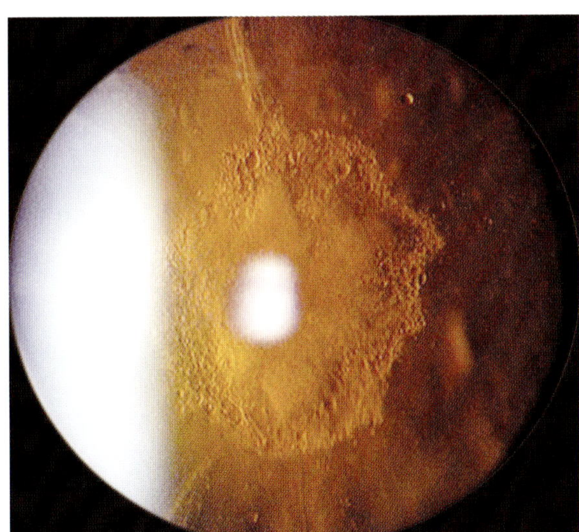

Figs 5 and 6: Posterior subcapsular cataract

CLINICAL SIGNS AND SYMPTOMS

A mild degree of posterior subcapsular cataract can produce a severe reduction in visual acuity with near acuity affected more frequently than distance vision, maybe as a result of accommodative miosis. Glare is a very important symptom particularly with posterior subcapsular cataracts, in comparison with cortical cataracts. They are less associated with nuclear sclerosis. The visual significance of small posterior subcapsular cataracts, affecting the visual axis is better evaluated with a normal-sized pupil to determine if the visual axis is compromised. After dilation, subcapsular opacities can be seen, but also the nuclear density, determined their status prior to phacoemulsification surgery. The lens position and integrity of the zonular fibers also should be checked. The importance of direct and indirect ophthalmoscopy in evaluating the integrity of the posterior pole must be underscored; frequently the fundus can be seen easily with indirect ophthalmoscope, even a total subcapsular opacity is present.

INVESTIGATIONS

Some investigators have demonstrated that cortical and posterior subcapsular cataracts were related closely to environmental stresses, such as ultraviolet (UV) exposure, diabetes, steroids use and drug ingestion. Histology studies shows that a posterior subcapsular cataract is associated with posterior migration of the lens epithelial cells in the posterior subcapsular area, with aberrant enlargement of the epithelial cells (Wedl or bladder cells).

DIAGNOSIS

Ocular imaging studies, like Mode-B echography are requested when posterior pole pathology is suspected and an adequate view of the back of the eye is obscured by the dense cataract; for some authors it is also helpful even when the posterior pole is visible. An accurate biometry also should be performed to calculate for the IOL power to be used. Corneal integrity, specifically the endothelial layer should be studied in some particular cases of suspected endothelial cells damage (specular microscopy).

TREATMENT

Conventional or microincisional phacoemulsification are the treatments of choice for cortical cataracts; because many times the nucleus remains unaffected, they are very soft cataracts very easy to emulsificate; also capsulorhexis performance is very easy because there is almost every time a nice red reflex. Rarely extracapsular procedures are needed.

PROGNOSIS

Frequently good if proper preoperative evaluation and surgical technique are performed.

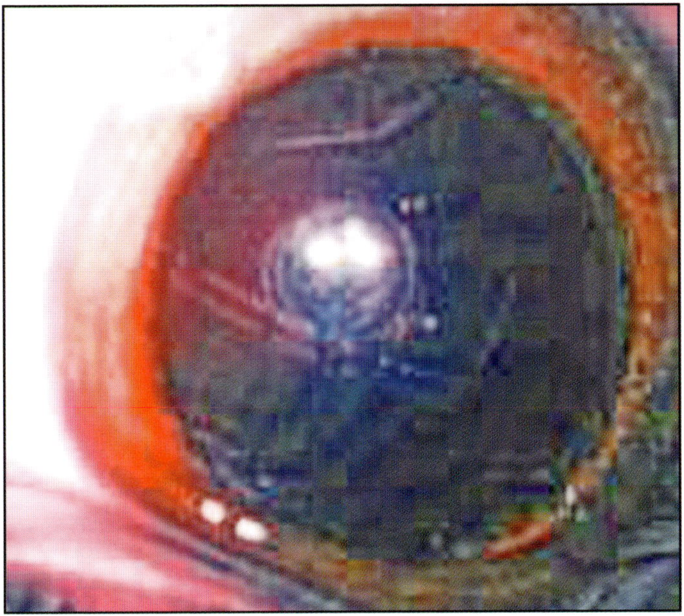

Fig. 7: Posterior polar cataract

Posterior Polar Cataract

INTRODUCTION

A posterior polar cataract is a round, discoid, opaque mass that is composed of malformed and distorted fibers of the crystalline lens, located in its central posterior part. This location is its main feature, in addition to its proximity to and possible adherence with the posterior capsule. Moreover, the capsule itself may be weakened because a malformation. As such, posterior polar cataract removal is a challenge to the surgeon because of its adherence to or the associated weakness or rupture of the posterior capsule.

CLINICAL SIGNS AND SYMPTOMS

- Decreased visual acuity: A diminution in the visual acuity is the most common complaint. The cataract is considered clinically relevant, and so indicative of surgery, if visual acuity is affected significantly. Central subcapsular posterior cataracts may have impaired vision since the early stages.
- Glare: This complaint may include an entire spectrum from a decrease in contrast sensitivity in brightly lit environments or disabling glare during the day to glare with oncoming headlights at night. Some patients report better vision at night in comparison with the bright of the day light.
- Monocular diplopia: At times, the subcortical changes are highly concentrated, resulting in a refractive area in the center of the lens, which conforms a second index of refraction of the lens.
- This distinctive subtype of lens opacity presents as an area of degenerative and malformed lens fibers that form opacity in the central posterior subcapsular area of the lens. Often, this opacity is adherent to the lens capsule, thereby making uncomplicated surgical removal problematic.

INVESTIGATIONS

The etiology of this congenital condition has been studied for many years. For some time, it has been recognized that posterior polar cataracts seemed to follow an autosomal dominant inheritance pattern with an occasional sporadic mutation. The direct cause of the lenticular fiber malformation during lens development has not been well understood. Genetic analysis has focused attention on a mutation on the *PITX3* gene, which was found to control the development of the anterior segment of the eye. The duplicate on of the 17 base pairs in this gene apparently alters the normal development of the anterior segment, leading to a posterior polar cataract.

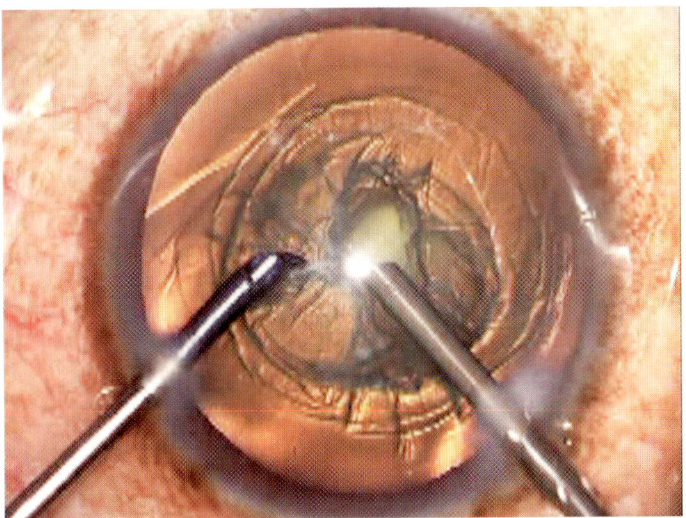

Fig. 8: Posterior polar cataract

DIFFERENTIAL DIAGNOSIS

The diagnosis of a posterior polar cataract is self-evident on slitlamp examination and does not require special diagnostic procedures beyond a full ophthalmic examination. Slit lamp examination and pupillary retroillumination allow a good evaluation of the visual significance of the opacity. The anterior vitreous should be examined carefully to ensure that it is free of opacity or capsular adherence.

TREATMENT

The histological changes of the malformed lens fibers are now recognized to be associated with an adherence of these degenerative lens fibers to an area of the weakened posterior capsule. Therefore, the surgical approach must be aimed at reducing the stress on the weakened posterior capsular. For this reason, various approaches have been suggested, including limited hydrodissection, viscodissection, and posterior capsulorhexis. Still, the reported rate of capsular rupture in the procedure is too high, sometimes 25% or more. Some other techniques suggested to minimize complications, include a bimanual microincisional approach (MICS or Phakonit), the use of viscodissection, a pars plana approach, and posterior capsulorrhexis. These approaches all address the weakness of the posterior capsule with its tendency to rupture. Since this challenge will continue to persist, different surgical approaches will continue to be offered.

PROGNOSIS

Frequently good according to the presentation of complications during surgery and the surgical management.

4

Complicated Cataract

Boris Malyugin (Russia)

Introduction

Cataract defined as any opacity of the natural lens, is a leading cause of blindness worldwide. Senile or age related cataract is referred as the lens opacity that occurs after the age of 50 without any evident cause. Cataract is considered "complicated" when it is developed due to some diseases or environmental factors.

Lens has a complex structure that may be affected both on the cellular or ultrastructural levels. Complicated cataract is usually posterior subcapsular. Histological such kind of opacities is associated with enlargement and migration of the epithelial cells in the posterior subcapsular region.

TRAUMA

Mechanical injury, radiation, electrical current and chemicals can cause traumatic lens damage. The reaction of the lens varies greatly with the origin of traumatic insult: sharp object, blunt contusion, electrical shock, etc.

Perforating and Penetrating Injury

In perforating or penetrating injury aqueous humor enters the lens through the capsular defect. This results in lens swelling, local opacification rapidly progressing to complete cataract formation. If the capsule defect is small it sometimes can heal spontaneously or can be blocked by the iris. In this cases localized lens opacity develops.

Contusion

In blunt trauma pigment epithelium can be imprinted in the anterior surface of the lens forming a Vossius ring. It is usually gradually resolves with time.

Blunt injury can cause acute or late cataract formation. Opacities usually localized in the anterior and/or posterior subcapsular region. Rosette-shaped cataract is often an early manifestation of lens contusion. It is located axially, involves posterior lens capsule, and can either improve spontaneously or progress to opacification of entire lens.

Blunt injury of the eye can also cause lens dislocation and subluxation . The leading mechanism of this is the compression of the globe in axial direction with expansion in the equatorial plane leading to zonular rupture. The lens may be dislocated in the anterior chamber or in the vitreous cavity.

Surgical Trauma

In cases of surgical trauma for instance after pars plana vitrectomy even if the lens capsule was not injured directly, posterior subcapsular cataract may form. The cause of this cataract is osmotic lens fibers insult leading to their hydration and subsequent transient or permanent opacification.

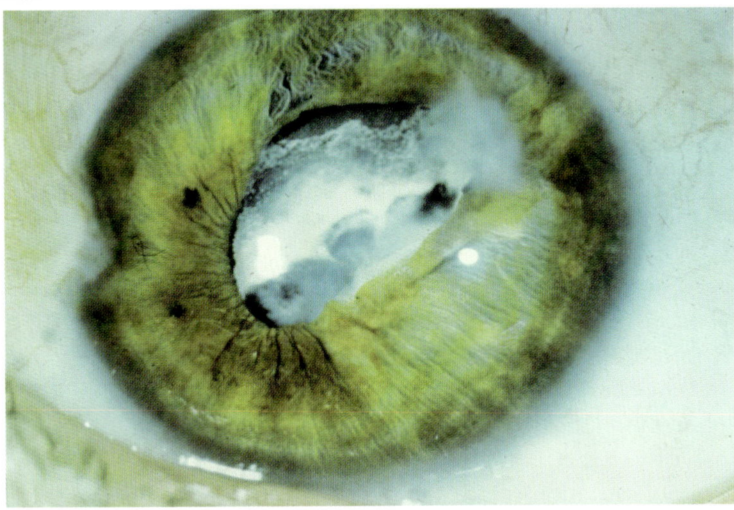

Fig. 1: Complete cataract after perforating corneal injury with iris and lens capsule damage

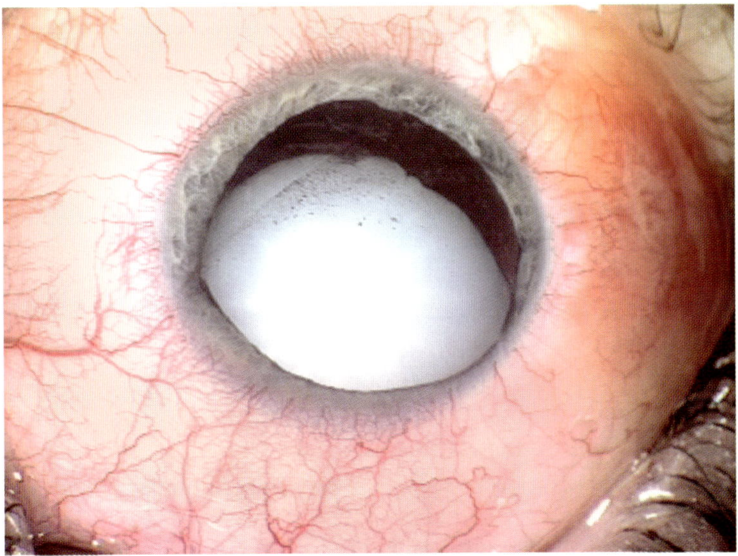

Fig. 2: Dislocated cataractous lens following blunt trauma

Electrical Trauma

Electrical shock leads to small vacuoles formation in the midperiphery of the lens that may disappear or transform to the grayish-white opacities in the anterior subcapsular region. Changes of the lens may progress, regress or remain stationary. Mechanism of lens opacification is protein coagulation.

RADIATION

The lens is very sensitive to ionizing radiation but cataract formation may take up to 2-3 decades depending on the dose of radiation and patient's age. Sources of ionizing radiation include natural (cosmic rays, gamma-rays) or artificial (X-ray stations, industrial devices, etc).

Different modalities of radiation vary in the energy required to cause cataract. The cause of cataract is the lens proteins damage by free radicals. Typical appearance of radiation cataract is the posterior subcapsular opacities.

Infrared radiation used to be a frequent cause of cataract in glassblower and furnace workers. The main leading factor is temperature rise in the anterior segment of the eye. Not frequent nowadays, typical appearance of this type of cataract include posterior subcapsular opacities with true exfoliation of the anterior capsule, which coils up in the anterior chamber.

UV radiation is also known as a predisposing factor of cataract formation leading to the nuclear and cortical changes via the mechanism of the free radical formation.

SYSTEMIC DISORDERS

Diabetes Mellitus

Mechanisms of diabetic cataract formation include protein damage due to glication and oxidative stress. As the result of the increased glucose blood level its concentration in the aqueous humor increases. Glucose enters the lens by diffusion and some of it is converted to sorbitol, which is not metabolized. Osmotic pressure causes the water influx in the lens leading to the lens swelling. This process can lead to transient refractive changes (induced myopia).

Frequency and progression of cataract depends on duration of diabetes and control of the disease. However, morphologically diabetic cataracts are indistinguishable from the senile cataracts.

In young diabetic patients with poorly controlled glucose blood level true diabetic cataract may occur. Lens opacify quickly with typical "snowflake" appearance: bilateral, dense gray-white anterior and posterior subcapsular opacities in the cortex. Intumescence and maturity of the cortical opacities follow the appearance of multiple subcapsular opacities. With appropriate treatment of diabetes opacities progression may be slowed down with development of lamellar cataract.

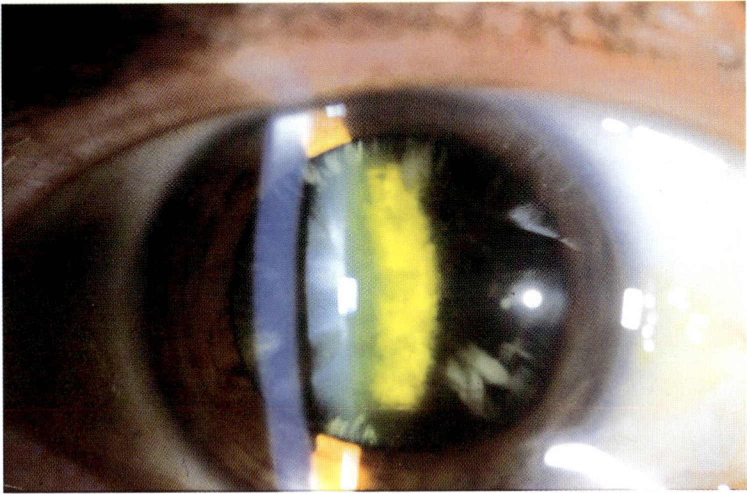

Fig. 3: Radiation cataract with posterior subcapsular opacities

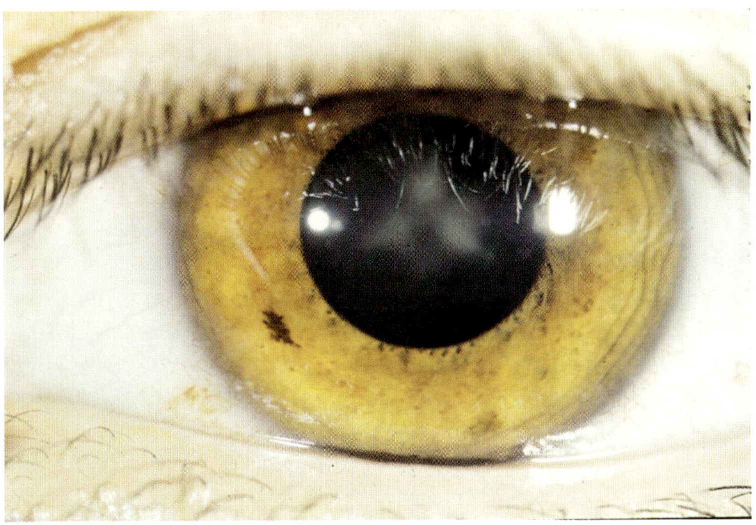

Fig. 4: True diabetic cataract (snowflake cataract)—gray-white subcapsular opacities

In patients with severe proliferative diabetic retinopathy cataract is not infrequently associated with iris rubeosis and neovascular glaucoma.

In adult diabetic patients cataracts are much more frequent than in the same age population. Different type of lens opacities can be observed—cortical, nuclear, and subcapsular.

Galactosemia

Galactosemia is an autosomal recessive disorder caused by absence of ferments responsible of conversion of galactose into glucose. Accumulation of galactose and galaction within the lens leading to osmotic swelling is the cause of lens opacities. Water influx is leading to the nucleus and cortex opacification has typical "oil droplet" appearance. Opacification of the lens may also occur in anterior and posterior subcapsular regions. In classic galactosemia within a few weeks of life the symptoms of mental deficiency, malnutrition, hepatomegaly and jaundice appear.

Hypocalcemia

Hypocalcemia is a well known cause of cataracts. It may be idiopathic or aquired (unintended destruction of parathyroid glands during surgery). The appearance: punctuate opacities located in the anterior and posterior cortex adjacent to the capsule but separated from it with the layer of clear cortex.

Wilson's Disease

Hepatolenticular degeneration (Wilson's disease) is inherited disorder of copper metabolism. Characteristic ocular manifestation is a brown discoloration of Descemet's membrane in the periphery of the cornea (Kayser-Fleisher ring). Sunflower cataract not infrequently develops with brown deposits consisted of cuprous oxide in the anterior lens capsule and subcapsular cortex in a stellate shape.

Myotonic Dystrophy

This inherited disease is characterized by delayed contracted muscles relaxation. Symptoms: ptosis, facial musculature weakness, cardiac pathology, and frontal balding. Typical cataract: polychromatic iridescent crystals in the lens cortex progressing to posterior subcapsular and then to complete cortical opacification.

Other predominantly inherited disorders including Alport syndrome, oculocerebral syndrome, etc. can lead to cataract formation as well.

DERMATOLOGICAL DISORDERS

Atopic dermatitis or eczema is associated with bilateral cataract in up to 25% of cases. Characteristic "shield" cataract is a dense anterior subcapsular plaque with cortical riders and wrinkled anterior capsule.

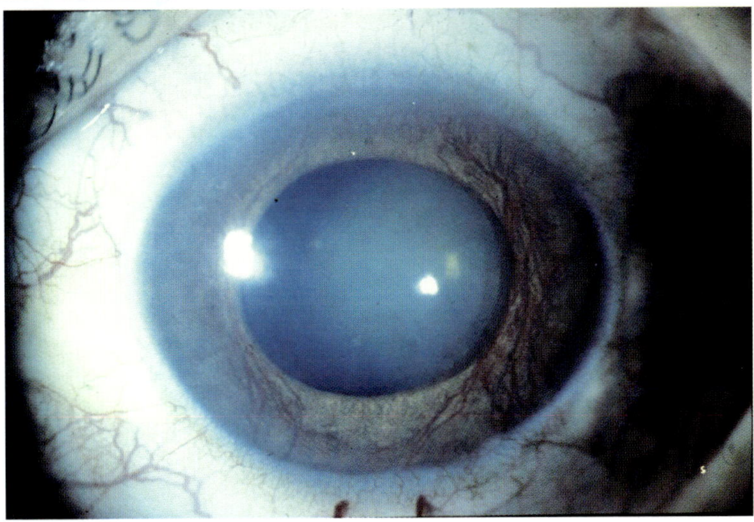

Fig. 5: Diabetic cataract with iris rubeosis and secondary glaucoma

Other dermatological diseases associated with cataract formation include ichthyosis, Werner's syndrome, Cockayne's syndrome, etc.

CENTRAL NERVOUS SYSTEM DISORDERS

CNS disorders—neurofibromatosis, Zellweger syndrome, Norrie's disease—are usually inherited. Cataract is only one of the symptoms of these diseases.

LOCAL OCULAR DISEASES

Local ocular diseases leading to cataract formation include glaucoma, uveitis, retinitis pigmentosa, degenerative myopia, tumors, gyrate atrophy, and ischemia.

Glaucoma

Chronic open angle glaucoma is not infrequently associated with cataract. The main predisposing factors of anterior subcapsular changes include use of miotics and other antiglaucoma drugs, glaucoma surgery leading to hypotony and anterior chamber shallowing.

Glaukomfleken – gray-white epithelial and anterior cortical lens opacities that occur following elevated IOP in acute angle-closure glaucoma. Characteristic white localized lens opacities appear under the anterior lens capsule. Histologically they composed of necrotic lens epithelium and degenerated subepithelial cortex.

Pseudoexfoliation Syndrome (PES)

In PES gray fibrillo-granular material is deposited on the cornea, lens, ciliary processes, zonular fibers and trabecular meshwork. This condition is associated with iris pigment atrophy, capsular fragility, poorly dilated pupil, zonular weakness, trabecular meshwork pigmentation, open-angle glaucoma. PES is associated with increased prevalence of senescent cataracts.

Tumors

Ciliary body tumors can also lead to the cortical lens opacifications usually localized in the affected region.

Uveitis

Inflammation can cause posterior subcapsular cataract changes that can arise from the disease itself as well as from the medications (corticosteroids). Chronic uveitis is often associated with lens changes. In some patients development of fibrovascular membrane covering the pupil secondary to uveitis can be observed.

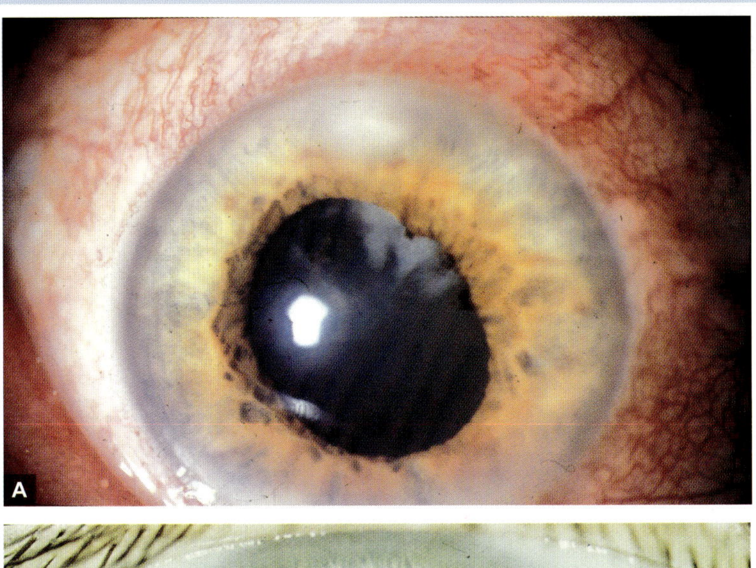

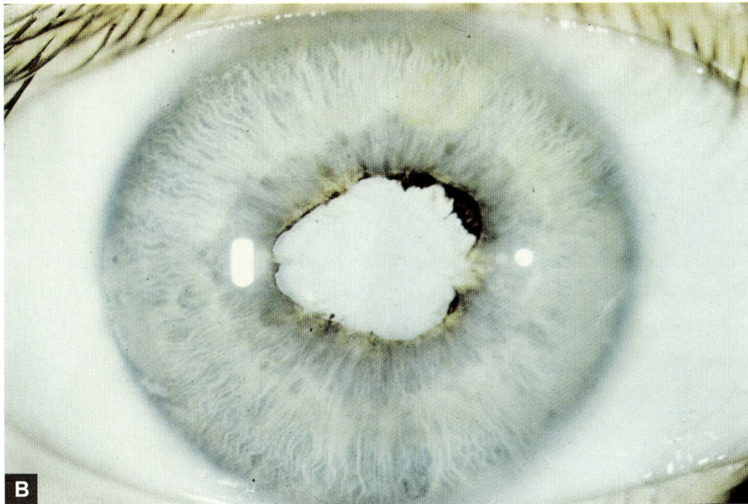

Figs 6A and B: Cataracts in patients with acute (A) and chronic (B) uveitis, note posterior synechiae formation

Fuchs heterochromic uveitis is a unilateral disease. Affected eye has iris discoloration associated with lens opacification.

Phacoantygenic uveitis is initiated by lens proteins leaked through the damaged lens capsule. It is usually occurs following traumatic lens rupture or retained cortical material after cataract surgery. In these patients symptoms of inflammation in the anterior segment (red eye, pain, anterior chamber flare and cells, corneal precipitates) are usually discovered.

Degenerative Ocular Disorders

In retinitis pigmentosa, essential iris atrophy, chronic hypotony, and absolute glaucoma cataracts begin as posterior subcapsular and gradually progress to total lens opacification.

ISCHEMIA

Posterior subcapsular cataracts can be caused by ocular ischemia due to the Takayasy arteritis (pulseless disease), Buerger disease (thromboangiitis obliterans) and anterior segment necrosis.

TOXIC CASES

Several drugs are known to cause cataract formation. Prolonged therapy with corticosteroids either topical or systemic is associated with posterior subcapsular cataract formation. The incidence is dose-dependent and related to duration of treatment as well as the individual susceptibility. Corticosteroid cataracts show centrally located posterior subcapsular opacity of about 3 mm in diameter that gradually increases in size.

Chronic use of anticholinesterase drugs for open-angle glaucoma treatment can lead to the anterior subcapsular vacuoles that may progress to nuclear and posterior cortical cataracts as well. Cataract formation is more likely in patients receiving miotic therapy over a long period of time.

The other drugs leading to cataract formation include: phenothiazines, antimitotic and antimalarial agents, amiodarone, and some others. Phenothiazines (psychotropic medications) lead to pigmented deposits accumulation in the anterior lens epithelium. Changes in visual acuity are mostly insignificant.

Toxic chemicals causing corneal burns can cause anterior punctuate lens opacities. Alkali compounds penetrate the cornea causing the change in pH of aqueous humor and subsequent cataract formation. Acid burns are less prone to intraocular damage because of their less prone tendency to penetrate the eye than alkali.

Copper that is deposited in the eye from the intraocular foreign body, eye drops or as the result of Wilson's disease results in development of sunflower cataract. The latter is a deposition of yellow or brown pigmentation in the lens capsule that goes from the anterior pole of the capsule to its equator.

Iron accumulation in the eye from the foreign body cause iris brown discoloration and flower-shaped cataract. The condition is called siderosis bulbi. Lens opacification gradually become complete with time.

HEREDITARY CATARACTS

Hereditary cataracts may be discovered in infancy or later on. They are associated with systemic syndromes such as dystrophia myotonica, Down's syndrome, Patau's syndrome, Edward's syndrome and some other hereditary diseases.

Clinical Signs and Symptoms

SYMPTOMS

Visual acuity and contrast sensitivity reduction, myopic shift, monocular diplopia, glare, color shift, visual field loss.

Symptoms of traumatic lens subluxation include decreased visual acuity, fluctuation of vision, monocular diplopia, high astigmatism. Irido- and phacodonesis are often present in traumatic cataract cases.

As opposed to the age-related cataracts with predominantly nuclear changes, in complicated cataracts subcapsular and cortical layers are involved in most cases. Some cataracts may have specific appearance (true diabetic cataracts, cataracts in myotonic dystrophy, etc.). Nevertheless most of complicated cataracts are indistinguishable one from another.

Investigations

Medical history and current therapeutic status are very important issues. Patient should be evaluated generally to reveal systemic disorders, diabetes mellitus, hereditary diseases. Special attention should be paid to the cardiac, bronchopulmonary and cerebrovascular disease.

Slitlamp microscopy is a major method to establish the diagnosis of cataract. However the image of the cataractous lens can poorly correlate with the patient's visual acuity. During examination pupil should be maximally dilated.

Specific preoperative ophthalmic tests include: refraction, visual acuity, keratometry, biometry, B-scan ultrasonography, specular microscopy, gonioscopy.

Physician has to evaluate not only affected eye but also the fellow eye when possible.

Differential Diagnosis

Differential diagnosis should be done between the main diseases causing cataracts in order to provide proper treatment. The surgeon has to establish the link between the coexistent ophthalmic pathology and its influence on the pre- and postoperative pharmacological regimen, recovery and outcome.

Treatment

The main treatment method of visually disabling cataract is extraction. In general, the majority of complicated cataracts can be safely removed with phacoemulsification followed by posterior chamber intraocular lens implantation. Indications for the surgical tactics in each particular case vary extensively. The surgeon should take in the consideration the visual needs of the patient according to his age, occupation, life style. Risks of the modern small incision cataract surgery are few if technically performed well. So the main source of complications is the ocular and systemic comorbidity. In complicated cataract surgery higher complication rate is anticipated.

Special surgical techniques (vitrectomy, capsular tension rings, pupil expansion devices) and alternative methods of IOL fixation (i.e. scleral and iris fixation) should be considered since zonular dehiscence, loss of capsular integrity, small pupils and some other clinical findings and intraoperative events are not common in complicated cataract cases.

Systemic conditions may negatively influence both the surgery and postoperative course. General factors influence surgeons and anesthesiologist decision about the type of anesthesia and sedation required. In systemic disorders good understanding of the therapeutic measures used in its treatment is essential for the success of the surgery.

Prognosis

Cataract removal usually leads to the visual rehabilitation. Nevertheless, ophthalmic disorders may prejudice good visual outcome. Uveitis may cause increased prolonged postoperative inflammation, atopic disease – predispose to infection, diabetes mellitus – to postoperative macular edema, etc. Risk factors include prolonged postoperative corneal edema, exuberant postoperative inflammation, increased risk of cystoid macular edema, IOP spikes, retinal detachment, etc.

The visual outcome of patients with complicated cataracts who undergo surgery depends on a couple of factors including amount of the initial eye damage, degree of surgical trauma of the ocular structures, and degree and duration of postoperative inflammation. Proper medical management of operated patients is essential for a successful outcome of treatment.

5

Traumatic Cataract

- **Traumatic Cataract**

  Arturo Perez Arteaga (Mexico)

- **Management of Traumatic Cataract**

  Rupesh V Agrawal, Satish Desai (India)

Traumatic Cataract

Arturo Perez Arteaga (Mexico)

Introduction

Traumatic opacification of the lens occur secondary to blunt or penetrating ocular trauma. Infrared energy (Glass-Blower's cataract), electric shock, and ionizing radiation are other rare causes of traumatic cataracts.

Clinical Signs and Symptoms

CLINICAL HISTORY

Mechanism of injury (sharp versus blunt); past ocular history including previous eye surgery, glaucoma, retinal detachment, diabetic eye disease. Visual complaints:

- Decreased vision—Cataract, lens subluxation, lens dislocation, ruptured globe, traumatic optic neuropathy, vitreous hemorrhage, retinal detachment.
- Monocular diplopia—Lens subluxation with partial phakic and aphakic vision
- Binocular diplopia—Traumatic nerve palsy, orbital fracture
- Pain—Glaucoma secondary to hyphema, pupillary block, or lens particles; retrobulbar hemorrhage; iritis.

CLINICAL FINDINGS

A complete ophthalmic examination is mandatory.

- Vision and pupils—Presence of afferent pupillary defect indicative of traumatic optic neuropathy
- Extraocular motility—Orbital fractures or traumatic nerve palsy
- Intraocular pressure—Secondary glaucoma, retrobulbar hemorrhage
- Anterior chamber—Hyphema, iritis, shallow chamber, iridodonesis, angle recession
- Lens—Subluxation, dislocation, capsular integrity (anterior and posterior), cataract (extent and type), swelling, phacodonesis
- Vitreous—Presence or absence of hemorrhage, posterior vitreous detachment
- Fundus— Retinal detachment, choroidal rupture, commotio retinae, preretinal hemorrhage, intraretinal hemorrhage, subretinal hemorrhage, optic nerve pallor, optic nerve avulsion.

PARACLINICAL FINDINGS

B-scan—If posterior pole cannot be visualized. A-scan—Prior to cataract extraction. CT scan orbits—Fractures and foreign bodies. Planning surgical

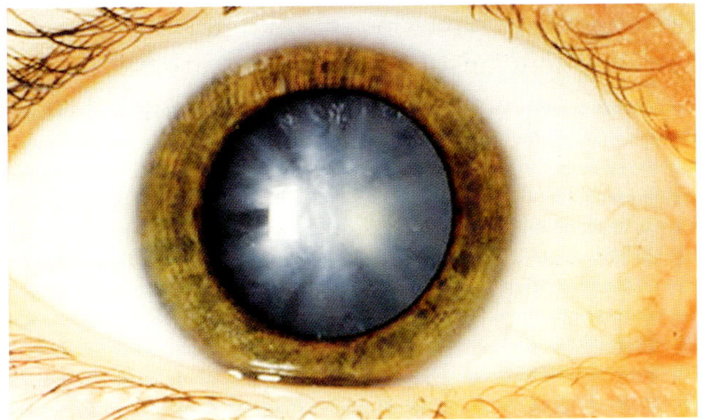

Fig. 1: Traumatic cataract

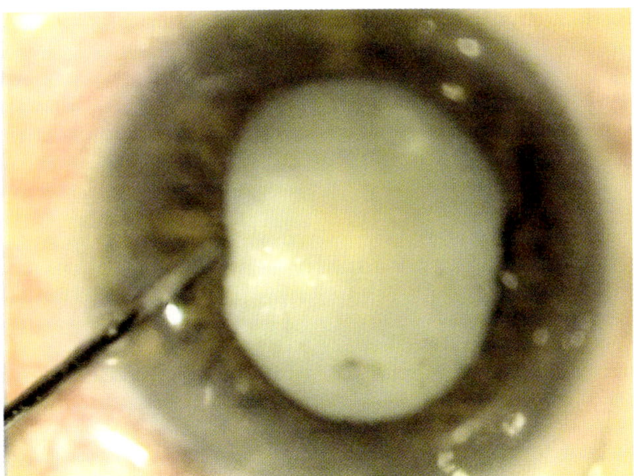

Fig. 2: Traumatic cataract

approach is of utmost importance in cases of traumatic cataract. Preoperative capsular integrity and zonular stability should be surmised. In cases of posterior dislocation without glaucoma, inflammation, or visual obstruction, surgery may be avoided.

Investigations

Blunt trauma is responsible for coup and countercoup ocular injury. Coup is the mechanism of direct impact. It is responsible for Vossius ring (imprinted iris pigment) sometimes found on the anterior lens capsule following blunt injury. Countercoup refers to distant injury caused by shockwaves traveling along the line of concussion. When the anterior surface of the eye is struck bluntly, there is a rapid anterior-posterior shortening accompanied by equatorial expansion. This equatorial stretching can disrupt the lens capsule, zonules, or both. Combination of coup, countercoup, and equatorial expansion is responsible for formation of traumatic cataract following blunt ocular injury. Penetrating trauma that directly compromises the lens capsule leads to cortical opacification at the site of injury. If the rent is sufficiently large, the entire lens rapidly opacifies, but when small, cortical cataract can seal itself off and remain localized.

Differential Diagnosis

Cataracts caused by blunt trauma have classically the form of stellate- or rosette-shaped; posterior axial opacities may be stable or progressive; in penetrating trauma with disruption of lens capsule forms cortical changes that may remain focal if small or may progress rapidly to total cortical opacification. Lens dislocation and subluxation are found commonly in conjunction with traumatic cataract. Other associated complications include phacolytic, phacomorphic, pupillary block, and angle-recession glaucoma, phacoanaphylactic uveitis, retinal detachment, choroid rupture, hyphema, retrobulbar hemorrhage, traumatic optic neuropathy and globe rupture. Traumatic cataract can present many medical and surgical challenges to the ophthalmologist. Careful examination and a management plan can simplify these difficult cases and provide the best possible outcome. The complete diagnosis of the damage caused to the whole globe must be done.

Treatment

a. In cases of posterior dislocation without glaucoma, inflammation, or visual obstruction, surgery may be avoided.
b. Indications for surgery include the following:
   — Unacceptable decreased vision

— Obstructed view of posterior pathology
— Lens-induced inflammation or glaucoma
— Capsular rupture with lens swelling
— Other trauma-induced ocular pathology necessitating surgery.

c. Standard phacoemulsification may be performed if lens capsule is intact and sufficient zonular support remains.
d. Intracapsular cataract extraction is required in cases of anterior dislocation or extreme zonular instability. Anterior dislocation of the lens into the anterior chamber requires emergency surgery for its removal, because it can cause pupillary block glaucoma.
e. Pars plana lensectomy and vitrectomy may be best in cases of posterior capsular rupture, posterior dislocation, or extreme zonular instability.

Prognosis

Prognosis is dependent on the extent of the injury.

Management of Traumatic Cataract

Rupesh V Agrawal, Satish Desai (India)

Introduction

Cataract is by far the commonest complication causing loss of vision following any type of ocular injury. The management of such cases is an important problem in ophthalmology and prognosis is variable. Extent of associated damage to anterior and posterior segment, time of intervention, operative and post-operative complications go a long way in determining the ultimate prognosis. The type of trauma, extent of lenticular involvement and associated secondary rise of intraocular pressure are factors of paramount importance which could dictate the exact time of management of traumatic cataract. Cataracts caused by blunt trauma classically form stellate or rosette shaped posterior axial opacities that may be stable or progressive, whereas penetrating trauma with disruption of lens capsule forms cortical changes that may remain focal if small or may progress rapidly to total cortical opacification. Lens dislocation and subluxation are found commonly in conjunction with traumatic cataract.

Pathophysiology

Blunt trauma is responsible for coup and contrecoup ocular injury. Coup is the mechanism of direct impact. It is responsible for Vossius ring (imprinted iris pigment) sometimes found on the anterior lens capsule following blunt injury.

When the anterior surface of the eye is struck bluntly, there is a rapid anterior-posterior shortening accompanied by equatorial expansion. This equatorial stretching can disrupt the lens capsule, zonules, or both. Combination of coup, contrecoup, and equatorial expansion is responsible for formation of traumatic cataract following blunt ocular injury.

Penetrating trauma that directly compromises the lens capsule leads to cortical opacification at the site of injury. If the rent is sufficiently large, the entire lens rapidly opacifies, but when small, cortical cataract can seal itself off and remain localized.

SEX

Male-to-female ratio in cases of ocular trauma is 4:1.

AGE

Work- and sports-related eye injuries most commonly occur in young adults and children.

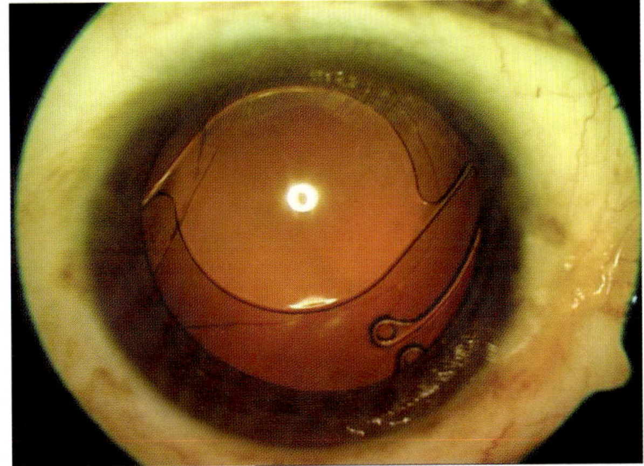

Fig. 1: CTR in bag

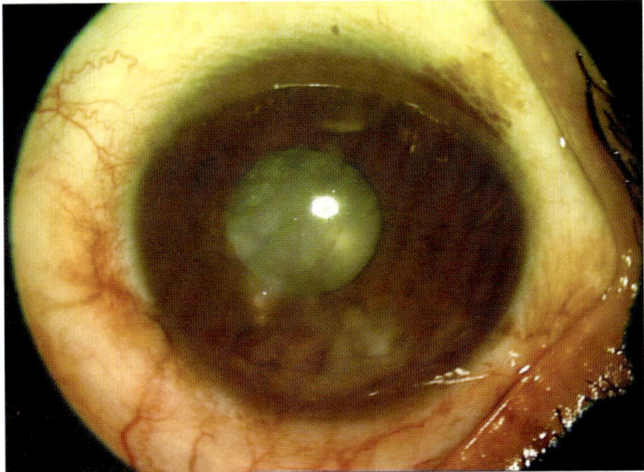

Fig. 2: Traumatic cataract with torn anterior capsule

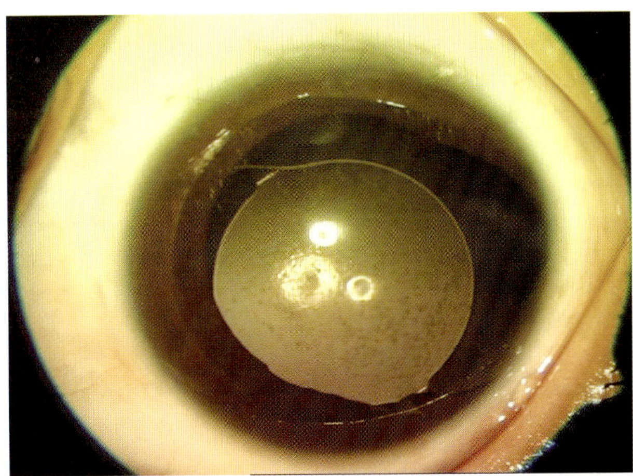

Fig. 3: Deposits on IOL

HISTORY

- Mechanism of injury—Sharp versus blunt
- Past ocular history—Previous eye surgery, glaucoma, retinal detachment, diabetic eye disease
- Past medical history—Diabetes, sickle cell, Marfan's syndrome, homocystinuria, hyperlysinemia, sulfate oxidase deficiency
- Visual complaints
  - Decreased vision—Cataract, lens subluxation, lens dislocation, ruptured globe, traumatic optic neuropathy, vitreous hemorrhage, retinal detachment
  - Monocular diplopia—Lens subluxation with partial phakic and aphakic vision
  - Binocular diplopia—Traumatic nerve palsy, orbital fracture
  - Pain—Glaucoma secondary to hyphema, pupillary block, or lens particles; retrobulbar hemorrhage; iritis.

Physical Examination

- Complete ophthalmic examination (tailored in cases of globe compromise)
  - Vision and pupils—Presence of afferent pupillary defect (APD) indicative of traumatic optic neuropathy
  - Extraocular motility—Orbital fractures or traumatic nerve palsy
  - Intraocular pressure—Secondary glaucoma, retrobulbar hemorrhage
  - Anterior chamber—Hyphema, iritis, shallow chamber, iridodonesis, angle recession
  - Lens—Subluxation, dislocation, capsular integrity (anterior and posterior), cataract (extent and type), swelling, phacodonesis
  - Vitreous—Presence or absence of hemorrhage, posterior vitreous detachment
  - Fundus—Retinal detachment, choroidal rupture, commotio retinae, preretinal hemorrhage, intraretinal hemorrhage, subretinal hemorrhage, optic nerve pallor, optic nerve avulsion.

Traumatic Cataract (types)

- Penetrating
- Concussion (Rosette cataract)
- Infrared irradiation (Glass Blower's cataract)
- Electrocution
- Ionizing radiation.

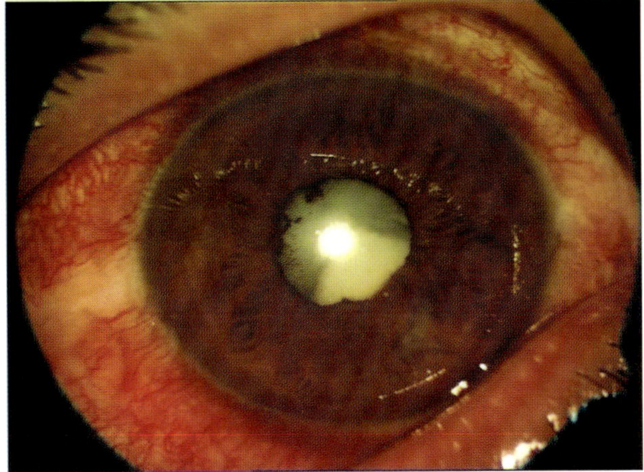

Fig. 4: Partial lens abscess

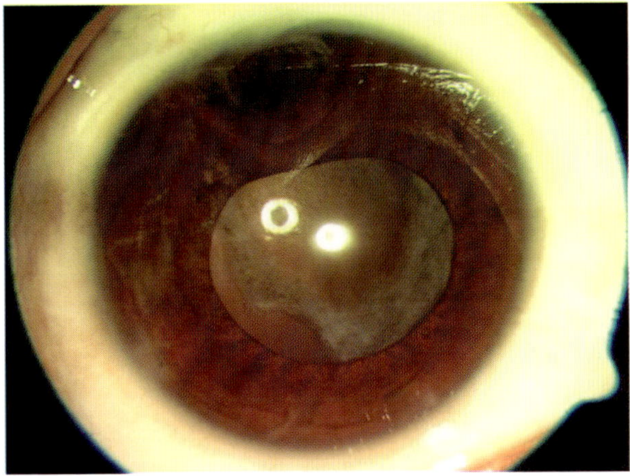

Fig. 5: Postcataract surgery with partially repaired iris

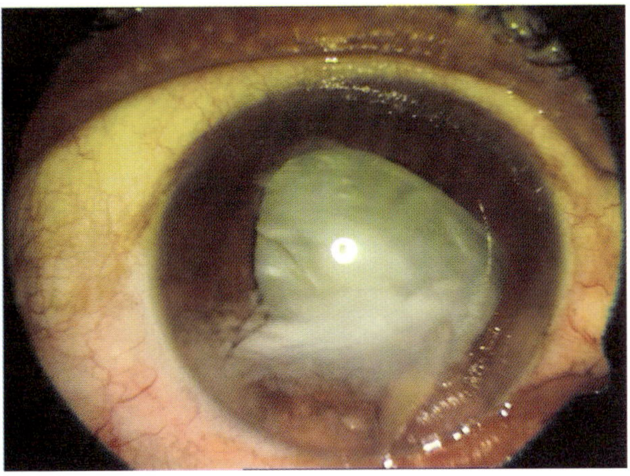

Fig. 6: Traumatic cataract with breached AC

CAUSES

- Traumatic cataracts occur secondary to blunt or penetrating ocular trauma.

OTHER PROBLEMS TO BE CONSIDERED

- Globe rupture
- Orbital fractures
- Retinal detachment
- Secondary glaucoma
- Traumatic optic neuropathy.

FACTORS TO BE ANALYZED

- Corneal involvement
- Preoperative and postoperative BCVA
- Visual axis involvement
- Breach in anterior capsule
- Lens matter in anterior capsule
- Pre-existing posterior capsular rent on ultrasound
- Subluxation of the traumatic cataractous lens
- Associated iridodialysis.

IMAGING STUDIES

- B-scan—If posterior pole cannot be visualized
- A-scan—Prior to cataract extraction
- CT scan orbits—Fractures and foreign bodies.

CAUSES OF POSTOPERATIVE NONIMPROVEMENT OF BCVA IN TRAUMATIC CATARACT

- Amblyopia
- Corneal scar involving visual axis
- Cortex in papillary area
- Subluxation of IOL
- IOL tilt
- CME
- Traumatic optic neuropathy
- Pupillary capture.

MEDICAL CARE

- If glaucoma is a problem, control intraocular pressure with standard medications; add corticosteroids if lens particles are the cause or if iritis is present.

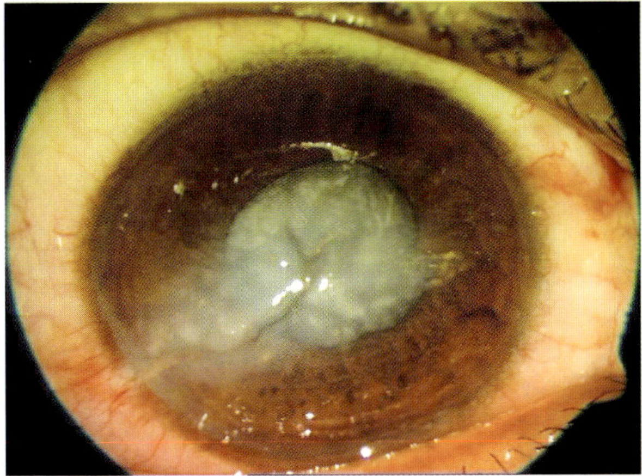

Fig. 7: Traumatic cataract with foreign body

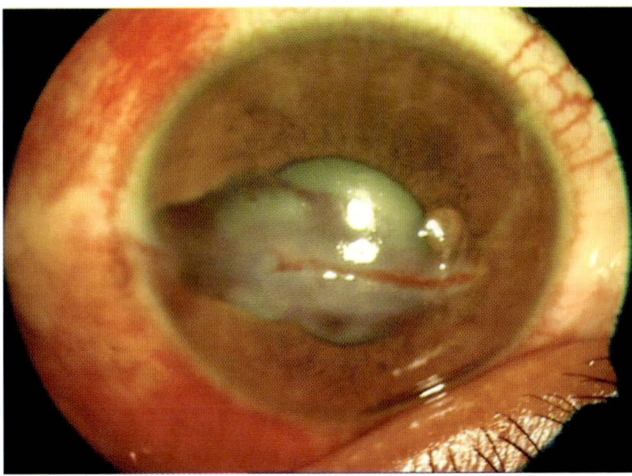

Fig. 8: Traumatic cataract with heme

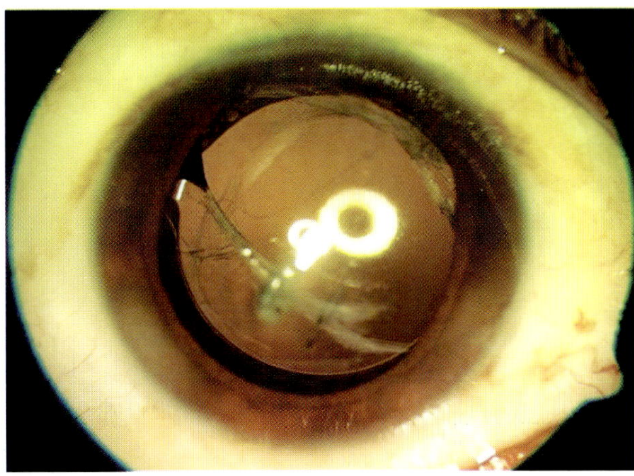

Fig. 9: Traumatic cataract with IOL in torn bag

- Focal cataract
  - Observation if cataract is outside the visual axis
  - Miotic therapy may be of benefit if the cataract is close to the visual axis.
- In some cases of lens subluxation, miotics may correct monocular diplopia; mydriatics may allow for vision around the lens with aphakic correction.

Practical Points in Management of Traumatic Cataract

- Corneoscleral integrity
- Meticulous restoration of normal relationships
- Sufficient release of posterior synechiae
- Capsular and zonular integrity
- Vitreoretinal changes

SURGERY

Depending on the clinical situation, the surgical management of a traumatic cataract is performed either a standard anterior limbal or posterior pars plana approach. An anterior approach is best for a traumatic cataract unless there is complete lens dislocation or capsular rupture with significant lens material incarcerated in the vitreous.

PRACTICAL TIPS WHILE PERFORMING TRAUMATIC CATARACT SURGERY

- Planning surgical approach is of utmost importance in cases of traumatic cataract.
- Preoperative capsular integrity and zonular stability should be surmised.
- In cases of posterior dislocation without glaucoma, inflammation, or visual obstruction, surgery may be avoided.
- Indications for surgery include the following:
  - Unacceptable decreased vision
  - Obstructed view of posterior pathology
  - Lens-induced inflammation or glaucoma
  - Capsular rupture with lens swelling
  - Other trauma-induced ocular pathology necessitating surgery
- Standard phacoemulsification or manual small incision cataract surgery may be performed if lens capsule is intact and sufficient zonular support remains.
- Intracapsular cataract extraction is required in cases of anterior dislocation or extreme zonular instability. Anterior dislocation of the lens into the anterior chamber requires emergency surgery for its removal, as it can cause pupillary block glaucoma.

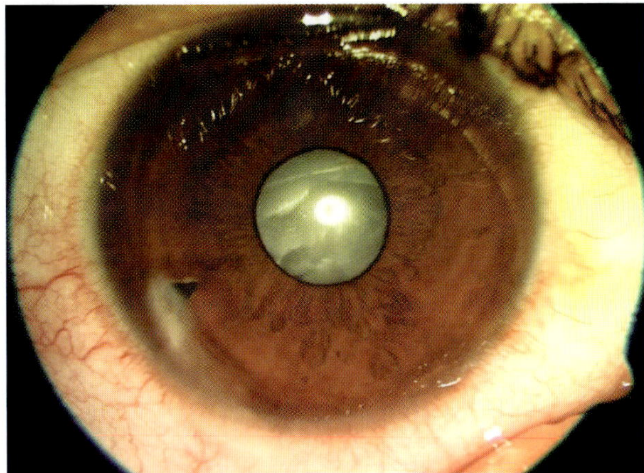

Fig. 10: Traumatic cataract with iris hole

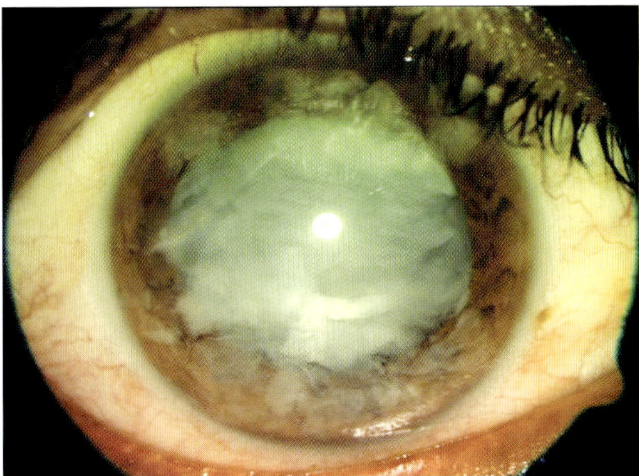

Fig. 11: Traumatic cataract with loose lens matter in AC

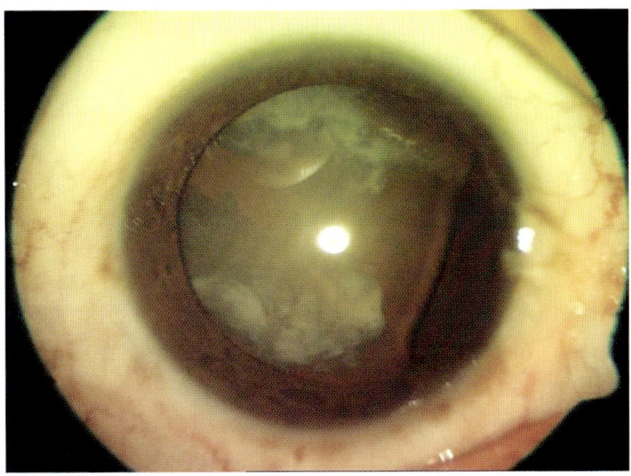

Fig. 12: Traumatic cataract with subluxation of lens

- Pars plana lensectomy and vitrectomy may be best in cases of posterior capsular rupture, posterior dislocation, or extreme zonular instability.
- Automated irrigation/aspiration can be used in patients younger than 35 years. Look for the posterior capsular support preoperatively, should be careful while performing automated irrigation aspiration and while switching the anterior chamber maintainer on as the fluid flow inside the eye can enlarge the pre-existing posterior capsular dehiscence and can result in lens matter drop or nucleus drop.
- Lens implantation
    - Capsular fixation is the preferred placement if lens capsule and zonular support are intact.
    - CTR may be implanted before or after phacoemulsification. Although early insertion provides support during phacoemulsification, it may create additional zonular trauma. The use of iris or capsule retractors at the capsulorhexis' edge or the use of a capsular tension segment (CTS; Morcher GmbH, Stuttgart, Germany [not currently approved by the FDA]) during phacoemulsification are other alternatives that do not induce significant capsular torque during insertion. The CTS is a partial PMMA ring segment containing an anteriorly offset eyelet through which an iris retractor or suture may be placed.
    - Capsular tension ring should never be implanted in cases with broken capsulorrhexis and in eyes with pre-existing posterior capsular rent.
    - Polymethyl methacrylate (PMMA) capsular tension rings allow capsular fixation in cases of zonular dialysis less than 180 degrees.
    - Sulcus fixation is safe if posterior capsule is compromised but zonular support is maintained.
    - Suture fixation is chosen if both capsular and zonular supports are insufficient and the angle is damaged minimally.
    - Anterior chamber placement is an option if no posterior support remains and iris or ciliary body trauma prevents suture fixation.
    - Aphakia may be a better choice in young children and patients with highly inflamed eyes; they may experience better outcomes if lens implantation is deferred.

Complications

Surgery for traumatic cataract is associated with high incidence of complications and surgeon should anticipate and be prepared for complications during the surgery. The different complications during traumatic cataract surgery can be:

- Posterior capsular rent
- Zonular dialysis

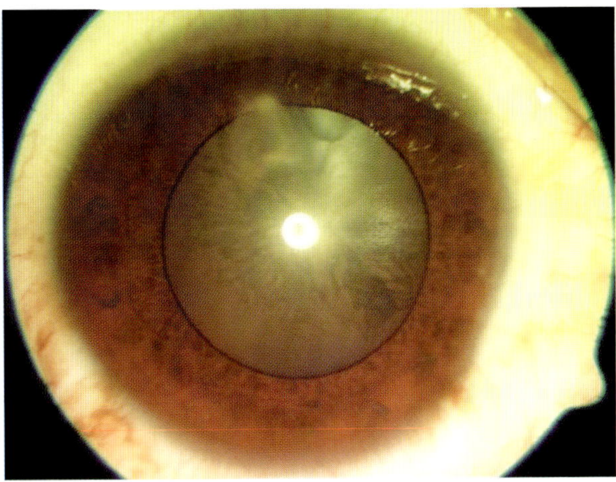

Fig. 13: Early Rosette cataract

- Nucleus or lens matter drop
- Postoperative unusual inflammation
- Posterior capsular opacification
- Pupillary capture of IOL
- Postoperative refractive surprise

6

Dismetabolic Cataracts

GM Cavallini, C Masini, L Campi,
C Chiesi, S Pelloni (Italy)

Introduction

Dismetabolic cataract is a loss of lens transparency due to an insult to the nuclear or lenticular fibers, caused by a metabolic disorder. The lens opacification may occur early or later in life, and may be isolated or associated to particular syndromes. The exact incidence of this kind of cataract is not known, as it is often numbered in the group of congenital cataracts. Actually, metabolic and systemic disease are found in as many as 60% of bilateral congenital cataracts. Screening for metabolic disorders in all children with bilateral cataracts is essential, as in some inherited metabolic disorders progressive and severe symptoms can be avoided with timely initiation of treatment.

The metabolic disorders that are more frequently associated to cataract formation are reported in table.

Table 1: Various metabolic disorder associated to cataract formation
Galactosemia
Mucolipidosis type I
Mucolipidosis type II
Fabry disease
Galactokinase deficiency
Glucose-6-phosphate dehydrogenase deficiency
Mannosidosis
Refsum disease
Lowe's syndrome
Alport's syndrome
Familiar hypoparathyroidism
Cholesterol biosynthesis defects (Smith-Lemli-Opitz syndrome, lathosterolosis...)
Metabolic syndrome
Diabetes

We describe some of these metabolic conditions associated with cataract formation, and in particular we report our experience with a patient affected by lathosterolosis that presented bilateral cataracts.

Cataract in Galactosemia

Classical galactosemia is an autosomal recessive disorder caused by a severe compromission of galactose utilization due to deficiency of the enzyme galactose-1-phosphate uridyltransferase (GALT). The GALT enzyme is responsible for the conversion of galactose-1-phosphate with UDP glucose to glucose-1-phosphate and UDP galactose. The gene encoding for GALT is located on chromosome 9p13. Patients present with hepatomegaly, liver failure, food intolerance, hypoglycaemia, muscle hypotonia, sepsis and cataract. The typical appearance of galactosemic cataract is an "oil-drop" central opacity, caused by the accumulation of galactitol in the lens. This causes an increase in the osmotic pressure within the lens, with a subsequent osmotic water inflow and lens

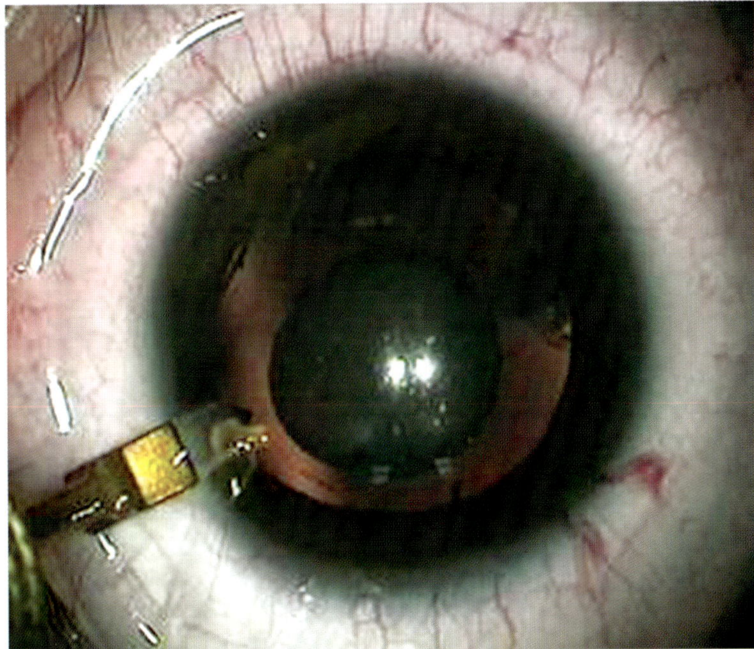

Fig. 1: Galactosemic dismetabolic cataract

opacification. The ophthalmologist may play an important role in this disease, since early recognition of cataract development followed by the initiation of a galactose-free diet may lead to clearing of lenticular opacities. Treatment involving the total restriction of lactose-containing foods is also life-saving but many patients develop late complications such as problems of mental development, disorders of motor function, disorders of speech and hyper-gonadotrophic hypogonadism.

Cataract in Galactokinase Deficiency

Galactokinase (GALK1) deficiency is an autosomal recessive disorder, which involves the first enzyme of galactose metabolic chain. Galactokinase deficiency results from mutation in the GALK1 gene mapped on 17q24. Cataract and, rarely, pseudotumor cerebri caused by galactitol accumulation seem to be the only consistently reported abnormalities in this disorder. Cataracts may develop during infancy or may be presenile in the adult population. The lens opacity has typically a lamellar shape.

As cataract and pseudotumor cerebri appear to be the only complications of galactokinase deficiency, the outcome for patients with galactokinase deficiency is much better than for patients with classical galactosemia.

Cataract in Lowe's Syndrome

The oculo-cerebro-renal syndrome of Lowe (OCRL) is a rare X-chromosomal disorder characterized by the triad of congenital cataracts, renal tubular dysfunction, and mental retardation. The mutation of the gene OCRL1 localized at Xq26.1, coding for the enzyme phosphatidylinositol bisphosphate 5 phosphatase, PtdIns P2, in the Trans-Golgi network is responsible for the disease. Bilateral cataract and severe hypotonia are present at birth. In the subsequent weeks or months the ocular picture may be complicated by glaucoma and cheloids. Psychomotor retardation is evident in childhood, while behavioural problems prevail and renal complications arise in adolescence.

Typically complete opacification and discoid deformation of the lenses (microphakia) are seen, indicating a developmental defect in early embryogenesis Patients with mild Lowe's syndrome phenotype may show incomplete lenticular opacities without visual impairment.

Cataract in Mannosidosis

Mannosidosis is a rare disorder of glycoprotein metabolism. The primary metabolic defect in mannosidosis is the deficiency of the acidic alpha-

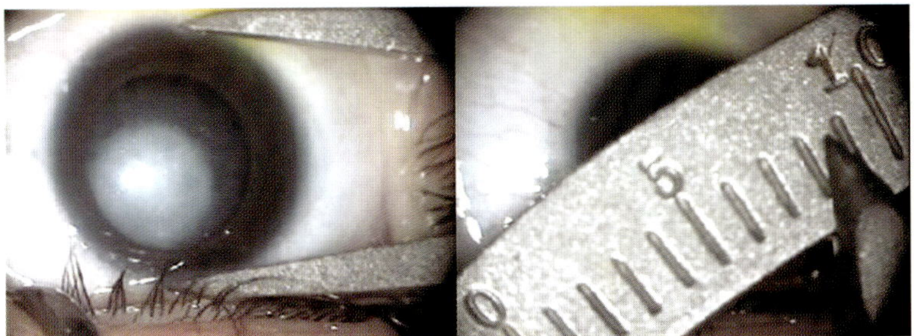

Fig. 2: Cataract in microphakia in a patient with Lowe's syndrome

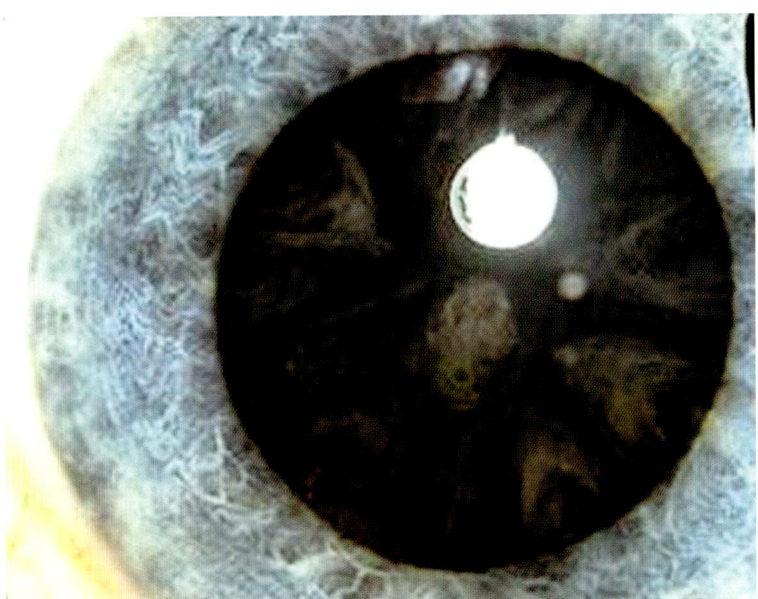

Fig. 3: Cataract in hypoparathyroidism

mannosidase A and B activities which results in the lysosomal accumulation of Mannose-Rich substrates. People with mannosidosis appear normal at birth and that their typical phenotype develops by two years of age. This is characterized by a distinctive coarse facies and dysostosis multiplex. Although recurrent infections, hearing loss and mental retardation occur, the course in this storage disorder generally is stable and is compatible with adult life. Alpha-mannosidosis in the human has been associated with cataract development in infancy. The lens opacities do not have typical appearance, but may be nuclear or capsular, or total.

Cataract in Hypoparathyroidism

Cataract is a well-known complication of hypoparathyroidism, albeit the mechanism is obscure. The typical appearance is characterized by cuneate radial opacities. The progression of cataract is typically slow in patients with idiopathic hypoparathyrodism. Anyway, there are also cases in which the typical hypocalcemic cataracts have an extremely rapid evolution, in particular when hepatic and renal failure occur, with alteration in the serum calcium and phosphorus levels. Physicians and ophthalmologists must be aware of cataracts developing rapidly in the setting of such metabolic derangements.

Cataract in Lathosterolosis

Lathosterolosis is a singular defect of cholesterol biosynthesis due to the lack of lathosterol-5-desaturase (SC5D), the enzyme that catalyzes the conversion of lathosterol to 7-dehydrocholesterol in the cholesterol synthetic pathway. Cholesterol is an abundant lipid in eukaryotic membranes, implicated in different structural and functional capacities, and its partial or complete lack as well as the accumulation of precursors, may lead to a group of malformative syndromes of recent identification. Lathosterolosis is a rare disorder that leads to developmental abnormalities, including mental retardation, and to date has only been identified in two patients one of which died at 18 weeks of age with diffuse intracellular storage.

We describe a unique case of cataract in a lathosterolosis patient who underwent cataract surgery. Our patient was a 7-year-old little girl diagnosed with lathosterolosis at age 2 years, through gas cromatography/mass spectrometry method for plasma sterol profile, that revealed a peak corresponding to cholest-7-en-3β-ol (lathosterol). The biosynthesis of cholesterol in her fibroblasts was defective, showing a block in the conversion of lathosterol into 7-dehydrocholesterol. Physical examination revealed dismorphic features, including severe microcephaly, receding forehead, anteverted nares,

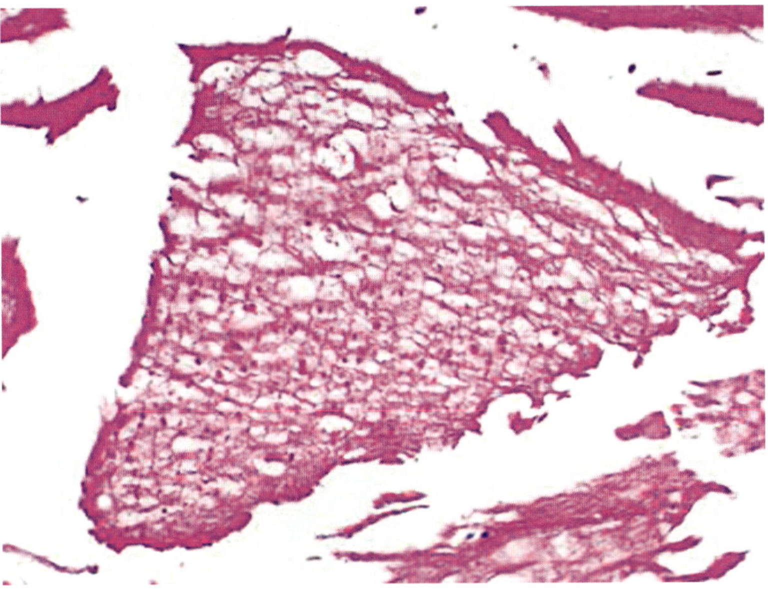

Fig. 4: Fragments of lens characterized by the presence of fibers disposed in a honeycomb way

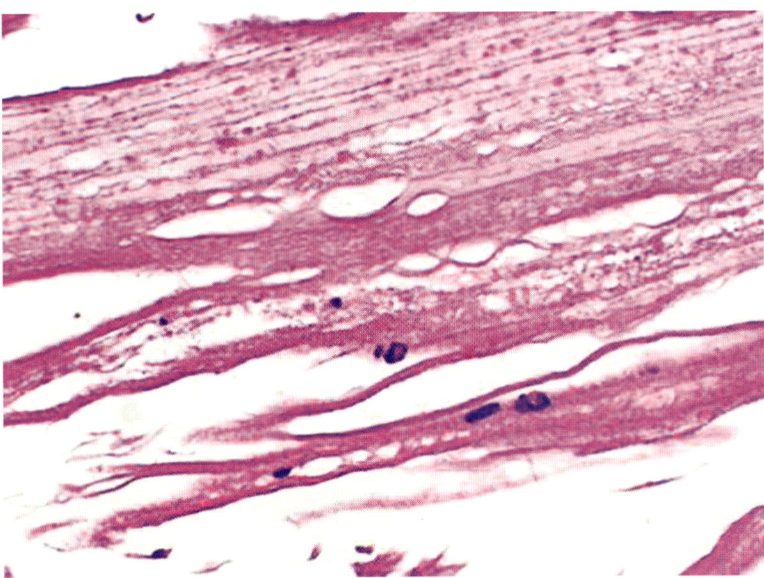

Fig. 5: Fragments characterized by bulgy elements referable to cortical fibers with degenerative characteristics

micrognathia, prominent upper lip, high arched palate, haxadactyly and syndactyly of the left foot. Severe psychomotor delay became increasingly evident with age; conductive deafness was found at the auditory evoked potentials. She also had liver disease with signs of cholestasis. At the first ophthalmic evaluation, carried out in June 2005, the little patient presented with bilateral posterior subcapsular cataracts at byomicroscopy and bilateral pale optic nerve head at fundus examination. In November 2005, after a severe gastroenteric Rotavirus infection with subsequent metabolic decompensation, a marked worsening in the lens opacity of the left eye occurred. There was no history of ocular trauma reported by parents, and Eco-B-scan examination revealed normal vitreous-retinal structures. A marked subconjunctival jaundice was evident at biomicroscopy, due to a severe intrahepatic cholestasis. After metabolic improvement, the little patient was encouraged to surgery for left cataract extraction. Surgery was performed on February 2006, under general anesthesia. We performed a bimanual microphacoemulsification mainly working in aspiration mode; an acrylic hydrophobic flexible IOL was inserted (Acri.Smart 48S- Acri.Tec, Co. Berlin, Germany) and manual posterior continuous curvilinear capsulorhexis (PCCC) and optic entrapment of the IOL were performed.[13] No intraoperative or postoperative complications occurred. After surgery, refraction was +0.75 sph with an astigmatism of + 0.50 (90°) diopter, remaining stable during the whole follow-up; biomicroscopic evaluation revealed absence of significant inflammation and good IOL centration; no posterior capsule opacification occurred 2 years after surgery. Visual acuity was not assessable due to complete lack of patient's collaboration; anyway, we noted a better orientation of the proband during the subsequent control visits, and parents referred a greater confidence and autonomy in her daily life attitudes.

The lens samples obtained during surgical removal were sent to the Department of Pathology and routinely processed and stained with hematoxylin-eosin and PAS; then, they were examined under a light microscope. Histological examination revealed lens fragments with the presence of fibers disposed in a honeycomb way, samples characterized by the presence of homogeneous eosinophilic lens fibers, and other fragments characterized by bulgy elements referable to cortical fibers with degenerative characteristics. These findings were compatible with cortical dismetabolic cataract.

The relationship between abnormal cholesterol metabolism and disturbed morphogenesis have been extensively studied in recent years, and it has been questioned whether cholesterol deficiency or increased levels of intermediate sterols are responsible for the abnormal functioning of the pathway in these syndromes. The prototypical example is the Smith-Lemli-Opitz syndrome (SLOS), a complex malformation syndrome including the presence of congenital cataracts. Our proband presented with bilateral subcapsular posterior cataracts, with rapid worsening in the left eye after a severe metabolic decompensation.

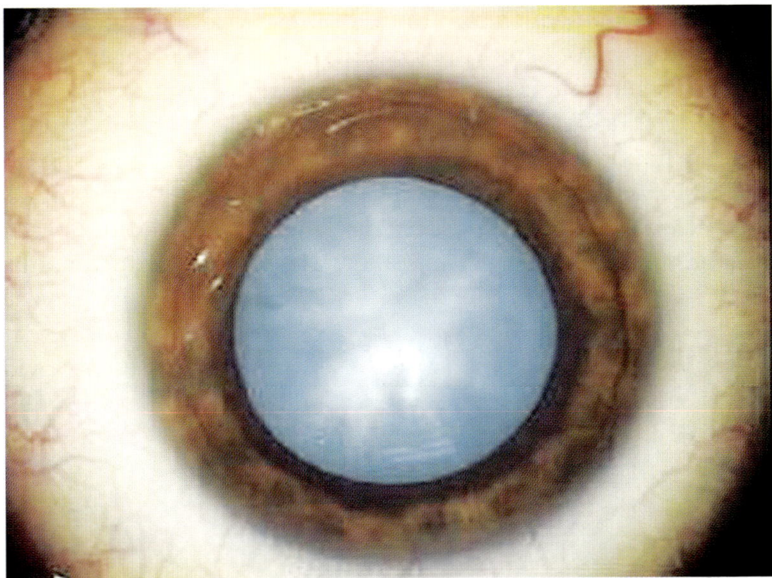

Fig. 6: Dismetabolic cataract in lathosterolosis

Hystopathologic examination confirmed the presence of a dismetabolic cortical cataract. We don't really know the exact pathologic mechanism involved; in two cases of dismetabolic cataracts in patients with SLO syndrome, it has been advocated a dysfunction or rupture of the lens capsule leading to acute osmotic shifts. We can hypothesize the same pathogenetic mechanism for our case. We conclude that lathosterolosis is a complex malformative syndrome that can lead to dismetabolic cataract development. This unique case of cataract in such a patient, has been successfully managed with cataract extraction and IOL implant.

7

Management of Pediatric Cataract

AK Grover, Gauri Nagpal, Shaloo Bageja (India)

Introduction

Congenital pediatric cataract is the commonest cause of treatable blindness in childhood.

The surgical management of the condition has undergone rapid strides over the last few decades making a profound difference to the prognosis in these cases yet it presents a profound challenge to the ophthalmic surgeon.

The Magnitude of Problem

It is estimated that of the total blindness in the world 5% is childhood blindness. The total number of blind children in the world is 1.4 million. An estimated 0.2 million children are blind from cataract. Approximately 3/4th of world's blind children live in poorest regions of Africa and Asia. **In India 60,000 children are blind** because of bilateral cataract.

Causes

In 50% of bilateral cataracts and in virtually all unilateral cases the underlying cause cannot be determined. Approximately 20% have a positive family history with autosomal dominant disease more commonly diagnosed than x linked or autosomal recessive disease. In the remaining 30% chromosomal abnormalities, Systemic abnormalities, metabolic disorders, intrauterine infections, prematurity or other ocular abnormalities are the underlying causes.

A study conducted in South India showed that 26% of cataracts in the first year of life were due to congenitally acquired Rubella. Therefore, Rubella immunization of girls aged 12-13 years or of all children younger than one year can be considered. Advice to the families with autosomal dominant congenital cataract is important and can help patients decide about family planning and ensure that affected children are diagnosed and treated early.

Examination

A thorough history, examination and clinical investigations are important in all cases of cataract. A positive family history and examination may show that cataract is hereditary. History of trauma both blunt and penetrating is important cause of childhood cataract. The morphology of the lens opacity may elucidate its origin.

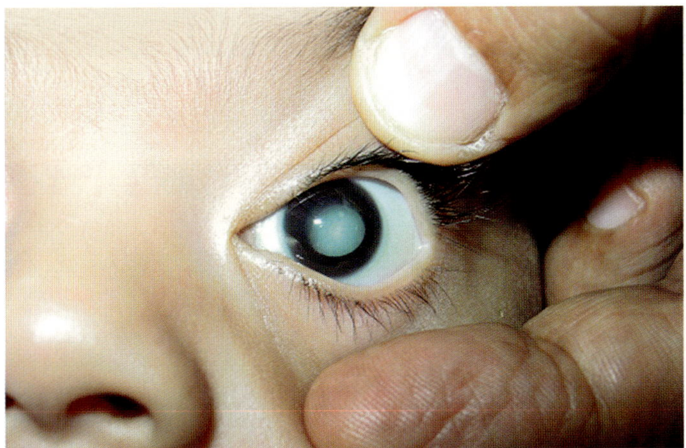

Fig. 1: Congenital Cataract

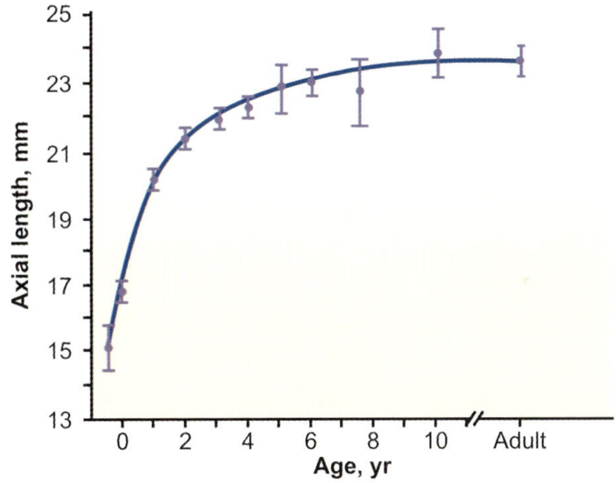

Fig. 2: Axial growth of the eyeball in mm with age

TABLE 1: Causes of congenital cataract

50%	Unknown or idiopathic
20%	Autosomal dominant
30%	Chromosomal abnormalities (trisomy 21, trisomy 13-15, trisomy 16-18, turners, cri du chat)
	Systemic abnormalities (skeletal, CNS, renal, dermatological, musculodigital)
	Metabolic abnormalities (galactosemia, galactokinase def, hypocalcemia, hypoglycemia)
	Intrauterine infections (rubella, CMV, varicella-zoster, herpes simplex, toxoplasma)
	Prematurity (PHPV, ROP, anirirdia, anterior cleavage syndrome,intraocular tumor)

TABLE 2: Morphology of lens opacity

Type of cataract	*Possible origin*
B/l posterior polar cataracts with or without lenticonus	Familial
Unilateral posterior cortical	Sporadic malformation of posterior capsule
B/l or u/l anterior polar opacities	idiopathic
B/l anterior lenticonus	Alport's syndrome
B/l anterior subcapsular	Atopic dermatitis
Nuclear, lamellar and multipunctate	Chromosomal abnormalities, metabolic and hereditary

Associated ocular abnormalities of anterior and posterior segments should be sought for A raised IOP may be associated with rubella or Lowe's syndrome.

TABLE 3: Associated ocular abnormalities

Anterior segment	*Posterior segment*
Microcornea	choroidemia
Corneal dystrophy	Retinitis pigmentosa
Anterior cleavage syndrome	PHPV
Iris atrophy	Norries disease
Aniridia	Stickler syndrome
Uveitis	Favre vitreoretinal degeneration

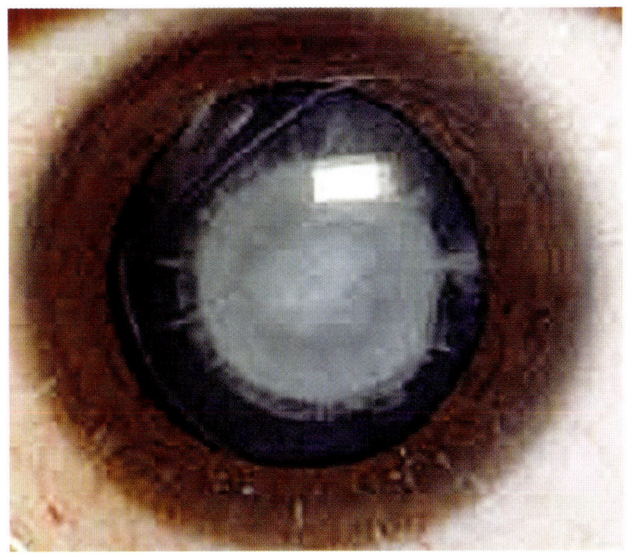

Fig. 3: Cataract involving the central 3 mm of the visual axis

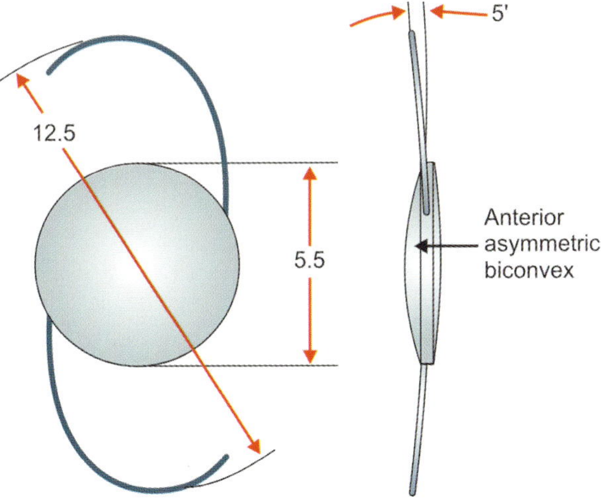

Fig. 4: Appropriate size of the IOL

LABORATORY EVALUATION

Laboratory evaluation for congenital infection should be done. TORCH titres, serological testing for syphilis, serum calcium and glucose for metabolic disorders,urine testing for reducing substances (especially after milk feeding) for galactosemia are done. Elimination of lactose from the diet may reverse or arrest lens opacification and is critical to general health and development in cases caused by galactose transferase enzyme deficiency. If urine tests are positive or equivocal, quantitative testing of RBCs for galactokinase can be done to confirm diagnosis. Urine for protien and amino acids along with serum electrolyte and bicarbonate levels are abnormal in lowes oculocerebrorenal syndrome.

TABLE 4: Laboratory evaluation

	Result	*Possible diagnosis*
URINE	**+ reducing substance** aminoaciduria Hematuria, proteinuria Maltase cross figures	**Galactokinase deficiency** Lowe's syndrome Alport's syndrome Fabry's disease
BLOOD	**Erythrocyte enzymes** glucose TORCH titres, VDRL tests Calcium, phosphorus	**Galactokinase deficiency** Hyper/hypoglycemia Rubella,toxoplasmosis,CMV hypo/psuedohypoparathyroidism

Management

THE PEDIATRIC EYE

The eye of the newborn is constantly in a state of growth both anatomically and functionally. A clear visual axis is necessary for the development of all its visual function. The **average axial length of eyeball at birth is 16.2 mm** which becomes 23.5 mm when the child is 2 years old. The **fixation reflex develops by 2-3 months** of age, **fusion and stereopsis by 6 months** and **color vision by 3 months**. Therefore, the **most critical period for visual development is between 4 weeks to 4 months**. A cataract during this period of growth will hamper the visual development due to visual deprivation. These changes can be reversed if there is early restoration of visual clarity. Therefore, an early intervention to all visually significant pediatric cataracts is essential for visual recovery.

VISUALLY SIGNIFICANT CATARACTS

Although it is difficult to assess vision in **infants** but in many cases it can be estimated with a fair degree of accuracy using **preferential looking test** (Teller cards) or **VEP recording**. The quality of fixation is also of importance in infants older than 3 months. The presence of unsteady fixation,nystagmus and strabismus are indicators of poor vision. In children **older than 2 years** of age

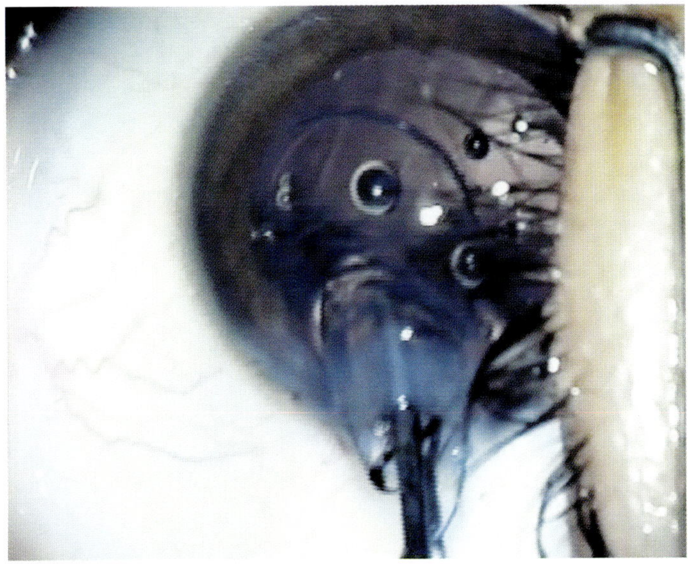

Fig. 5: Foldable IOL being inserted through a 3 mm incision

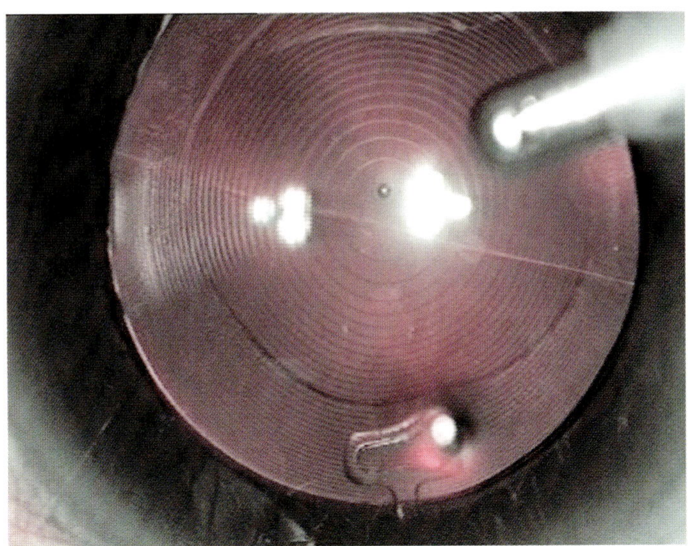

Fig. 6: In the bag multifocal IOL

picture or letter optotypes resembling standard Snellen notation can be used reliably. Such tests include **Landolt C test , tumbling E test** or picture naming **Allen Cards**.All the cataracts that occupy the **central 3 mm of the lens** are visually significant. Bilateral or unilateral **total cataracts** are obviously visually significant . **Unilateral partial cataracts** are generally visually significant due to not only visual deprivation but also due to binocular rivalry giving rise to earlier and denser amblyopia.

TIME OF SURGERY

It is generally accepted practice is to perform surgery**, for visually significant cataracts as early as possible**,even few days after birth to prevent irreversible ambylopia. In significant bilateral cases, the second eye should be operated on within a week of the first. Older children presenting with severe opacities are somewhat less demanding of urgent attention and can be prolonged for a week or two for surgery. Children with partial cataract and nonamblyogenic cataract may benefit from instillation of mydriatic drops to permit vision through a larger unopacified area of the lens. **Elective surgery can be planned after the age of 4** when the eye has grown and postoperative care will not be difficult. However, it is important to ensure that they are reassessed on a regular follow up basis. In Infancy, examination should be repeated every few months. Older children can be seen once or twice a year.

IOL IMPLANTATION

IOL implantation provides the best means of optical correction of aphakia. Implanting an IOL in the eye of a child older than 1-2 years is a safe and successful procedure as most of the ocular growth has occurred. However, implanting an IOL in children less than one year is controversial. The reason is the difference in size of the newborn and adult eye and the pediatric eye is highly reactive to accept the foreign material. Therefore a regular size IOL in small eyes could cause many complications like retardation of ocular growth, raised IOP ,uveitis, decentration and PCO formation. However, various studies done by *Michael O Keef, Anna Lundvall et al, Trivedi et al* and *Grover et al* have shown long term safety of IOLs with newer designs, materials and sizes and are tolerated well by children not only more than one year old but also less than one year old infants.

Size of IOL

IOLs were specially made to fit the pediatric eyes from 1988. They have an **overall diameter of 10.50–12.0 mm and optic plate diameter of 5.5–6.5 mm (Fig. 4)** as compared to adult 12.5-13.75 overall diametre. However,these lenses are always not available.

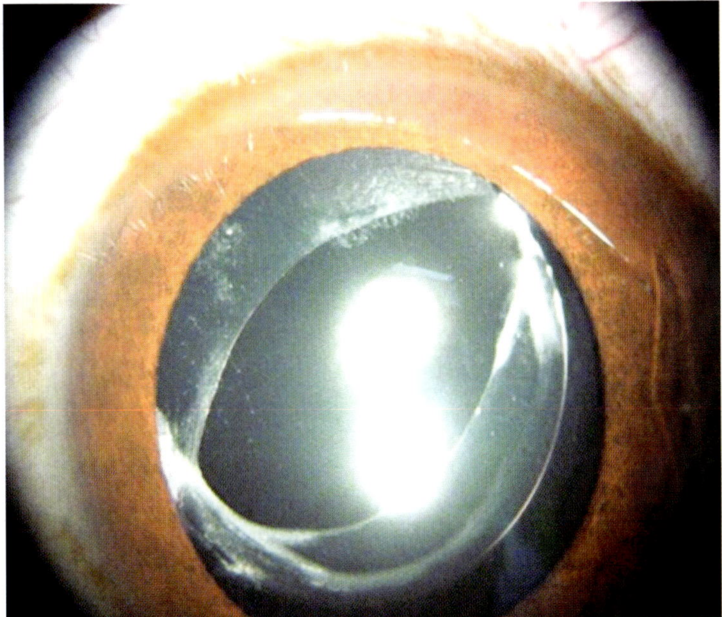

Fig. 7: Capture of the IOL in the posterior capsule (IOL optic behind the post. Capsule and haptics in front of the post Capsule)

Material of IOL

PMMA lenses that are **heparin surface modified** are advantageous in children with intense postoperative inflammatory response. The incision must be extended when implanting a PMMA IOL and this is a disadvantage because larger incisions result in more pronounced postoperative inflammation. Acrylic lenses are well tolerated in highly reactive Pediatric eyes. Acrylic lenses are soft, adhere to the capsule snugly inhibiting the proliferation of LECs (lens epithelial cells). **Acrylic hydrophobic** is even better than hydrophilic because of greater contact angle.

Design of IOL

C loops have been shown to prevent the central migration of LECs and create a more symmetrical radial stretch of the posterior capsule. The **insertion angle** between the haptic – optic junction should be 90 degree in case of PMMA lenses as there is more complete apposition of anterior or posterior leaflets as compared to oblique insertion.

Power of IOL

The axial length, the corneal curvature and the power of the lens of the infant eye is different from the adult eye. An infant would need **IOL power 30±3 D** compared to 20±2 D in an adult eye. **BenEzra** suggested implanting a standard adult IOL of 21 D in all cases. This would be acceptable in most children older than 2 years, however, in infants the induced hypermetropia would be 10 diopter or more. Implanting a standard adult IOL in an infant would mean leaving the patient with a large amount of hypermetropia that could be highly amblyogenic and its correction with heavy glasses or contact lenses will have their inherent limitations. Aiming for emmetropia in an infant means risking a large myopic shift that would necessitate an exchange of IOLs, a refractive

DAHAN'S GUIDELINES TO DETERMINE IOL POWER

For children younger than 2 years
Do biometry and undercorrect by 20%
Or
use axial length only

Axial length (mm)	IOL power
17	28
18	27
19	26
20	24
21	22

for children between 2 and 8 years
do biometry and undercorrect by 10%

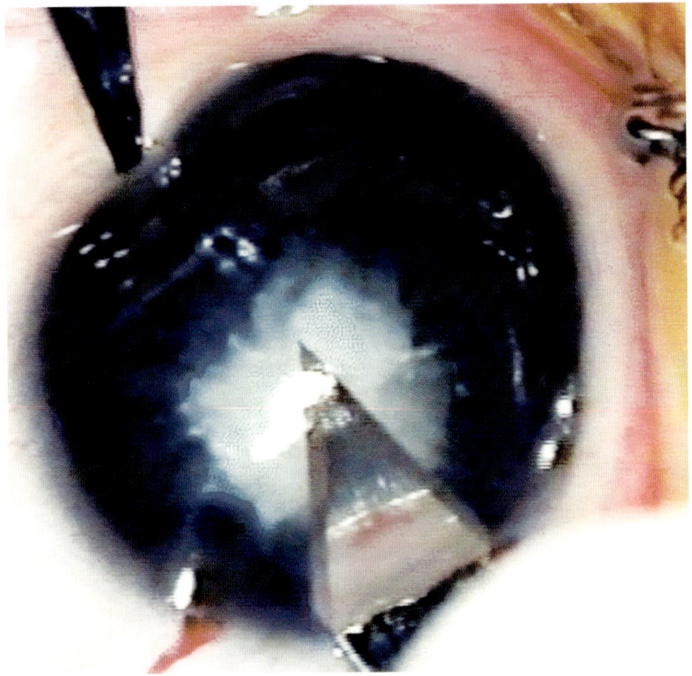

Fig. 8: A 3 mm triplanar corneal incision being made

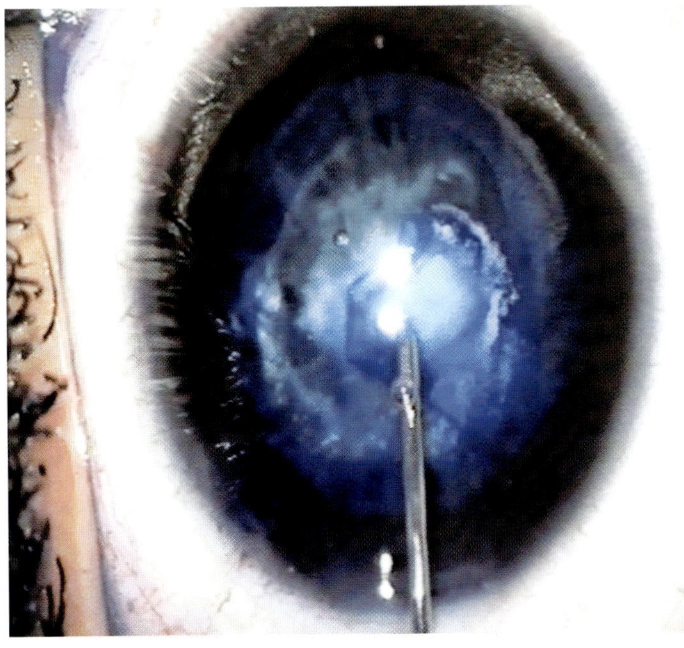

Fig. 9: Capsulorhexis done after staining of anterior capsule

procedure like lasik or a piggyback IOL before adolescence. The solution probably lies in finding a compromise between these two extremes as suggested by **Dahan et al** who aim for an undercorrection of 20% in infants and 10% in toddlers. In other words, an infant should receive 80% of the IOL power needed for emmetropia while a toddler or a young child the IOL power should correct 90% of aphakia. The K reading in children younger than one year can be ignored as theses readings rapidly change, therefore, can be replaced by average adult K reading,that is 44. The induced initial hypermetropia is correctable with spectacles which can be adjusted throughout life according to patients refractive development. Thus emmetropia will develop in late childhood while a moderate degree of myopia may be reached in adolescence or in adulthood.

Hiles and Atkinson suggested 20-50% undercorrection from the calculated till 2 years of age and emmetropic correction for older children.

Type of IOL

Not only **monofoca**l but also **multifocal IOLs** have been used sucessfully in the pediatric age group. Better uncorrected near visual acuity and stereopsis were observed in comparison to monofocal implantees an comparison to monofocal implantees. However, long-term results using multifocal IOLs are not yet available.

TYPE OF SURGERY

Lens Aspiration and IOL Implantation

Cataract in pediatric eyes is soft and can be easily aspirated. Pediatric eyes are very reactive and may be associated with anomalies of angle and anterior chamber. They lack scleral rigidity and are also small giving rise to various technical difficulties. Therefore, lens aspiration and IOL implantation in young can lead to higher incidence of inflammation and PCO formation.

Various studies show that in the bag IOL leads to less inflammation and best visual rehabilitation.

Primary Posterior Capsulectomy and Anterior Vitrectomy

PCO is still the most common and serious complication and is caused by proliferating anterior lens epithelial cells and scaffolding on the posterior capsule, anterior vitreous face and the anterior and posterior IOL surfaces.

Studies undertaken by Vasavada et al has led to the concept of performing a primary posterior capsulotomy and anterior vitrectomy at the time of cataract extraction to prevent PCO formation in children under 5 years of age. In children above the age of 5 there is no need for anterior vitrectomy as the vitreous is less

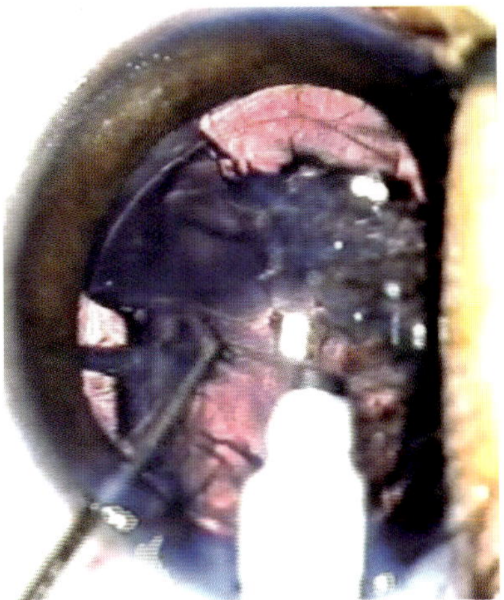

Fig. 10A: Phacoaspiration of nucleus being done

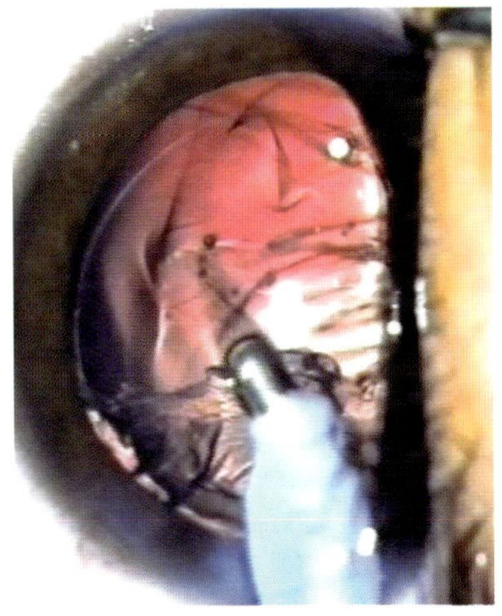

Fig. 10B: Irrigation aspiration of the cortical matter being done cortical matter

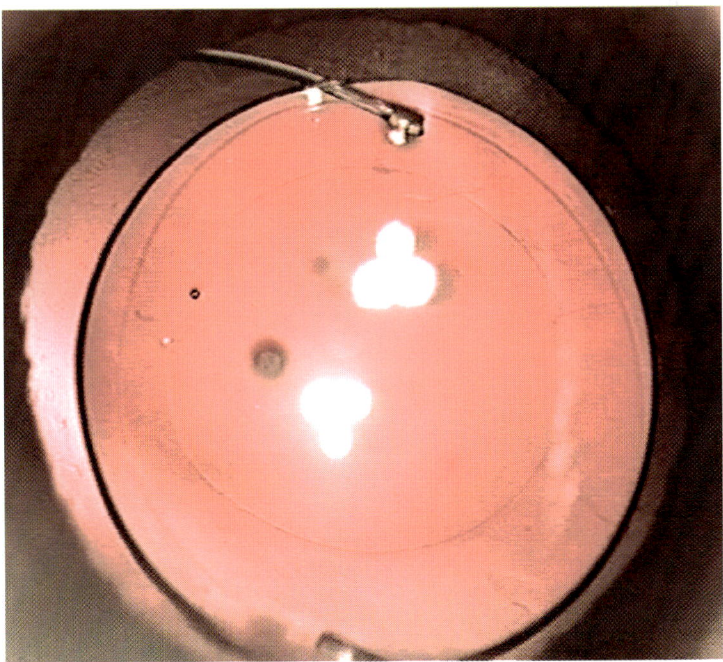

Fig. 11: In the bag IOL without optic capture. Posterior capsulotomy is smaller than the ant. capsulotomy

reative and the child will be cooperative to get a yag capsulotomy done if at all it develops.

Optic Capture

Howard V Gimbel et al proposed that if PCC and optic capture are done there was no need to do anterior vitrectomy to reduce the PCO formation.

The technique of optic capture in the posterior capsule consists of haptics remaining in the bag, whereas the optic lies behind the posterior capsule. The apposition of anterior and posterior leaflets 360 degree except the optic – haptic junction seals the lenticular epithelial cells (LECs) to grow centrally onto the visual axis.

However, it was seen that LECs can migrate through the optic- haptic junction where the leaflets are not apposed and obscure the visual axis, therefore in children younger than 5 years when the vitreous is highly reactive anterior vitrectomy along with optic capture should be done.

On the contrary if anterior vitrectomy is done, it may not be necessary, especially with acrylic hydrophobic lenses to do an optic capture as it has not shown, to further lessen the PCO formation.

One advantage of optic capture is that with a well centered PCC, IOL centration can be enhanced.

TECHNIQUE OF SURGERY

It is possible to have an anterior or posterior approach to achieve a clear visual axis.

Anterior Approach

Using anterior approach, anterior capsulorhexis, phacoaspiration or irrigation aspiration, posterior capsulorhexis ,anterior vitrectomy with IOL implantation is done.

Posterior Approach

In the posterior approach, Pars plana vitrectomy and posterior capsulolectomy is done after lens aspiration and IOL implantation.

Using an anterior or posterior approach is a matter of surgeons preference and experience with the procedure.

Both have their advantages and disadvantages. Using the posterior approach, it is important to remember that the length of pars plana is 0.5 –1.5 mm and becomes 2.5 mm till the first year, thus pars plana incision in infants increases the risk of creating a retinal break. Anterior vitrectomy if not done properly through the anterior route can cause vitreous adhesion and incarceration in the wound thereby increasing the risk of CME and retinal detachment.

Age of child	Type of surgery recommended
Infants <1 year	Lens aspiration + PCCC +Ant. Vitrectomy ± IOL (ant. Or post. Approach)
1-5 years	Lens aspiration + PCCC + Ant. vitrectomy + IOL, ± optic capture (ant. or post. Approach)
>5 years	Lens aspiration + PCCC + IOL

STEPS OF SURGERY

The authors preference is to do an anterior approach. All the precautions that are to be taken will be mentioned briefly step by step.

Incision

The tendency towards collapse of anterior chamber and the prolapse of iris tissue can be countered by constructing wounds that snugly fit instruments and permit essentially closed chamber techniques. 3 mm triplanar corneal wound minimizes the chamber shallowing.

Wound closure usually is self sealing but if fishmouthing is seen a 10-0 monofilament nylon suture can be applied in the end.

Anterior Capsulorhexis

The anterior capsule in children is thick and elastic. It can easily extend especially in presence of a positive vitreous pressure that causes the anterior chamber to collapse. Use of high molecular wt. Viscoelastics like Healon and Healon GV are very helpful in deepening the anterior chamber and relaxing the zonules. A central puncture is made with a cystotome and the leading edge of the capsule is grasped with forceps. Several repeated grasps are done for better control of the rhexis. The force applied should be centripetal and a small capsulorhexis should be aimed forl as it usually enlarges due to its inherent elasticity.

Lens Aspiration

The lens is soft and can be aspirated either by a phaco probe or an irrigation probe. All the lens nucleus and cortex should be removed in order to reduce the postoperative inflammation.

Posterior Capsulorhexis

Posterior capsulorhexis is made in the similar way as the anterior capsulorhexis is made. The diameter should not be less than 3.0 mm or it will tend to close and should not be more than the optic of the IOL.

Anterior Vitrectomy

Atleast 1/3 rd of the anterior vitreous should be eliminated. Care should be taken to avoid leaving vitreous in the anterior chamber, in the capsule bag or close to the opening of the posterior capsule.

IOL Implantation

The foldable IOL is inserted into the capsular bag with the help of either a holder folder forceps or a lens insertor optic capture is done by pushing the optic of the IOL with the help of a blunt repositor very gently. A study done at our center showed that there was no significant difference in PCO with Acrylic hydrophobic lenses (Acrysof) with or without optic capture.

Conclusion

Management in Pediatric cataract has improved with the advances in the microsurgical techniques in cataract surgery. There are increasing numbers of pediatric cataract surgeons who opt for IOL implantation rather than leaving the infant aphakic. We hope that the accuracy of formulas for predicting postoperative and final refraction will continue to improve, or that modifiable implants or refractive surgery will advance to a level which will enable us to maximize the visual outcome for children with cataracts.

Lens Diseases (Surgical)

Section 2

8

Pearls and Tricks in Congenital Cataract Surgery

Simonetta Morselli, Roberto Bellucci (Italy)

Introduction

The definition of congenital cataract is the evolutive opacification of the crystalline lens that causes limitation of the visual acuity. This type of opacity can be present at birth or it can develop in the first 3 months of life. This type of cataract is called "early developmental" cataract. The incidence of the congenital cataract is 0.4% of the total population. It is an important blindness factor for babies, that accounts from 20 to 38% of the total blindness. The management of this disorder has long challenged clinicians, but the past few decades have seen significant changes in the approach and in the management, due to the information gathered from basic scientific and clinical research. The most important visual loss is mainly attributable to amblyopia, that is caused from stimulus deprivation with the additional factor of ocular rivalry in unilateral disease. Thus, enhanced understanding of critical periods of visual development led to surgical intervention for dense cataract being deemed necessary within the first 3 months of life, and possibly as early as the first 6 weeks in unilateral disease. The need to ensure early detection and to allow prompt treatment, has resulted in the implementation of various strategies, it is recommended to carry out population screening examinations of newborn examination in many countries.

Diagnosis

The diagnosis is very easy when a complete cataract is present at birth because of the visible leukocoria. When the cataract is posterior and not progressing to the anterior lens layers, the white color of the pupil cannot be detected easily and the diagnosis can be very late, when nistagmus or strabismus appears. Unfortunately, the visual deprivation in the first month of life creates a sensorial obstacle that causes amblyopia, nistagmus and strabismus.

Preoperative Pearls

PUPIL DILATION

The dilation of the pupil is a very important factor for congenital cataract surgery. The mydriasis is very difficult to obtain and to maintain during surgery. In our experience this type of mixture works very well: 1 mL of phenylephrine 10 % and tropicamide 0.5 % + 1 mL of atropine 1% diluted in the same syringe with 8 cc of saline water. Apply 1 drop every 15 min, starting two hours before surgery and until the pupil is dilated. To maintain the mydriasis inject 0.5 mL of adrenaline into the 500 mL BSS bottle used during surgery.

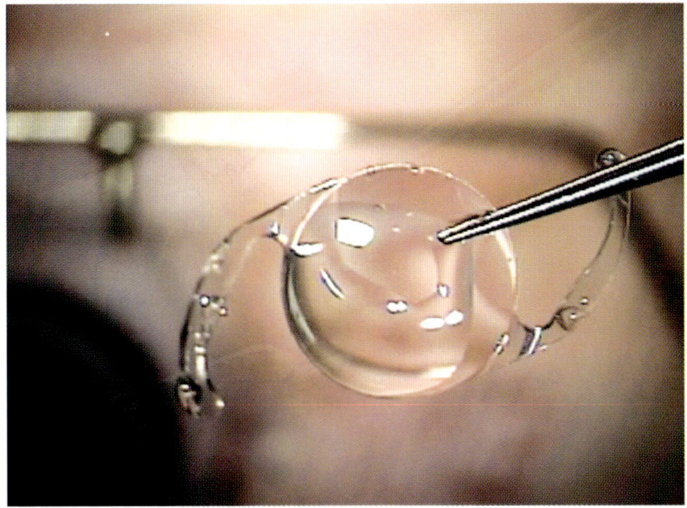

Fig. 1: AcrySof SA30AL IOL is available. This model has a 12.5 mm overall diameter and 5.5 mm optic diameter

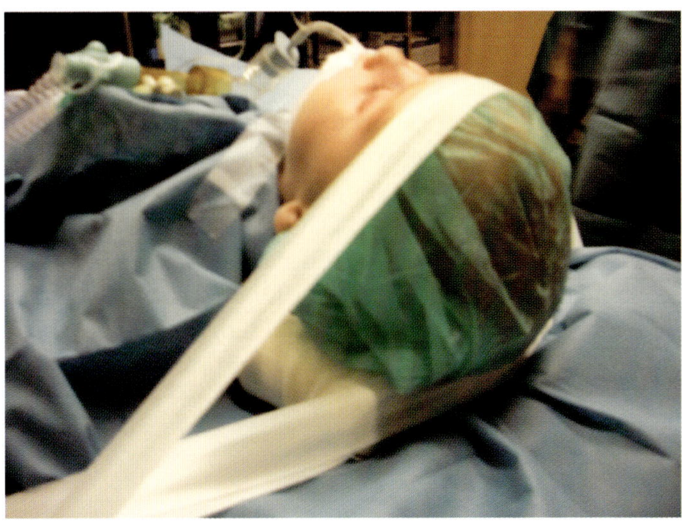

Fig. 2: The baby head must be fixed with an adhesive strip to the operating bed

IOL IMPLANTATION

We plan to implant in babies from birth and onwards, because we had negative experiences in the compliance with glasses or with contact lenses after surgery. The type of IOL implantation at the time of cataract surgery is one of the most critical points in congenital cataract surgery. Polymethylmethacrylate (PMMA) IOLs have been successful in pediatric eyes; however, the capsular and inflammatory responses remain a problem. Now the AcrySof IOLs made of flexible hydrophobic acrylic material are available (Alcon Laboratories, Forth Worth, Texas), with favorable outcome when used in children. Out of the AcrySof family, the 5.5 mm optic lens seems the most apt to small babies. Until recently, the 5.5 mm optic AcrySof IOL was available only in a 3-piece design with PMMA haptics (MA30 BM), with a total diameter of 12.5 mm. Now also the single piece AcrySof SA30AL IOL is produced, with the same optic diameter and overall length.

IOL POWER CALCULATION

Preoperative values of axial length and corneal curvature are rarely available in patients with congenital cataracts. Therefore, these values have to be obtained under general anesthesia immediately before surgery. K readings are not easy to obtain even under general anesthesia because a portable corneal topographer is necessary. In addition, the K readings can change during the growth of the eye. Therefore, it could be convenient to base the IOL power calculation not on the K readings but only on the axial length. We select the IOL power with reference to the rules of Dr Dahan for babies less than one year old. If the axial length is about 20 mm we select a +25 D IOL, if it is about 19 mm we implant a +26 D, if the length is about 18 mm we implant a +28 D IOL. If the axial length is between 21 and 23 mm the power of the IOL will be equal to the axial length value +1D per mm exceeding 21. If the axial length is longer than 24 mm the power implanted will be equal to the axial length value -1D per mm exceeding 24.

GENERAL ANESTHESIA

The anesthesiologist must be skilled in general anesthesia in very young patients. The use of curare is mandatory to have the eye in natural position and not in the "Bell phenomenon position". The baby's head must be fixed with an adhesive strip to the operating bed; two rolled cloths help to immobilize the head.

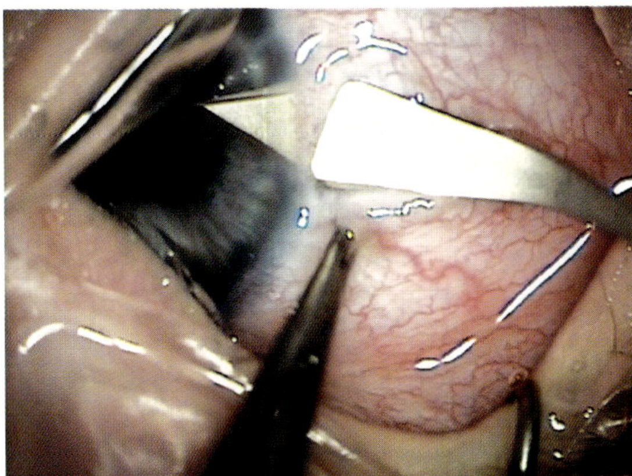

Fig. 3: The incision is created at 12 o'clock under a conjunctival flap

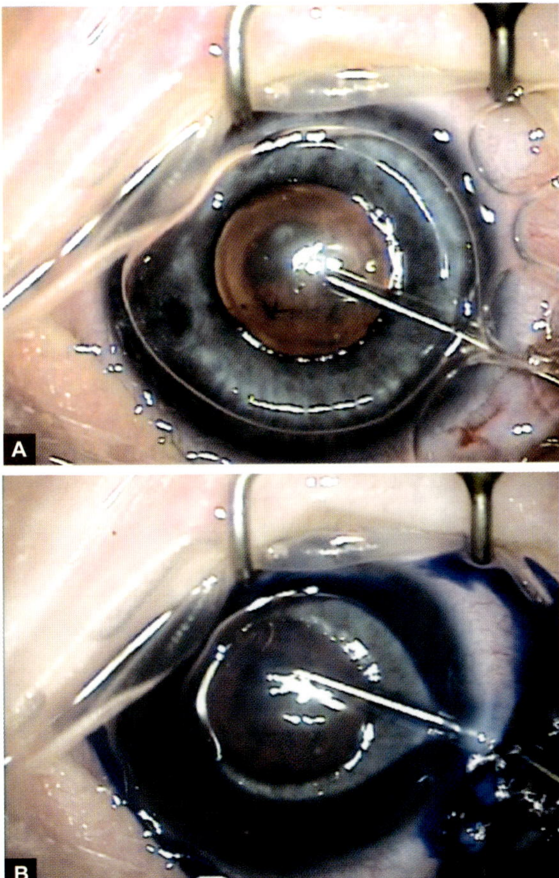

Figs 4A and B: Aspirate 1 ml of methylene blue in an insulin syringe with an air bubble, inject the air bubble first and then methylene blue, with the same syringe through the side port incision

Surgical Pearls and Tricks

We pass a suture through the superior rectus muscle and fix it with 'Pean forceps' to modulate the position of the eye as the surgeon requires during the various steps of the surgery.

The main incision is created at 12 o'clock under a conjunctival flap.

At least one side-port incision is also created. At the end of the surgery it is mandatory to close the incisions with 10/0 vicryl.

The use of methylene blue under an air bubble is very helpful to color the anterior capsule before performing anterior capsulorhexis. Aspirate 0.5 mL of the methylene blue dye into an insulin syringe, followed by 0.5 mL of filtered air. Inject the air bubble first and then the methylene blue, to avoid any collapse of the anterior chamber: the air will empty the anterior chamber and the dye will be injected onto the capsule without touching the endothelium.

Use high molecular weight and cohesive viscoelastic substance to help performing capsulorhexis. The newborn capsule is very elastic and needs to be perforated by a 30 G needle. The rhexis tear tends to escape toward the equator because of this elasticity, like it happens in pig eyes in wet-labs.

Posterior capsulorhexis is easier if you do not overfill the capsular bag with viscoelastic substance. A small hole in the center of the posterior capsule with a 30 G needle helps creating space to inject allows viscoelastic injection between the anterior hyaloid surface and the posterior surface of the posterior capsule.

The posterior capsulorhexis is completed with 'Corydon forceps'. Anterior vitrectomy is mandatory.

The IOL is inserted with the injector or with the forceps trying to inject the first loop into the ciliary sulcus.

This is usually difficult because the operated eye is very soft at this moment. The second loop is positioned in the sulcus with a manipulator. The optical plate is then pushed under the posterior capsulorhexis, so while the loops remain in the sulcus, the optical plate is incarcerated behind the two capsules.

Doing this maneuver the capsular bag remains closed and there is less opportunity for the remaining lens cells to proliferate and to create secondary cataract. The IOL remains stable and centered into the eye. The vitreous body stays behind the IOL and the capsular bag. With this method of IOL implantation, we experienced less inflammation and less synechiae between the IOL and the iris. In the postoperative, it is mandatory to maintain the pupil dilated with omatropine applied twice a day at least for one month to reduce inflammation and to prevent posterior synechiae.

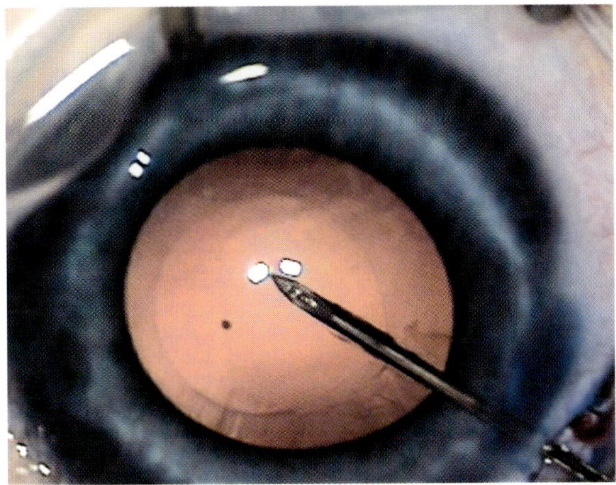

Fig. 5: A small hole in the center of the posterior capsular bag with a needle

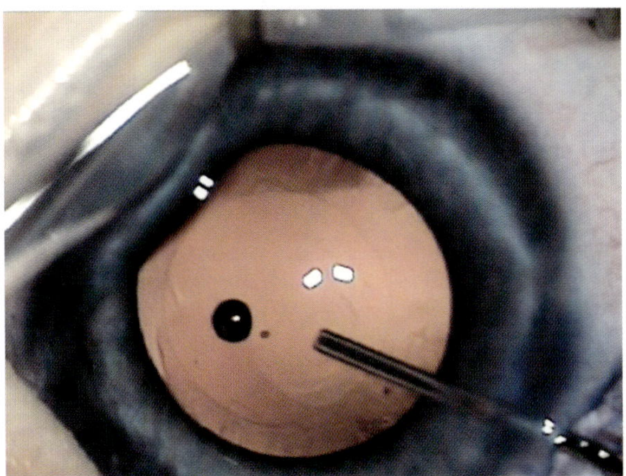

Fig. 6: Inject the viscoelastic between the anterior surface of hyaloid and the posterior surface of the capsular bag

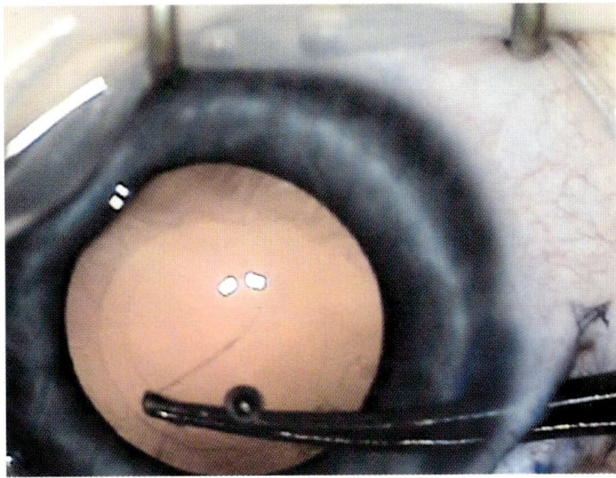

Fig. 7: The capsulorhexis is completed with 'Coridon forceps'

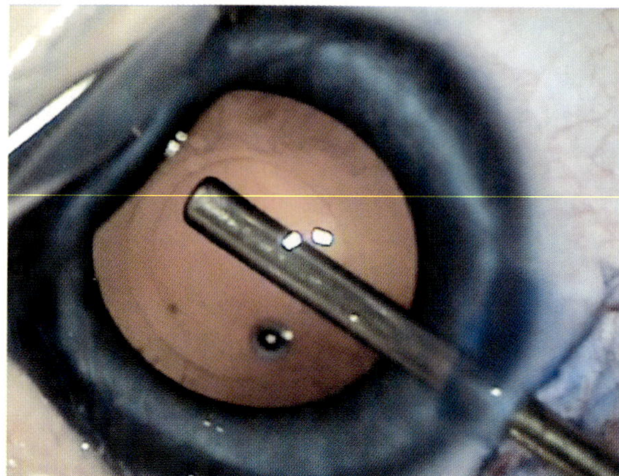

Fig. 8: Anterior vitrectomy is mandatory

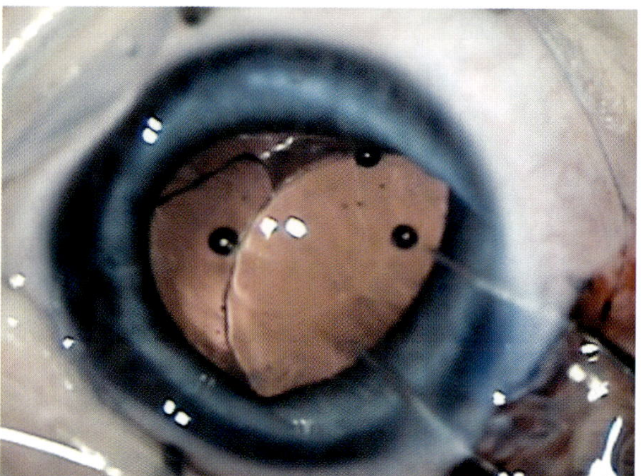

Fig. 9: The IOL is inserted with the injector or with the forceps trying to inject the first in the sulcus

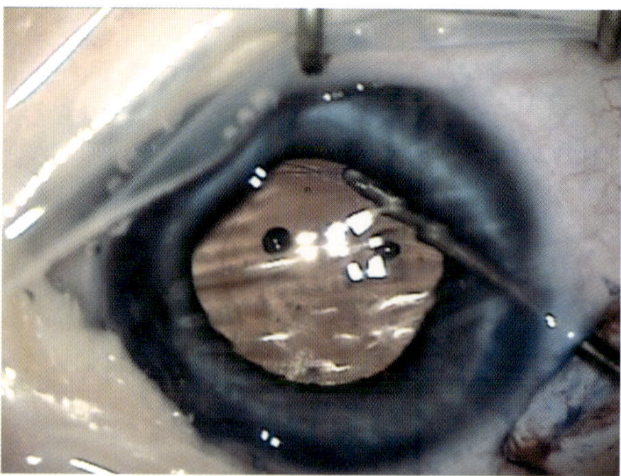

Fig. 10: The optical plate of the IOL is incarcerated behind the two capsules

9

Microphakonit in Pediatric Cataract Surgery

L Felipe Vejarano, Alejandro Tello (Colombia)

Introduction

Cataract surgery has been evolving at a very rapid way during the last decades, passing from extracapsular extraction to ultrasonic phacoemulsification, which has become progressively the standard method for cataract surgery around the world, because it affords less astigmatism induction, rapid astigmatism stabilization, less postoperative inflammation and less possibility of postoperative complications than extracapsular cataract extraction. One of the latest crucial breakthroughs in phacoemulsification has been to perform the phacoemulsification surgery through a microincision with a bimanual approach, using a sleeveless phaco tip. The idea of removing the crystalline lens through two microincisions has been proposed since the 1970s, however, it was not until that independently Agarwal in India and Tsuneoka in Japan began that technique in 1998 and 1999, respectively, that it gained popularity, although it is still practiced by a small percentage of the world's surgeons. Agarwal coined the term "Phakonit", which initially stood for phacoemulsification (phaco) performed with a needle opening (N) via an ultrasmall incision (I) with the sleeveless ultrasound tip (T). Originally Agarwal described an incision as small as 0,9 mm, using a standard sleeveless Microtip. Although initially the theoretical possibility of a possible thermal burn was a concern, this fear was dispelled by several studies; Tsuneoka showed experimentally in a porcine eye that using a sleeveless ultrasound tip, the temperature of the cornea at the incision elevated only 8.4 °C without developing thermal burns. In other experiments Olson et al demonstrated that clinically unusual parameters were necessary to produce a wound burn in bimanual phaco and moreover, when using "cold phaco" with a bare 19-gauge aspiration needle in human cadaver eyes, a wound burn could not be produced at the highest energy settings unless all flow into the eye and all aspiration were occluded. These settings are well beyond clinically applicable conditions. The authors' explanation is that it is difficult to completely occlude a linear stab incision with a metal circular instrument, unlike the situation in standard coaxial phaco, where a flexible irrigation sleeve fills the wound and reduces the flow around the sleeve, particularly in a tight wound. The combination of a tight wound, filled by a flexible irrigation sleeve, and complete occlusion of aspiration and therefore complete blockage of irrigation results in a wound burn. So in fact, the risk of thermal burn may be less in Phakonit than in coaxial phaco.

Agarwal initially reported 305 eyes that underwent the technique successfully. He had the assistant continuously pouring cooled balanced salt solution (BSS®) over the phaco needle. The original incision had to be enlarged in order to implant the IOL. No one case of thermal wound occurred. Tsuneoka and coauthors also initially reported 637 cases that underwent cataract surgery through a 1.4 mm incision without a case of thermal burn. Likewise we have not found any case of corneal wound burn in our cases.

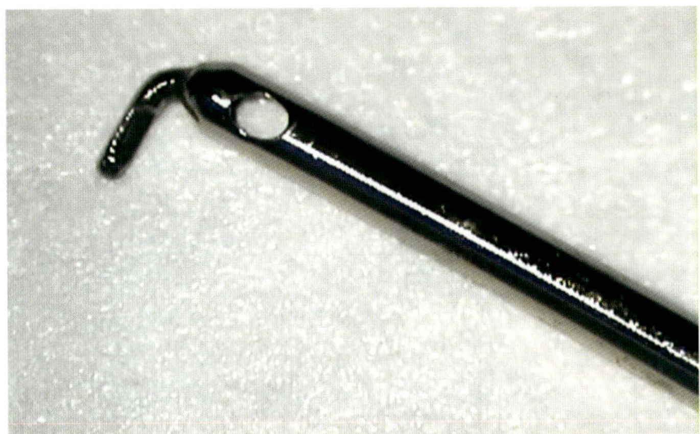

Fig. 1: Vejarano's irrigation chopper for Phakonit. It has 0.9 mm diameter, and two irrigation holes close to the tip

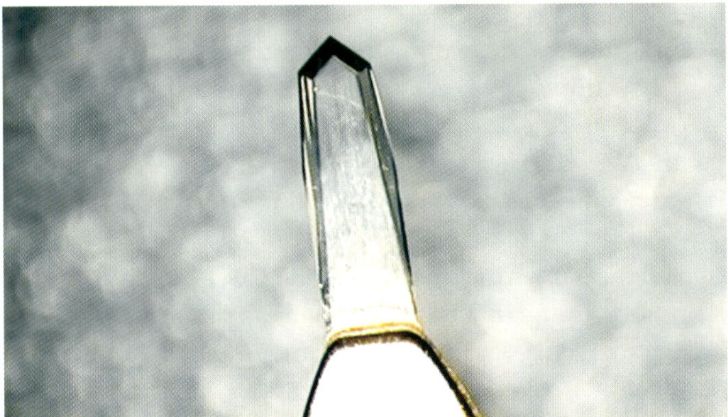

Fig. 2: 0.9/1.2 mm diamond knife (Accutome, Malvern, USA)

Around the world several other surgeons, including us, have reported their results using bimanual microincisional surgery with different phaco machines. Alió, coined the term Microincision Cataract Surgery (MICS), and has reported good visual performance of two availables IOLs, which may be implanted through microincisions. In a prospective randomized consecutive case series he reported that microincision cataract surgery significantly lowered mean phacoemulsification time, mean total phacoemulsification percent, mean effective phaco time, and surgically induced astigmatism when compared with coaxial phacoemulsification. Fine has highlighted the advantages of maintaining a more stable intraocular environment during lens removal. This advantage may be especially important in high myopes who are at a greater risk for retinal detachment following lens extraction or high hyperopes decreasing the possibility of a expulsive hemorrhage.

In 2002, Olson, was the first to use a 0.8 mm phaco needle and a 21 gauge irrigating chopper in bimanual cataract surgery and called this technique microphaco.

These techniques of performing phacoemulsification through incisions around 1.0 to 1.5 mm have been spreading around the world. Other names given to these techniques are bimanual phacoemulsification and sleeveless phaco. Recently Agarwal reported the microphakonit, a similar technique, but using a 0.7 mm needle and a 0.7 mm irrigating chopper through a sub-1 mm incision.

For match all the names that this technique has, I prefer to use MICS when I use only aspiration through microincision with no phaco needle like in pediatric cataracts, where with only aspiration you can remove it but if you going to use ultrasound power then called Phakonit, Microphakonit if the incision is smaller, Microphaco or Bimanual Phaco so indicates that the removal of the cataract is going to be by ultrasound (Phaco power).

Going from a 0.9-mm phaco needle to a 0.7-mm needle diminished the aspiration flow rate, the holding power and in general the efficiency of the tip, so in order to have a feasible procedure, a modified 30 degree tip was developed by Microsurgical Technology – MST (Redmond, USA), with thinner walls, allowing for an increased inner diameter thereby increasing efficiency close to that of a 0.9 mm tip. Agarwal uses his end-opening sharp irrigating chopper and gas forced infusion, initially he employed an external air pump and then the Anterior Vented Gas Forced Infusion (AVGFI) system of the Alcon's Accurus equipment, with the infusion pump preset to 100 mmHg. One of us (LFV) has been using the Phakonit technique for more than 4 years (since September 2002), with a personal chopping technique, the "Vejarano's safe chop" and the Vejarano's irrigating chopper. We have already published results with a phakonit technique through 1.2 to 1.5 mm, using the 20-gauge Microtip, or 19

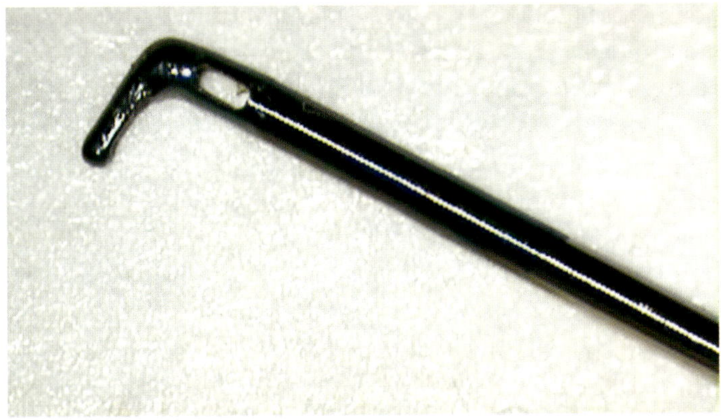

Fig. 3: Microphakonit 22 g Vejarano's irrigating chopper, (Microsurgical Technology – MST, Redmond, USA)

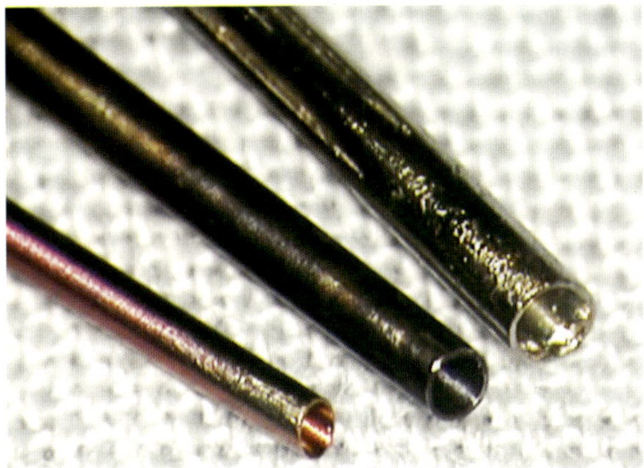

Fig. 4: Comparation of Phaco needles from Microflow (standard tip) (B and L), Microtip (Alcon) and Nanotip (Microsurgical Technology)

gauge Standard or MicroFlow® tips. Now we have available the special designed 0.7 mm Nanotip (MST) that allow us to perform the surgery through 0.8 mm incision. Because of the good results of these techniques we are using it in all our adult and pediatric cataract patients and we show our technique on these cases.

Surgical Technique

PHAKONIT

Before surgery, the pupil is dilated with tropicamide 1% and phenylephrine 10%. Povidone-iodine 10% is applied on the lashes and eyelids margins and Povidone-iodine 5% is applied in the conjunctiva, and washed out three to five minutes later, if the pupil does not dilate good enough, then use Epinephrine 1/10000 u in the anterior chamber.

In regard with the side port incision, it must be as watertight as possible when the instrument (irrigating chopper or irrigating device) is in position, but without compromising its maneuverability, and this is a very important issue, since in Phakonit this is the instrument that makes most of the movement necessary to emulsify the nucleus and in pediatric cataract to mobilize the opacified crystalline. For this reason we use a trapezoidal shape side port incision, which internally maintains very good water tightness, and externally has more room for a wider arch of movement of the instrument, if you feel the instrument gets stuck at the incision is a good idea to apply a small amount of viscoelastic on the chopper to make its movement easier.

We have found that performing a trapezoidal 0.8/1.2 mm (inner/outer size) incision let us to use the Vejarano's Irrigating Chopper® (AC7340, Accutome, Malvern,USA), which for Phakonit has 20 g (approximately 0.9 mm diameter), with almost no leakage and very good maneuverability. To achieve a good architecture we use a 0.8/1.2 mm diamond knife (Accutome, Malvern,USA) to perform this incision, but an alternative is to use 20 gauge vitreoretinal blades or 1.2/1.4 mm steel blades (Micro Surgical Technology -MST, Redmond, USA).

When performing the main incision, we use 1.2 mm diamond lancet or the same 0.8/1.2 mm diamond knife to avoid additional expenses (Both Accutome, Malvern,USA), if we are going to use a 20-gauge Microtip, and a 1.5 mm diamond blade (Natural Clear Cornea Vejarano's Microincision Knife. AK6018 Accutome, Malvern, USA) when using a 19 gauge Standard or MicroFlow® tip. We think that it is not indispensable that the main incision has a trapezoidal shape because in Phakonit the phaco needle does not move considerably, just back and forth. Moreover, in the wider (1.5 mm) incision a trapezoidal shape could lead to excessive leakage.

The incision width is not determined arbitrarily but is contingent upon the needle diameter. A common misconception is that a 0.9 diameter instrument

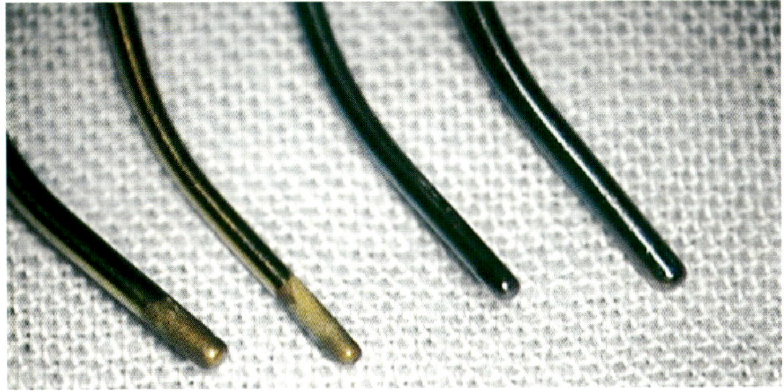

Fig. 5: Bimanual I/A tips (20 and 22 gauge) (Microsurgical Technology – MST, Redmond, USA)

will fit in a 0.9 mm incision. This will cause excessive stretching of the incision, and may tear it, compromising its water-tightness and due to the too tight contact between the tissue and the phaco tip, will increase the risk of thermal damage because the fluid going out helps to cool the needle's shaft. On the other hand a too big incision will increase the leakage and will compromise the anterior chamber stability. According to the gauges of the irrigating instrument and the phaco needle that you normally use, you can determine the proper size of your incisions. You calculate the circumference length of the instrument, using the formula $[2(\pi \times r)]$, where **r** means radius of the instrument in mm. Then, since each lip of the incision covers a half, not the whole length of the instrument's circumference is needed (and the incision length corresponds to one incision's lip length), you have to divide the result by two (in order to find out how long is half of the circumference of the instrument and therefore the incision length). Moreover, the cornea has elastic properties and so you have to take in account the tissue compliance that empirically, according with the true incision length measured in our procedures, we have calculated in 20%. Thus the final formula to decide upon the right length of the incision is:

$[2 (\pi r) / 2] - 20\%$. This may be simplified as: $\pi \times r \times 0.8$.

For instance for a 0.9 mm tip (approximately 20 g), the incision length should be:

$\pi \times r \times 0.8 = \pi \times 0.45 \text{ mm} \times 0.8 \approx 1.1 \text{ mm}$.

For a 1.1 mm tip (approximately 19 g), the incision length should be:

$\pi \times r \times 0.8 = \pi \times 0.55 \text{ mm} \times 0.8 \approx 1.4 \text{ mm}$.

Generally we use DUOVISC® (Alcon, Fort Worth, TX, USA) with the Arshinoff´s Soft Shell technique, in all the pediatric cases we stain the anterior capsule with trypan blue, before viscoelastic in regular cataracts with zonular integrity and after viscoelastic in those cases with anomalies in the shape of the crystalline as Marfan, agenesia and others in order to avoid the stain of the vitreous with the dye; this stain makes the capsulorhexis easier and gives a better sensation of control, also this dye gives to the capsule more rigidity and less elasticity.

A 5.0 mm or less continuous curvilinear capsulorhexis (CCC) is created because of the features of the capsule it increases its diameter, using the Micro Incision Capsulorhexis Forceps, 23 g (Accutome, Malvern, USA) or DUET Capsulorhexis Forceps with Fine grasping tip, 23 g (MicroSurgical Technology-MST, Redmond, USA), through microincisión the stability of the anterior chamber is amazing avoiding the draining of the viscoelastic material through the incisions and of course controlling the positive pressure of the vitreous in this infants cases preventing capsulorhexis lost, also you can use the vitrector to try to get a similar shape of CCC but with its edges wonot be really continuous.

In cases where there is not good red reflex (white pediatric cataracts) we always use trypan blue as described by Melles, but diluting the commercially available 0.1% solution to a 0.05% solution, with very good results in contrast and visualization.

Hydrodissection is performed using the Gimbel or Chang cannulae, previously depressing lightly the posterior lip of the incision, to allow that a small amount of viscoelastic goes out from the anterior chamber, thus avoiding a sudden arise of intraocular pressure during hydrodissection; hydrodelineation, may be performed rarely, according with surgeon's personal preferences but with only hydrodissection you obtain the luxation of the nucleus, so go underneath anterior capsule and direct toward the periphery of the crystalline, inject the BSS there and in other different places and immediately the nucleus goes to the anterior chamber where you can aspirate or emulsified it avoiding any contact with the posterior capsule.

The Vejarano's Irrigating Chopper® 20 g (Accutome, Malvern, USA), or 22 g (Micro surgical Technology -MST, Redmond, USA) is entered through the side port, in order to maintain adequate space in the anterior chamber. The features of the 20 g chopper are shown in. It has an outer diameter of 0.9 mm (approx. 20 gauge) that fits rather tightly in the 0.9/1.2 mm side port incision. We have found it to be very useful, and with a high safety profile in cases performed using the Infiniti Vision System (Alcon, Fort Worth., USA.).

A partially sleeveless phaco tip is entered to the anterior chamber, through the main incision (in those cases that you believe will need phaco power). A cut sleeve is used in the phaco needle, according with the description by Prakash, and we found that it is useful to diminish the amount of fluid splashed from the phaco needle during the application of ultrasound energy (like rain). We do not use any additional external fluid to cool the wound.

The parameters used in the phaco machines are related with the hardness of the nuclei, which in these cases is very low just to try to unclog the tip. We use gas forced infusion with the systems that has it incorporated, but we have found that with the Vejarano´s irrigating chopper we can perform the surgery with a stable anterior chamber, using the bottle with passive (gravitatory) infusion at an enough height, even in these cases where the vitreous push anteriorly in the whole procedure.

The parameters can be summarized as follows:

Infiniti® Vision System

Fixed Flow rate: 25 to 30 cc/min.

Lineal Vacuum: 250 - 300 mm Hg.

Dynamic Rise: 3 - 4

Lineal Power: 10%

Mode: Pulsed, 20 - 50 pps.

Modulation Power: 20 % ON

Mode: Burst: 50 msec.

Bottle High: 180 cm above the patient's head

Bimanual Irrigation/Aspiration of cortical remnants using bimanual handpieces and, if necessary, posterior capsule polishing are done also the aspiration and cleaning of the anterior capsule epithelial cells to try to avoid its fibrosis, in cases with soft nuclei (as the majority of them) since the beginning we use this Bimanual I/A to remove the whole crystalline avoiding any use of ultrasound.

Previously to the IOL insertion in every case, we implant a capsular tension ring (CTR) to gives scleral support in this cases with not enough rigidity and to try to stop the growth of the lens cells from the equator and the capsule contraction too, we had been doing this since two and a half years with excellent results avoiding that.

We prefer to make a new tunnel incision through the sclera superiorly to implant the IOL to prevent any leakage, anterior chamber collapse postoperative and infection because the lack of rigidity in this young eyes and always we use 10-0 nylon to suture closing the wound.

The decision of the IOL is still a point of discussion. Usually we implant acrylic hydrophobic IOLs [Acrysof SA60A, Acrysof Natural single-piece or Acrysof IQ IOLs (Alcon, Fort Worth, TX, USA)] using a Titanium Single Hand Injector EL-30 (EPSILON, Montclair, CA, USA), which makes possible the implantation through an 1,8 to 2,2 mm incision. It is important that the injector is a single hand instrument (with a plunger), since the second hand is use to exert contra-pressure with a second instrument through the side port incision, fixating the eye, and the injection through the incision must be fast and always in the bag.

At the end of the case always we leave a 0,3 cc of Kenalog (4,5 mg), can help to see any leakage through the incisions and we notice a big advantage in decreasing the postop inflammation, non any pupilary membrane and always a reactive pupil at next day, with this concentration we did not have had any elevation of the intraocular pressure.

MICROPHAKONIT

The microphakonit technique is very similar, but obviously the incisions' length is smaller. We use instruments 22 g, even irrigating choppers (Agarwal or Vejarano or Verges (Microsurgical Technology – MST, Redmond, USA) or I/A tips.

According with the formula explained above, for a 0.7 mm instrument (approximately 22 g), the incision length should be:

$\pi \times r \times 0.8 = \pi \times 0.35 \text{ mm} \times 0.8 \approx 0.9 \text{ mm}$.

We construct a 0.9 mm side-port incision with the 0.9 – 15° side port Diamod Knife (Accutome) to introduce the microphakonit 22 g Vejarano's irrigating chopper, (Microsurgical Technology – MST, Redmond, USA) which is approximately 0.7 mm in external diameter and 0,65 mm in internal diameter.

Like Dr Agarwal's microphakonit chopper, this instrument has thinner walls, allowing for an increased inner diameter, and moreover it features two lateral very elongated irrigation holes, thereby increasing inflow.

Main incision of 0.9 mm is performed using the same diamond blade or using the new MST 0,8 mm disposable lancets but with these the 23 g. Microutrata forceps fits very tightly which difficult its mobility. We use the MST nano tip, 0.7 mm diameter, and the Infiniti® system (Alcon). We have found that this tip has a very good performance and efficiency in emulsifying and aspirating the nuclear material, despite its very small outer diameter, because of its design of a very thin wall.

The parameters used on the Infiniti system are the same ones as for Phakonit.

When finishing the pediatric cases we prefer to put a suture in both, the main incision (always) and paracentesis if leakage is noted. Moreover, in order to diminish the possibility of capsular opacification, and hence the necessity of a posterior YAG-laser capsulotomy, and also to minimize the anterior capsule retraction as in Phakonit, we always use a capsular tension ring in these pediatric cases. Our experience after two and a half years of follow up is that 94% of the capsules are transparent, and we have not had any case of capsular phimosis.

Also as in Phakonit always we use the Kenalog at the end of the case.

Conclusion

There is an evident trend between leading ophthalmologists all around the world to perform microincision techniques, because of its advantages more in these pediatric cataracts where the inflammation is an issue to think. We think that smaller incisions are in fact safer, since we are working in an almost closed system. Using the right parameters the anterior chamber is much more stable than in coaxial Phaco with much less turbulence, endothelial cells trauma and less spend of BSS. Moreover during the phaco it is evident an improved followability, since currents rejecting fragments far from the phaco tip, such as in coaxial phacoemulsification, are avoided. In addition, the incoming irrigation flow can be used as a third intraocular instrument, which helps in directing fragments to the phaco tip and pulling structures away from it like posterior capsule or iris.

The availability of better instruments, including the MST nanotip designed in cooperation of Dr Agarwal and MST, along with the Vejarano's irrigating choppers (20 and 22 gauge) and bimanual I/A tips (20 and 22 gauge), let us to safely perform microincision cataract surgery, and even break the 1 mm frontier with the microphakonit, a really nano-surgery technique. We think that this several advantages make microincisional phacoemulsification techniques ideal also for pediatric cases.

The use of a capsular tension ring has improved our results in the sense that the posterior capsule is kept transparent and the anterior capsule retraction is avoided and the use of Kenalog has reduced the inflammation postop and improves the velocity of visual recovery.

10

Dynamics of the Capsulorhexis

Roberto Pinelli (Italy)

Introduction

When planning an extracapsular removal of the cataract, an opening of the anterior capsule has to be made in order to evacuate the opaque substance of the lens. The residual capsular tissue, the "capsular bag" can then host the artificial lens sequestrating it from the other ocular structures and giving it the best support for centration and stabilization. An intact capsular bag is more easily obtained by creating an anterior continuous curvilinear capsulorrhexis (CCC) as described by Drs Howard Gimbel and Thomas Neuhann.

The circular opening behave as a sphincter distributing the traction or dilating forces over all the circumference thus exhibiting a much higher resistance compared to an opening with a jagged margin.

A regular margin is best obtained using a continuous tear. The direction of the tear is determined by the interaction of forces exerted by

- The surgical maneuver
- The elastic properties of the capsular tissue
- The zonular attachments.

APPLYING A FORCE ON A THIN SHEET OF ELASTIC TISSUE

A tractional force applied on an elastic tissue *in the same direction of the elastic fibers* causes a deformation of the tissue. The amount of deformation is proportional to the ***stress*** that is the amount of force divided by the cross-sectional area where the force is being applied. The change in length of an elastic strip of material divided by its original length is called ***strain.*** With increasing levels of stress, the strain will increase up to the elastic limit of the tissue, than beyond it causing **permanent** deformation, than further on, up to the point of breaking.

Just before the breaking point, a smaller amount of stress will be needed to cause the same amount of strain.

If one wanted to tear apart a piece of elastic fabric, he could exert a traction on the two sides of the strip of material increasing the applied force until reaching the breaking point. The rupture will happen in an uncontrolled manner, starting in an unpredictable point of less resistance and the tear will unpredictably progresses even after the traction is no longer exerted because the force stored into the elastic fibres will continue to exert stress. If a more controlled rupture is wanted, it is better to start with creating a place of less resistance, like a small cut, in the desired location and then exert small amounts of traction making the line of rupture to progress in a controlled manner without allowing the elastic fibres to collect more than the energy just required to continue the tear. The direction of ripping will follow the rule of vectorial summation of direction and strength of the two forces.

If the same traction is exerted perpendicularly to the surface of the same thin sheet of fabric, with the points of application of traction opposite to the direction

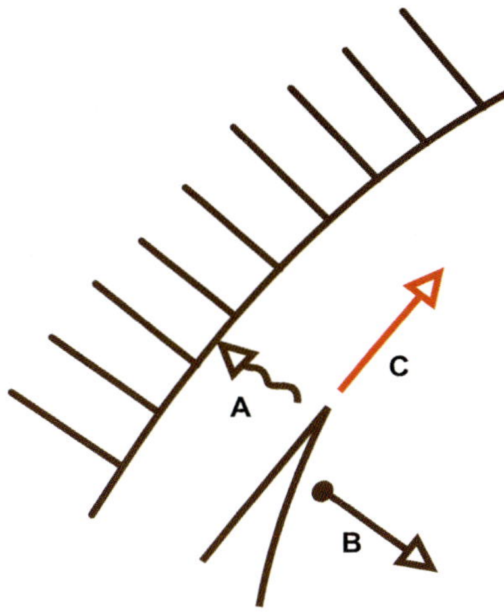

Fig. 1A: Swinging arrow A represents elastic resistance opposed by the capsular tissue plus elastic zonular traction. Arrow B is the pulling force. The effect is the direction of tear progression C resulting by two forces counteracting in the same line

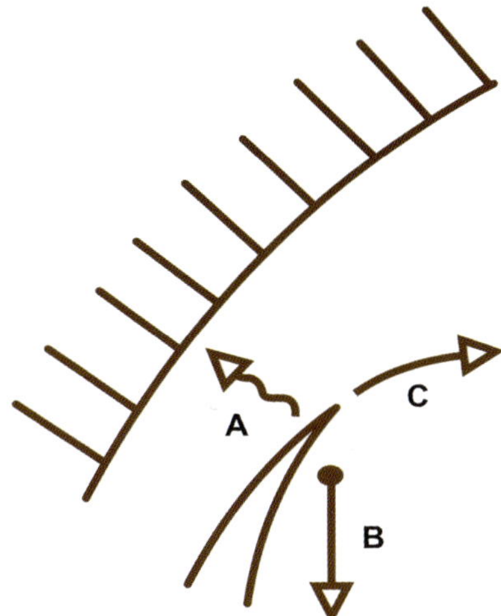

Fig. 1B: When the pulling force is exerted in a direction forming an angle different from 180° from the direction of resistance, the direction of the tear progression will tend to intersect that angle

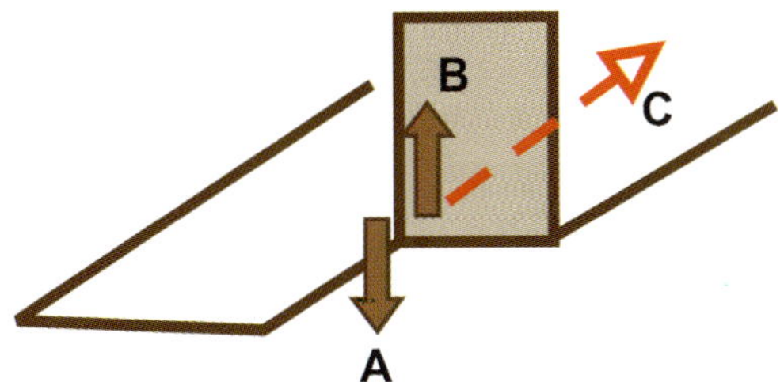

Fig. 2: B represents the shearing force, A represents the resistance. The breaking point lies inbetween the two forces and moves ahead in a very predictable and linear way

of resistance, the effect will be of shearing and the tissue will behave as a stiff substance, like a piece of paper. The breaking point is always located among the points of application of the two forces: traction and resistance.

RIPPING AND SHEARING

After creating a flap in the central portion of the capsule, the capsulorhexis can be continued in two ways:

Ripping: The flap is grasped with a forceps or engaged with the point of a curved needle very close to the origin of the tear. The pulling force is exerted mostly with a direction towards the center of the capsule, but changes of direction of the progression of the tear are easily and quickly done by small changes of the direction of the pulling force.

Remember: Before the pulling is able to make the tear progresses, elastic resistance of both the capsular tissue and the zonula has to be overcome. The effect of pulling will always be displacement followed by ripping. The amount of displacement is proportional to the elasticity so that it will be larger in a young capsule compared with an old or diseased capsule. The progression of the tear will happen along with recovery of the stretched tissue and such a return movement has to be considered when planning the direction of pulling. A continuous pull toward the centre of the capsule will result in a tear that extends to the periphery of the capsule, toward the zonular attachments. The tear has to be directed through continuous pull-release-pull movements changing direction of pulling according to the direction of the tear.

Shearing: The flap is folded over the intact capsule. Pulling the flap very close to the tear, most of the force is directed pointing upward while the adherence of the capsule to the cortical material and the overall stability of the capsular bag exerts counterforce in the opposite direction. The result is a tear that progresses in a very safe manner because almost independent from the elastic forces that exert their maximum effect tangentially while the breaking effect results from forces exerted perpendicularly to the tissue. The pure shearing movement, perpendicular to the tissue, has good "steering capability", but if the movement is continued without changing the point on application of traction, the fold will gradually start to "unfold" transforming a shearing movement in a ripping **movement** so that it is safer to release the flap and regrasp it close to the tear almost every 60 degrees.

The shearing movement is safer, but the steering action is slow so that when the tear is close to the zonular attachments a ripping technique will more efficiently redirect the tear.

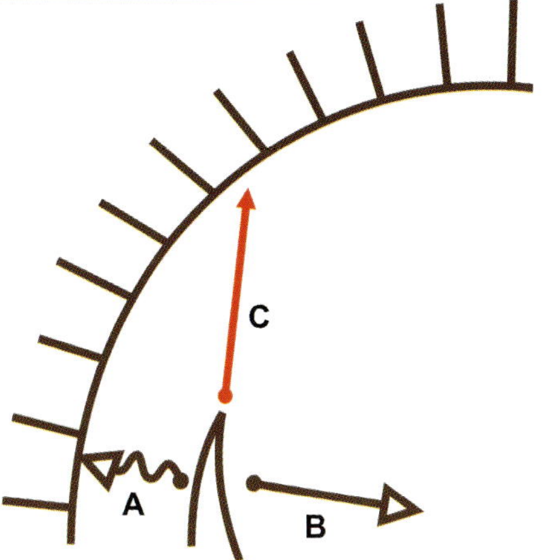

Fig. 3A: If the pulling force continues to be active in the same direction, the tear will progresses towards the zonula

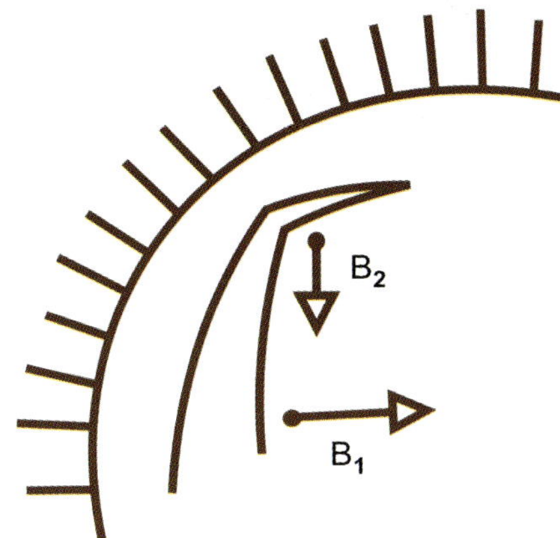

Fig. 3B: If a change of direction of the tear is wanted, traction has to be stopped and restarted in a new point with a new direction of pulling

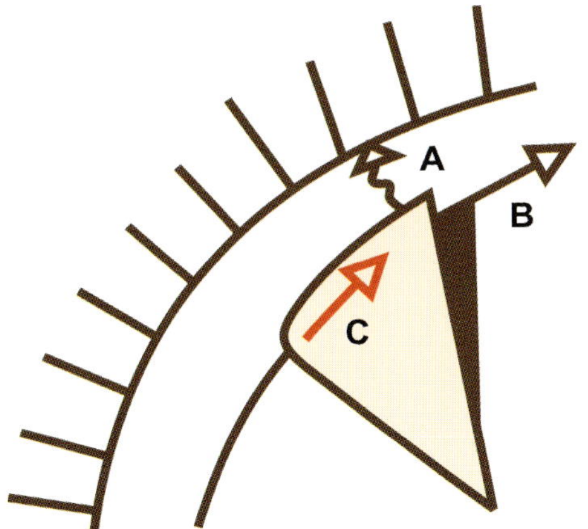

Fig. 4A: A pure shearing motion

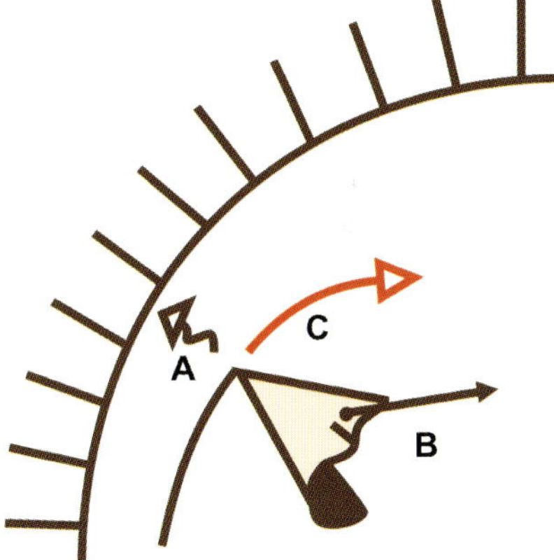

Fig. 4B: A mixed shear and rip technique used to change direction of tear progression

DEALING WITH THE CAPSULE

The capsule is an elastic envelope subjected to forces coming from:

- Anterior chamber pressure
- Lens substance pressure
- Vitreous pressure
- Zonular traction.

The elastic module of the capsule changes with age, being stiffer in an old patient and very elastic in a child.

Pressurizing the anterior chamber before starting the capsulorhexis is of paramount importance because it relaxes the zonular attachments on the anterior capsule (tightening those on the posterior capsule) decreasing an important counterforce able to direct the tear peripherally. On the contrary, an increased vitreous pressure tightens the anterior zonula.

A swollen lens substance (such as in an hypermature cataract) increases the tension of the capsule and increases the vectorial force directed towards the periphery.

A zonular insufficiency will make the capsulorhexis more difficult changing the ripping action in a displacement effect.

All these tissue components have to be taken in account when doing the capsulorhexis: adjusting the external forces (refilling the chamber or releasing pressure on the globe) or modifying the surgical strategy.

Dynamics of the Capsulorhexis

APPROACH A

Many techniques of capsulorhexis are available nowadays, and most of them are very personal. The main characteristics of the different techniques are changing proportionally with the experience of the surgeon.

A common approach is to begin the capsulorhexis from the centre of the capsule (point A) with a viscoelastic syringe using the needle carefully.

Once created a flap from point A to point B, we can continue the maneuver with the same needle, injecting viscoelastic if needed in order to see the flap better and its integrity, and perform capsulorhexis with the visco-syringe in a clockwise direction.

The same maneuver can be performed with the capsulorhexis forceps.

In order to better control the diameter and the regularity of the capsulorhexis it is better to stop the maneuver at every quadrant (from 9 h to 12 h, from 12 h to 3 h, etc.).

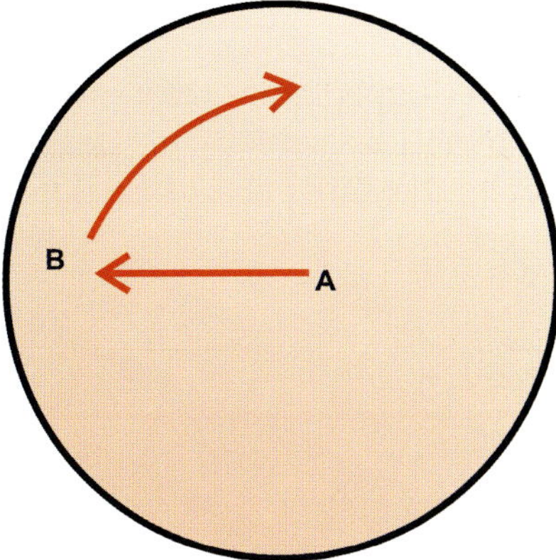

Fig. 5: Clockwise capsulorhexis

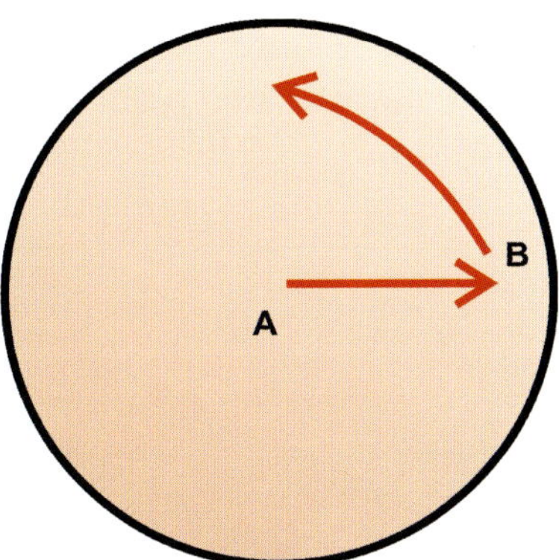

Fig. 6: Anticlockwise capsulorhexis

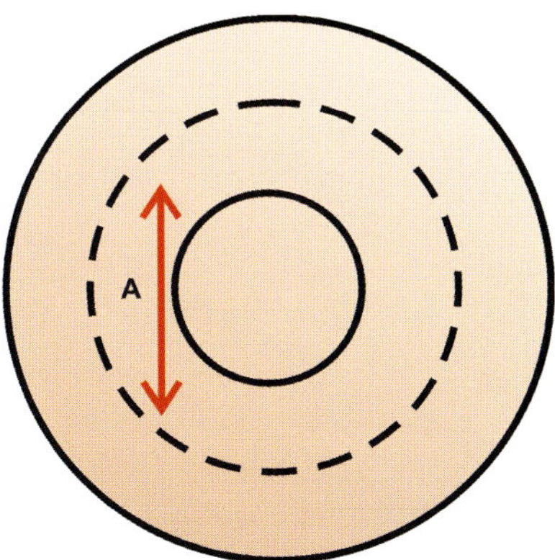

Fig. 7: Small capsulorhexis enlargement (see the tangential approach)

APPROACH B

The same approach can be performed in an anticlockwise direction. This decision is up to the surgeon, and mainly depends on his attitude (left-handed or right-handed surgeon) and in its dynamics shows no difference compared to the approach A.

Small Capsulorhexis

In case of small capsulorhexis, a careful approach can fix this problem considering the forces involved in the dynamics of this technique.

A small capsulorhexis enlargement can be performed prior to the phacoemulsification (should be) or after the insertion of the IOL in the bag (in this case, the clear red reflex through the IOL can help in clarity).

Starting from point A for the incision, it should be easier to manage the forces involved to create a new flap. Moreover, it would be also easier to perform and to manage this new flap to the diameter requested.

We consider this tangential approach safer and the most dynamically correct.

Viscoelastic injection under the small capsulorhexis can help during this maneuver.

Also in this case, the direction (clockwise or anticlockwise) can be chosen by the surgeon depending on his personal attitude.

11

Microphakonit: 700 Microns Cataract Surgery

Amar Agarwal, Athiya Agarwal,
Sunita Agarwal, Ashok Garg (India)

History

On August 15th 1998 the authors (Amar Agarwal) performed 1 mm cataract surgery by a technique called Phakonit (Phako being done with a Needle Incision Technology). Dr Jorge Alio (Spain) coined the term MICS or Microincision cataract surgery for all surgeries including laser cataract surgery and Phakonit. Dr Randall Olson (USA) first used a 0.8 mm phaco needle and a 21 gauge irrigating chopper and called it Microphaco.

On May 21st 2005, for the first time a 0.7 mm phaco needle tip with a 0.7 mm irrigating chopper was used by the authors (Am A) to remove cataracts through the smallest incision possible as of now. This is called Microphakonit.

Microphakonit (0.7 mm) Needle Tip

When we wanted to go for a 0.7 mm phaco needle the point which we wondered was whether the needle would be able to hold the energy of the ultrasound. We gave this problem to Larry Laks from MST, USA to work on. He then made this special 0.7 mm phaco needle. As you will understand if we go smaller from a 0.9 mm phaco needle to a 0.7 mm phaco needle the speed of the surgery would go down. This is because the amount of aspiration flow rate would be less.

It was decided to solve this problem by working on the wall of the 0.7 mm phaco needle. There is a standard wall thickness for all phaco tips. If we say the outer diameter is a constant, the resultant inner diameter is an area of the outer diameter minus the area of the wall.

The inner diameter will regulate the flow rate/ perceived efficiency (which can be good or bad, depending on how you look at it). In order to increase the allowed aspiration flow rate from what a standard 0.7 mm tip would be, MST (Larry Laks) had the walls made thinner, thus increasing the inner diameter. This would allow a case to go, speed wise, closer to what a 0.9 mm tip would go (not exactly the same, but closer). With the gas forced infusion it would work very well. Finally we decided to go for a 30 degree tip to make it even better.

Microphakonit (0.7 mm) Irrigating Chopper

In you will notice two designs of 20 gauge (0.9 mm) irrigating choppers which we designed. On the left is the Agarwal irrigating chopper made by the MST (Microsurgical Technology) company. This is incorporated in the Duet system. The irrigating chopper on the right is made by Geuder, Germany. Notice in the right figure the opening for the fluid is end opening, whereas the one on the left has two openings in the side. Depending on the convenience of the surgeon, the surgeon can decide which design of irrigating chopper they would like to use. There are advantages and disadvantages of both types of irrigating choppers.

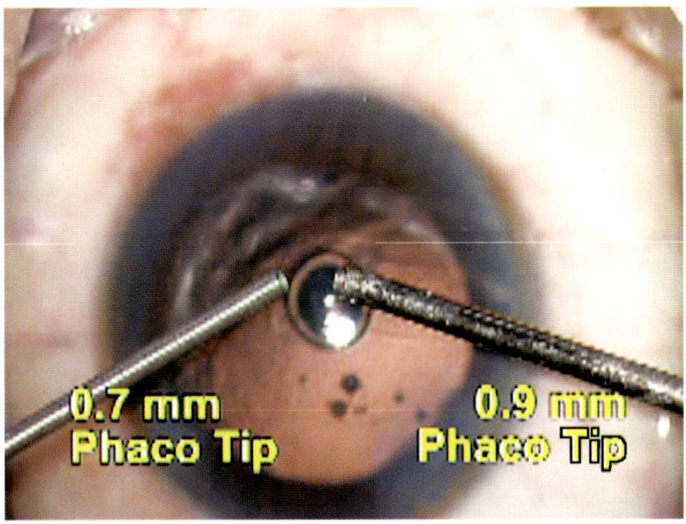

Fig. 1: 0.7 mm phaco tip (microphakonit) as compared to a 0.9 mm phaco tip (phakonit)

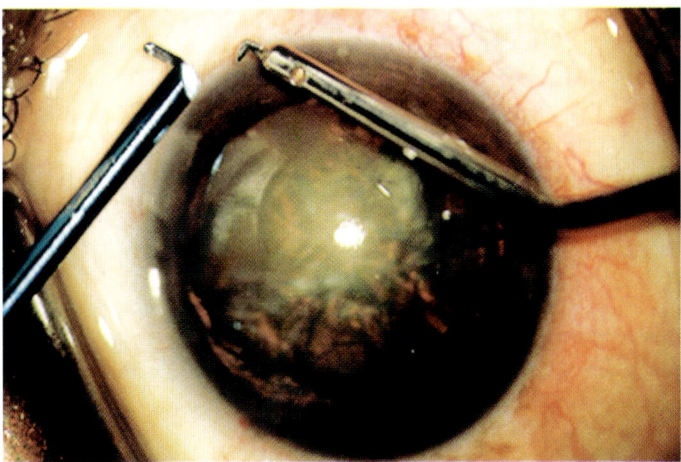

Fig. 2: Two designs of Agarwal irrigating choppers. The one on the left has an end opening for fluid (microsurgical technology). The one on the right has two openings on the sides (Geuder–Germany)

The end opening chopper has an advantage of more fluid coming out of the chopper. The disadvantage is that there is a gush of fluid which might push the nuclear pieces away. The advantage of the side opening irrigating chopper is that there is good control as the nuclear pieces are not pushed away but the disadvantage is that the amount of fluid coming out of it is much less. That is why if one is using the side opening irrigating chopper one should use an air pump or gas forced infusion.

The MST in their irrigating chopper increased flow by removing the flow restrictions incorporated in other irrigating choppers as a bi-product of their attachment method. They also had control of incisional outflow by having all the instruments to be of one size and created a matching knife of the proper size and geometry.

When we decided to go smaller to using a 0.7 mm irrigating chopper we decided to go for an end-opening irrigating chopper. The reason is as the bore of the irrigating chopper was smaller the amount of fluid coming out of it would be less and so an end-opening chopper would maintain the fluidics better. With gas forced infusion we thought we would be able to balance the entry and exit of fluid into the anterior chamber and that is what happened.

We measured the amount of fluid coming out of the various irrigating choppers with and without an air pump. We also measured the values using the simple aquarium air pump (external gas forced infusion) and the accurus machine giving internal gas forced infusion.

The microphakonit irrigating chopper which we have designed is basically a sharp chopper which has a sharp cutting edge and helps in karate chopping or quick chopping. It can chop any type of cataract.

TABLE 1: Fluid exiting from various irrigating choppers (values in ml/minute)

Irrigating chopper	*Without gas forced infusion*	*With gas forced infusion using the accurus machine at 50 mm Hg*	*With gas forced infusion using the accurus machine at 75 mm Hg*	*With gas forced infusion using the accurus machine at 100 mm Hg*	*Air pump with regulator at low*	*Air pump with regulator at high*
0.9 mm side opening	25	36	42	48	37	51
0.9 mm end opening	34	51	57	65	52	68
0.7 mm end opening	27	39	44	51	41	54

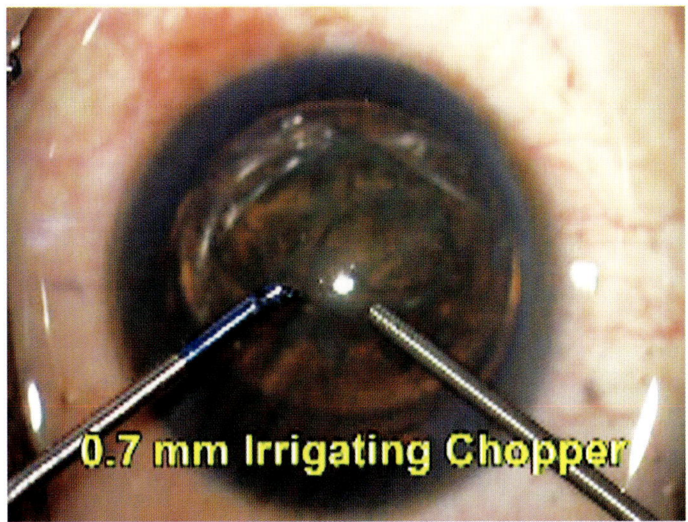

Fig. 3: 0.7 mm irrigating chopper

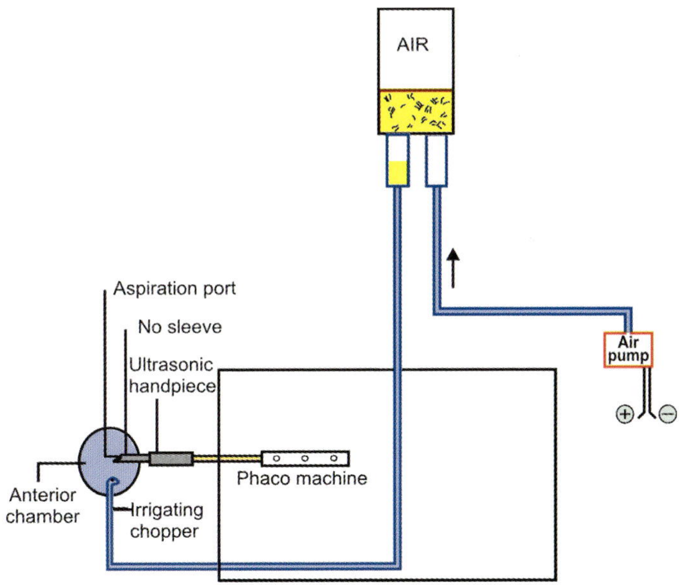

Fig. 4: Air pump

Air Pump and Gas Forced Infusion

The main problem in phakonit we had was the destabilization of the anterior chamber during surgery. We solved it to a certain extent by using an 18-gauge irrigating chopper. Then one of us (SA) suggested the use of an antichamber collapser, which injects air into the infusion bottle. This pushes more fluid into the eye through the irrigating chopper and also prevents surge. Thus, we were able to use a 20/21 gauge irrigating chopper as well as solve the problem of destabilization of the anterior chamber during surgery. Now with a 22 gauge (0.7 mm) irrigating chopper it is extremely essential that gas forced infusion be used in the surgery. This is also called external gas forced infusion.

When the surgeon uses the air pump contained in the same phaco machine, it is called internal gas forced infusion (IFI). To solve the problem of infection we use a millipore filter connected to the machine. The advantages of the Internal Forced Infusion over the External are:

1. The surgeon does not have to incorporate an external air pump to the surgical system to obtain the advantages of the forced infusion.
2. The surgeon can control all the parameters (forced infusion rate, ultrasonic power modulations and vacuum settings) in the same panel of the surgical system he or she is working with.
3. The forced infusion rate can be actively and digitally controlled during the surgery, adjusting the parameters to the conditions and/or the surgical steps of each individual case.

When we decided to use the 0.7 mm MST Duet set we decided to use the internal gas forced infusion of the accurus machine to measure the pressure of air exactly. This is from alcon. The advantage by this was that we could regulate the amount of air entering into the infusion bottle and thus titrate the system in such a way that there is no surge or collapse of the anterior chamber. When we are using a 0.7 mm irrigating chopper the problem is that the amount of fluid entering the eye is not enough. To solve this problem gas forced infusion is a must.

The anterior vented gas forced infusion system (AVGFI) of the accurus surgical system helps in the performance of phakonit. This was started by Arturo Pérez-Arteaga from Mexico. The AVGFI is a system incorporated in the Accurus machine that creates a positive infusion pressure inside the eye. It consists of an air pump and a regulator which are inside the machine; then the air is pushed inside the bottle of intraocular solution, and so the fluid is actively pushed inside the eye without raising or lowering the bottle. The control of the air pump is digitally integrated in the Accurus panel. We preset the infusion pump at 100 mm Hg when we are operating microphakonit.

As you will notice in Table 1 if we use the air pump at high it is equal to using the accurus machine at about 100 mm Hg pressure and if we use the air pump at low it is equal to using the accurus machine at 50 mm Hg pressure. Some air pumps come with such a regulator so that one can have more air

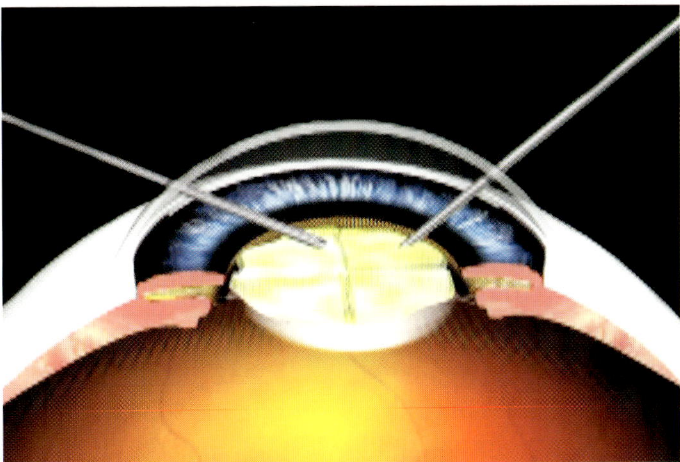

Fig. 5: Illustration showing normal anterior chamber when case is started. Air pump is not used

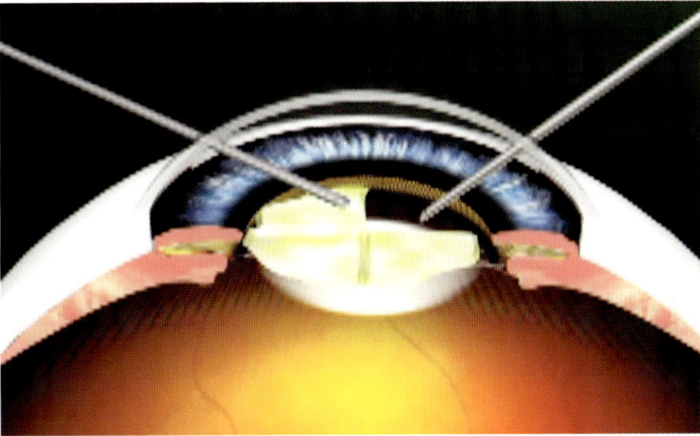

Fig. 6: Illustration showing surge and chamber collapse when nucleus is being removed. Air pump is not used. Note the chamber depth has come down. When we use the air pump this problem does not occur

coming out of them. The regulator has a switch for low and high pressure. The cost of the air pump is about US $ 2 to US $ 10/- depending on the country. This can be got from an aquarium shop. If one uses an air pump one can connect a millipore filter to it to prevent any infection. Alternatively one can use a gas forced internal infusion system using the accurus machine. In such a case preset the pump at 100 mm Hg.

Bimanual 0.7 mm Irrigation Aspiration System

Bimanual irrigation aspiration is done with the bimanual irrigation aspiration instruments. These instruments are also designed by Microsurgical Technology (USA). The previous set we used was the 0.9 mm set. Now with microphakonit we use the new 0.7 mm bimanual I/A set so that after the nucleus removal we need not enlarge the incision.

DUET HANDLES

All these instruments of the 0.7 mm set fit onto the handles of the Duet system. So if a surgeon has already got the handles and is using it for phakonit they need to get only the tips and can use the same handles for microphakonit.

Technique

INCISION

The incision is made with a keratome. This can be done using a sapphire knife or a stainless steel knife. One should be careful when one is making the incision so that the incision is a bit long as one would be using gas forced infusion in microphakonit. Before making the incision, a needle with viscoelastic is taken and pierced in the eye in the area where the side port has to be made . The viscoelastic is then injected inside the eye. This will distend the eye so that the clear corneal incision can be made easily. Make one clear corneal incision between the lateral rectus and inferior rectus and the other between the lateral rectus and superior rectus. This way one is able to control the movements of the eye during surgery.

RHEXIS

The rhexis is then performed of about 5-6 mm. This is done with a needle. In the left hand a straight rod is held to stabilize the eye. This is the Globe stabilization rod. The advantage of this is that the movements of the eye can get controlled if one is working without any anesthesia or under topical anesthesia.

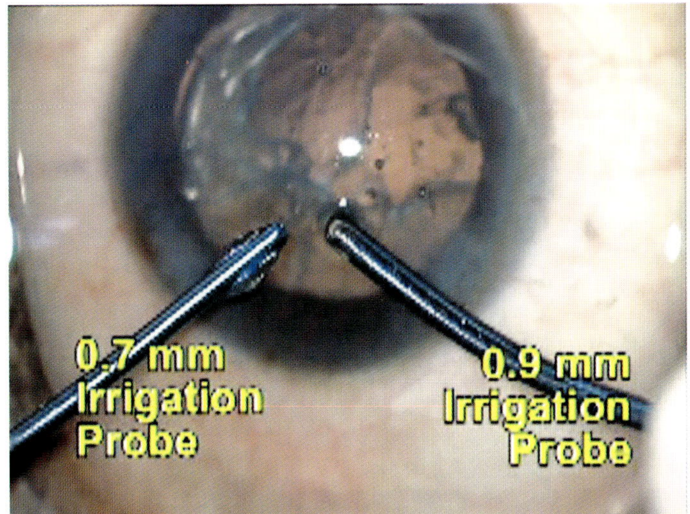

Fig. 7: 0.7 mm irrigation probe used for bimanual I/A compared to the 0.9 mm irrigation probe

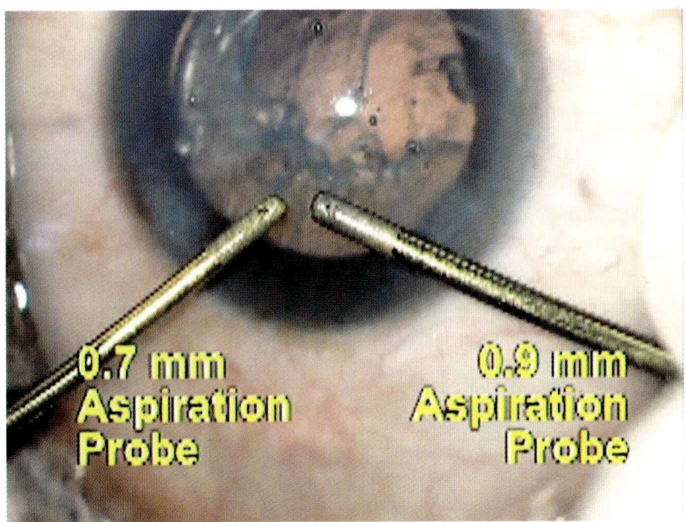

Fig. 8: 0.7 mm aspiration probe used for bimanual I/A compared to the 0.9 mm aspiration probe

HYDRODISSECTION

Hydrodissection is performed and the fluid wave passing under the nucleus checked. Check for rotation of the nucleus. The advantage of microphakonit is that one can do hydrodissection from both incisions so that even the subincisional areas can get easily hydrodissected. The problem is as there is not much escape of fluid one should be careful in hydrodissection as if too much fluid is passed into the eye one can get a complication.

MICROPHAKONIT

The 22 (0.7 mm) Gauge irrigating chopper connected to the infusion line of the phaco machine is introduced with foot pedal on position 1. The phaco probe is connected to the aspiration line and the 0.7 mm phaco tip without an infusion sleeve is introduced through the clear corneal incision. Using the phaco tip with moderate ultrasound power, the center of the nucleus is directly embedded starting from the superior edge of rhexis with the phaco probe directed obliquely downwards towards the vitreous. The settings at this stage are 50% phaco power, flow rate 24 ml/min and 110 mm Hg vacuum. Using the karate chop technique the nucleus is chopped. Thus the whole nucleus is removed. Cortical wash-up is then done with the bimanual irrigation aspiration (0.7 mm set) technique. During this whole procedure of microphakonit gas forced infusion is used.

Summary

With microphakonit a 0.7 mm set is used to remove the cataract. At present this is the smallest one can use for cataract surgery. With time one would be able to go smaller with better and better instruments and devices. The problem at present is the IOL. We have to get good quality IOL's going through sub 1mm cataract surgical incisions so that the real benefit of microphakonit can be given to the patient.

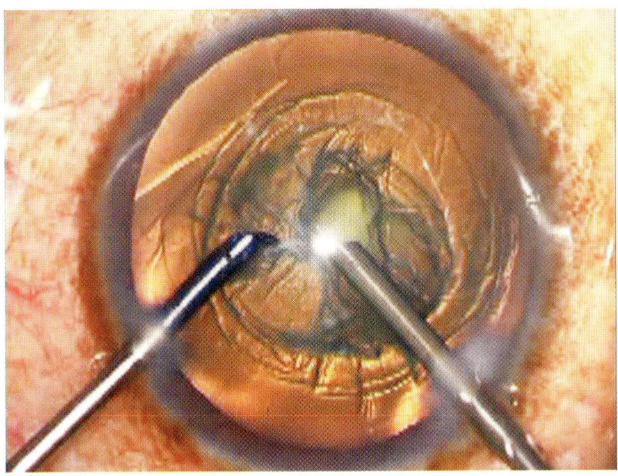

Fig. 9: Microphakonit started. 0.7 mm irrigating chopper and 0.7 mm phako tip without the sleeve inside the eye. All instruments are made by MST, USA. The assistant continuously irrigates the phaco probe area from outside to prevent corneal burns

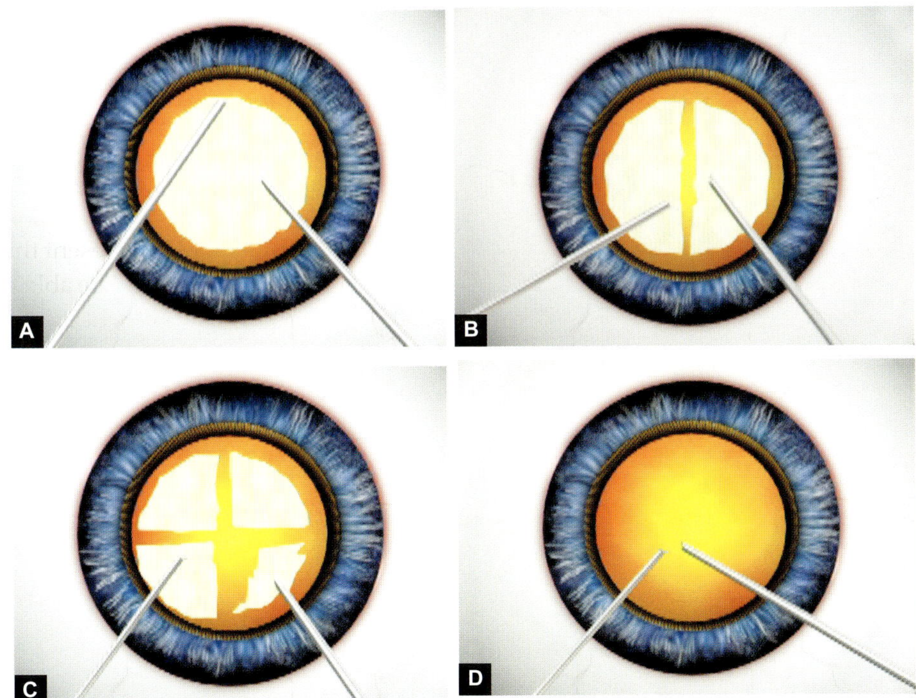

Figs 10A to D: Illustration showing the nucleus removal

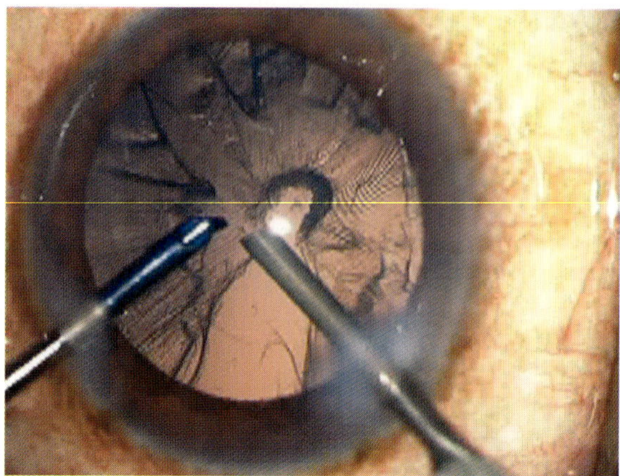

Fig. 11: Microphakonit completed. The nucleus has been removed

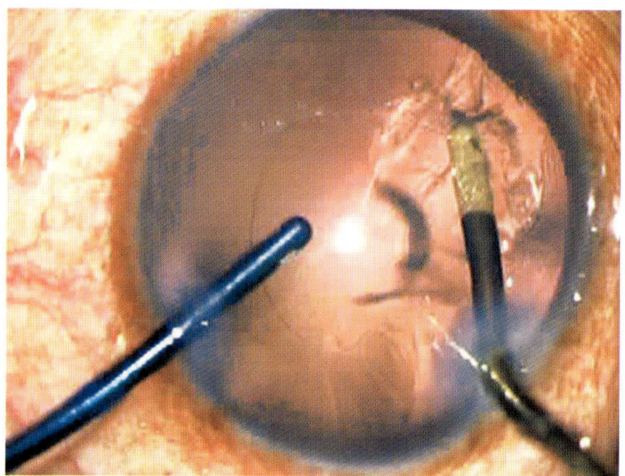

Fig. 12: Bimanual irrigation aspiration started with the 0.7 mm set

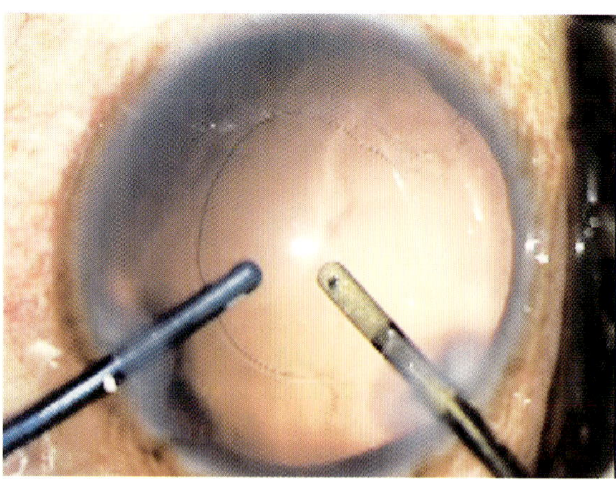

Fig. 13: Bimanual irrigation aspiration completed

12

Microincision Cataract Surgery (MICS)

Jorge L Alió, Pawel Klonowski,
José L Rodríguez Prats, Bassam El Kady (Spain)

Introduction: The Trends Towards Microincision Cataract Surgery (MICS)

Surgery techniques to remove the cataract lens has undergone revolutionary transformations over of hundreds years. Many years ago, cataract surgery was performed by pushing down nuclei lenses into the vitreous chamber. Then a corneoscleral incision was made in order to extract the lens from the eye. However, this caused considerable damage to the outside layers of the eye. The operating wound was approximately 180° around the limbus, which caused a large number of interoperation's and postoperative complications. The post-operative wound was closed by microsutures.

However, some problems still remained: postoperative astigmatism, bacterial infections, vitreous loss, iris inclusion, wound leakage, macular edema, expulsive hemorrhage, and the long period of patient convalescence.

The method of lens phacoemulsification with the help of ultrasound discovered by Charles Kelman in the late 1960s was a turning point. This method reduced the surgical wound by a few millimeters, a 5.5-6.0 mm intraocular lens (IOL) remained the limit. The Discovery of foldable lenses allows the incision to be smaller. The reduction of the incision has been 3.5-2.75 mm in 90 years. The limit remained connected with applying the end tip and sleeve for 2.5 mm breadths. Attempts to make the phacoemulsification tip breadth smaller caused the function of the irrigation-aspiration system to fail. The quantity of ultrasound energy passed into the anterior chamber remained on the high level, in spite of applying modern ultrasound generators with high efficiency aspiration pumps. Perioperative injury still occurred when using the mechanical, thermal and wave shock energy. The development of faster partition, breaking and aspiration of lens masses was a progress but it was not the main turning point in this field.

At the beginning of 1990 new possibilities in the field of cataract surgery were being explored: minimization of the incision, making intraoperative damage smaller, new IOLs, new techniques of IOL implantation. The possibility of developing the phacoemulsification standard technique and devices seemed to be impossible. However, the phacoemulsification tip with the sleeve were still considerably wide and it didn't allow the size of the operating wound to be smaller. The evolution in devices led to a change in the way of thinking regarding the lens phacoemulsification technique. Not only existing tools but also fluidics started to play an important part in the leading role.

Biaxial microincision clear corneal phacoemulsification was a new method which made the corneal incision smaller. This method was described by Shearing in1985. This procedure uses separate irrigations with an irrigating chopper, sleeveless phacoemulsification tip, and also requires pulsed phacoemulsification energy.

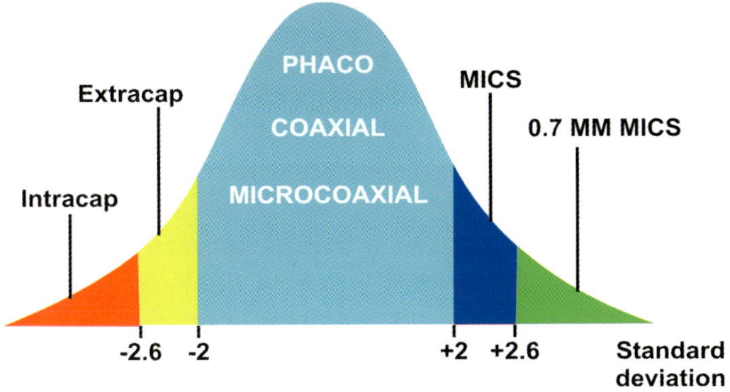

Fig. 1: Natural evolution of cataract surgery

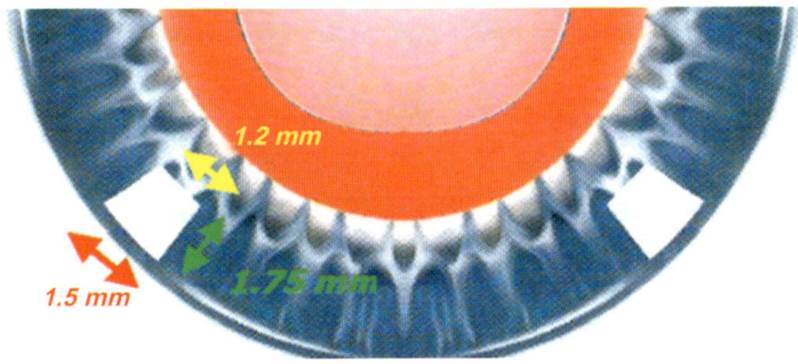

Fig. 2: MICS incision

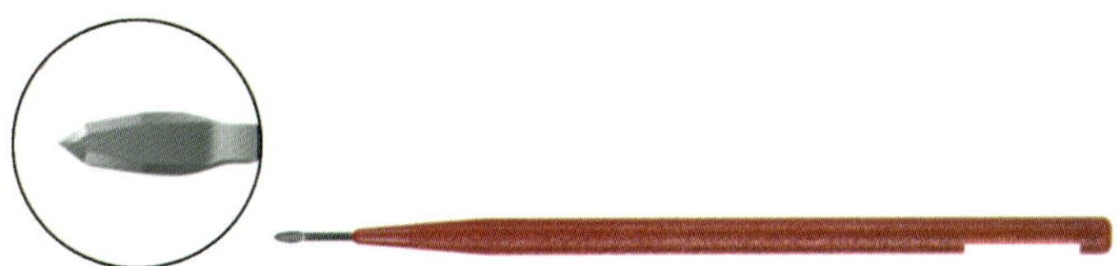

Fig. 3: Alio´s MICS Metal Knife (Katena Inc, Denville, NJ, USA)

The minimization of the incision is a consequence of a natural evolution of the cataract surgery technique in the search of excellence. When we place cataract surgery within the context of Gaussian distribution, it is clear that the standard of practice today is standard coaxial phacoemulsification. Extracapsular 6-mm surgery is a procedure still in practice today, but rarely performed, hence between -2 and -2.6 standard deviation. The Gaussian curve is like a wave. It moves from antient to new surgical techniques. Intracapsular cataract surgery causes a corneal wound length of over 10 mm. At present, this technique is almost never used. Extracapsular cataract extraction was then invented. This method allowed the removal of cataracts through a 7 mm surgical incision. It became a universal method during the 1960s and 1970s. Phacoemulsification technique was developed in early 70s and 80s. Nowadays standard coaxial technique is still one of the most popular types of cataract surgery in the world. However, the wound of the cornea was still 2.75 mm, in spite of the availability of foldable intraocular lenses. MICS should be considered beyond the 2 up to the 2.6 standard deviations of our Gaussian distribution. MICS will be the standard of practice in future, and what we could call sub 1-mm MICS or micro-MICS will be the next standard.

Cataract surgery is one of the most frequently performed surgeries in the world with approximately 4.5 million surgeries taking place annually in the USA and EU, and an increase of around 5 percent every year. Due to the increase in number of cataract surgeries performed each year, there is an increasing need to investigate various problems such as post operative astigmatism, problems with leaking wounds and also the risk of endophthalmitis.

The standard phacoemulsification technique is also limited due to the width of the surgical tools. Making the incision smaller without decreasing the parameters of the flow in the standard phacoemulsification technique isn't possible. New intraocular lenses exists, which allows to cross the barrier of the incision. Natural evolution of cataract surgery leads to making incisions smaller, smaller perioperative injuries, maximization of visual acuity and decreases the probability of postoperative infection. Nowadays, we can make the most of phaconit by Amar Agarwal, coaxial phacoemulsification, bimanual phacoemulsification.

Surgery technique meeting these conditions is MICS. MICS is the next stage in the evolution of cataract surgery. MICSs incisions additionally do not cause postoperative astigmatism in most cases.

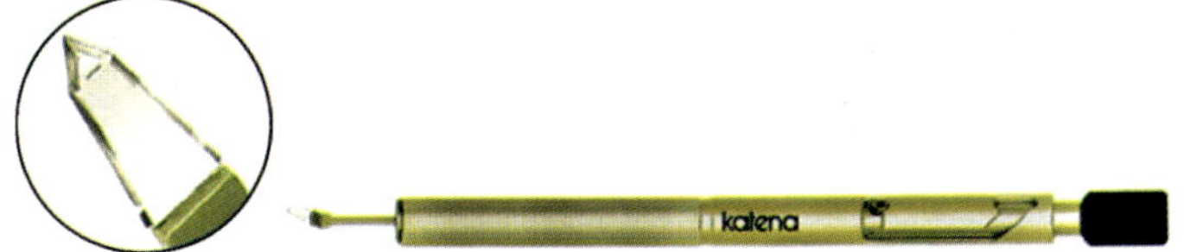

Fig. 4: Alio's MICS Diamond Knife (Katena Inc, Denville, NJ, USA)

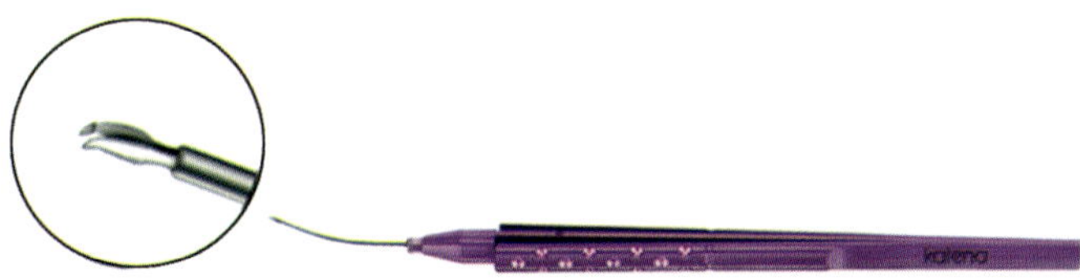

Fig. 5: Alio's MICS Capsulorhexis Forceps (Katena Inc, Denville, NJ, USA)

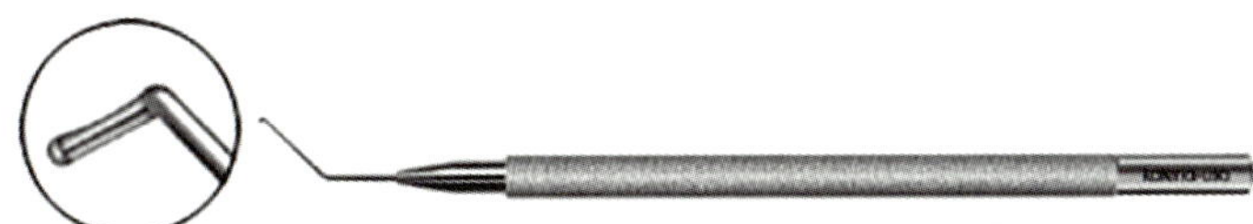

Fig. 6: Alio-Rosen Phaco PreChopper for Micro Incision Cataract Surgery (Katena Inc, Denville, NJ, USA)

ADVANTAGE OF MICS

1. Surgery
   a. I/A separation
      - With no leakage
      - Fluidics work as instrument
      - More flexible surgery, assisted by fluidics
      - Intraoperative control of intraocular pressure (IOP) in leakage free environment.

   b. Smaller incision
   c. Decreased Effective Phaco Time (EPT) – more efficient surgery.
2. Patient
   a. Minimal surgical induced astigmatism
   b. Minimal aberration unaltered
   c. Faster postoperative recovery
   d. Excellent visual acuity.

Ophthalmology surgeons who perform cataract surgery in standard phacoemulsification mode won't have a problem to change the operation technique to MICS because the principle idea of the manipulation inside the eye remains unchanged. The main aim of MICS is to understand the principles.

MICS Definition

In 2001, MICS was patented as a new operating method by Jorge Alio on the definition Microincisional Cataract Surgery (MICS) is the surgery performed through incisions of 1.5 mm or less. Understanding this global concept implies that it is not only about achieving a smaller incision size but also about making a global transformation of the surgical procedure towards minimal aggressiveness. In other words a transition from conventional small incision surgery to the more developed concept of MICS.

Microincision Cataract Surgery it is a new surgery for the removal of cataracts made by small incision in the cornea. It is operation technique, for which the principle aim is to remove cataracts a way that reduces the aggressiveness and trauma of the eye. The experienced surgeon who applies this procedure must be fully aware of the operation technique. The surgeon must be aware of the system of the lens fragmentation, have new tools, and have an active apply of fluidics and have foldable lenses adapted for such a small incision.

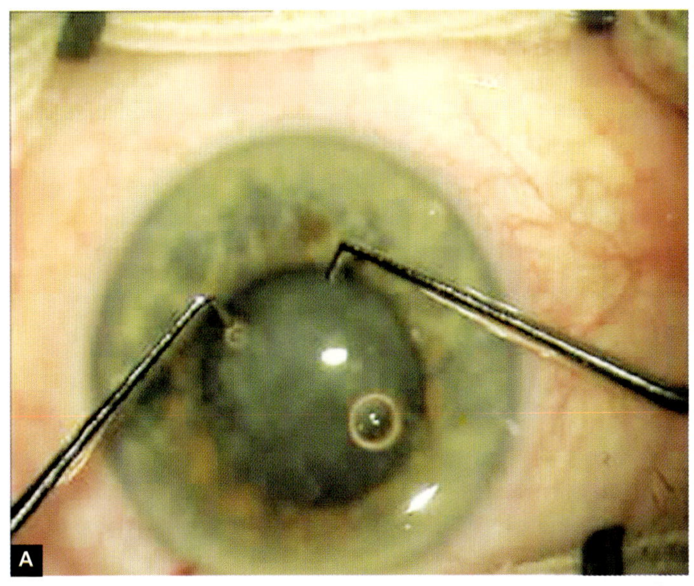

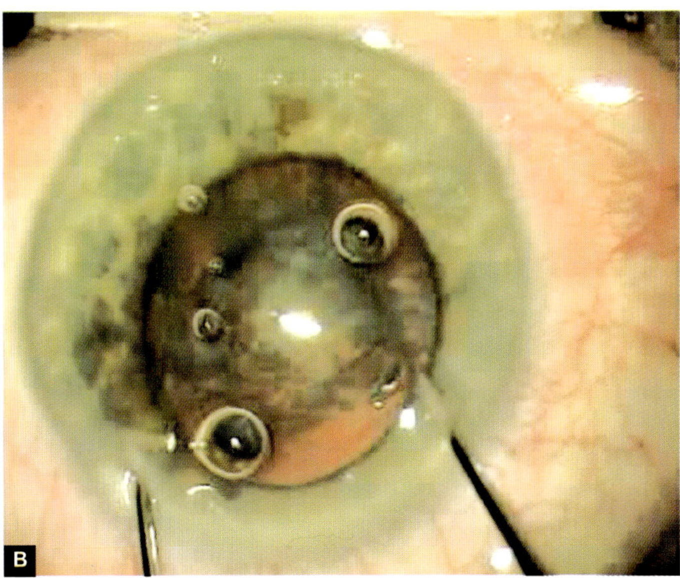

Figs 7A and B: MICS Prechopping with Alio-Rosen Phaco PreChoppers

Indication for MICS Surgery

There is no limitation of indication to MICS cataract operation. You can operate all gradient of cataract LOCS III, even hard cataracts. Subluxated lenses, post traumatic lenses, zonular laxity and congenital cataracts can also be operated with MICS, but with small doses of ultrasound. MICS is especially dedicated for "refractive cataract operation". Generally MICS doesn't induce astigmatism. MICS can be used for refractive cataract surgery by injecting multifocal lenses and toric lenses and after refractive surgery.

Surgical Technique Step by Step

MICS ANESTHESIA

After the incisions, intraocular anesthesia and mydriatics are applied to the eye. We use 1% Lidocaine local anesthesia by injecting it into the anterior chamber. Pupil dilatation is achieved by intraocular tropicamide 10% and fenilefrine 10% combination with no preservatives.

MICS INCISION

The incision optimization results from holding the constant of the anterior chamber depth, adapting for used tools, implantation of the lens and counter stretching in the route of manipulation. To be able to achieve the best visual acuity after surgery also requires the changes with the minimization of astigmatism. The minimization of the incision is required to carry out MICS correctly. Incisions lower than 1.5 mm don't normally induce postoperative astigmatism. It is needed for the faster postoperative rehabilitation and at the same time for getting the perfect visual acuity. Nowadays we use 19 G (1/1.1 mm) i 21 G (0.7 mm) tools to do MICS. The incision should be adapt to this dimensions.

The first stage of the operation is making two corneal incisions with a distance of 90°-110° angle steps. To assure the reduction of existing astigmatism, a dominant incision must be made in a positive meridian of astigmatism. Placement the incision at the positive meridian probably led to 30% reduction in the refractive cylinder. Relaxation incisions can also be made. Incisions should allow correct tool manipulation, be watertight and the wound should be correctly closed in the post-operative period. These basic conditions should be fulfilled.

Two or three steps of the incision should be carried out in order to have a correct lock wound mechanism. The shape of the wound is very important, it should have the trapezoidal shape with two breadths of the operating wound. Smaller measurement for 1,2 mm breadths inside the wound near the Descemet's membrane and the wider measurement 1.4 mm outside near the epithelium.

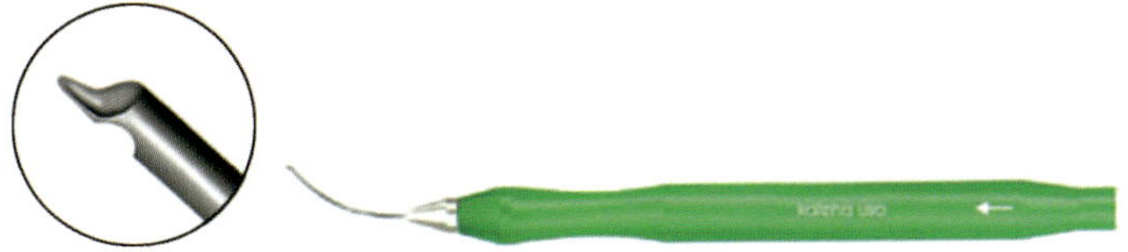

Fig. 8: Alio's original fingernail MICS irrigating hydromanipulator (Katena Inc, Denville, NJ, USA)

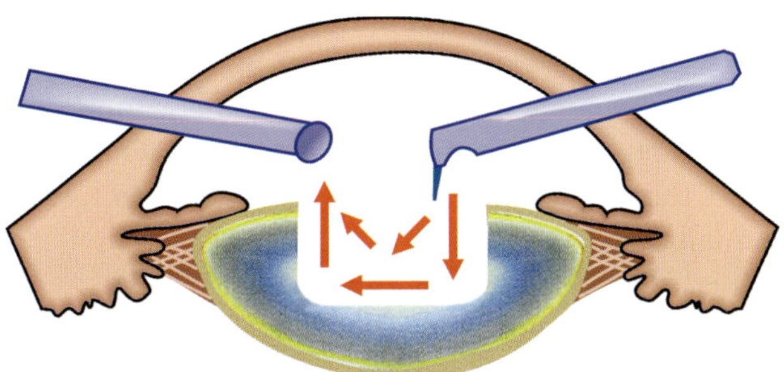

Fig. 9: Posterior irrigation helps to open capsular bag, doesn't induce turbulences, elevates nucleus fragments towards the phaco tip and helps in cortex cleaning

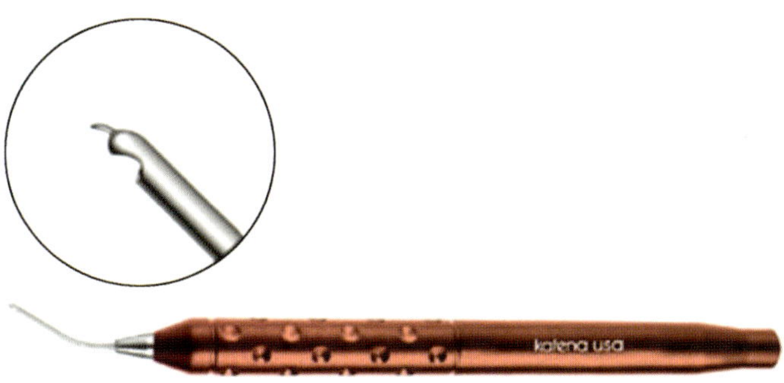

Fig. 10: Alio's MICS Irrigating Stinger (Katena Inc, Denville, NJ, USA)

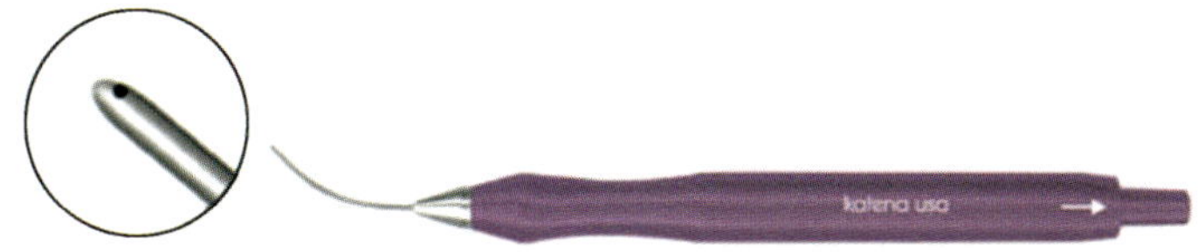

Fig. 11: Alio's MICS Aspiration Handpiece (Katena Inc, Denville, NJ, USA)

This shape is particularly important because of the necessity of the tools manipulation inside the anterior chamber. By forming the wound this way it enables quite a considerable transfer of tools without any anxiety of the distortion, deformation and macerate when coming into existence of the leakage in the wound. It also protects against the induce postoperative astigmatism. This is essential as the structure of the wound must be protected against the leakage and at the same time it provides an opportunity to work without anxiety and reduces tissues injury. The mechanical injury to tissues can suppress healing, extending healing and contribute to the uprising of the leakage, hypotony and increased risk of the endophthalmitis. It is also necessary to remember that too small incisions will prevent us to correct manipulations and a too big incisions will lead to the unchecked leakage from the wound.

To make the incision, we are used trapezoidal knives, which have changeable gauged breadth of the incision from 1,2 mm on the peak to 1,4 mm by the base (Katena Inc, Denville, NJ, the USA).

To achieve this target two kinds of knives can be used:

Alio´s MICS Knife (Katena Inc, Denville, NJ, the USA). Trapezoid shape 1.25 mm/1.4 mm/2.0 mm angled, double bevel.

MICS Diamond Knife (Katena Inc, Denville, NJ, USA) trapezoid shaped pale 1.25 mm / 1.4 mm/2.0 mm width laser etched line indicating 1.25 mm width.

The discussed breadth of the wound is adapted to phacoemulsification tip 0.9 mm breadths. For smaller phacoemulsification tips the breadth of the incision should be appropriately smaller. Through this incision we can inject anesthetics and ophthalmic viscoelastic devices (OVD) without any problems using standard infusion cannulas.

The watertightness of the wound guarantees the holding stability and the right depth of the anterior chamber. The value of such incision reduces the possibility of exchanging liquids between the anterior chamber and the conjunctiva sack. It is essential for the minimization the risk of the endophthalmitis.

MICS CAPSULORHEXIS

Correctly performed capsulorhexis is exquisitely important for keeping the MICS course. Well performed capsulorhexis will allow a safe operation.

OVD injecting with low viscosity dispersive (Viscoat) and medium viscosity dispersive (Celoftal) will allow the preservation of cells endothelium in more distant stages of the operation, but at the same time will deepen the chamber in the anterior chamber for correct tool maneuvering.

For this we used Alio's MICS Capsulorhexis Forceps (Katena Inc, Denville, NJ, the USA). It is an exquisitely delicate forecep with a 23G diameter.

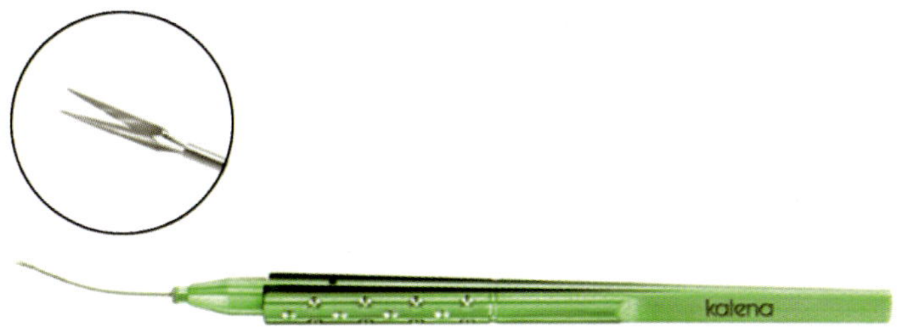

Fig. 12: Alio's MICS scissors (Katena Inc, Denville, NJ, USA)

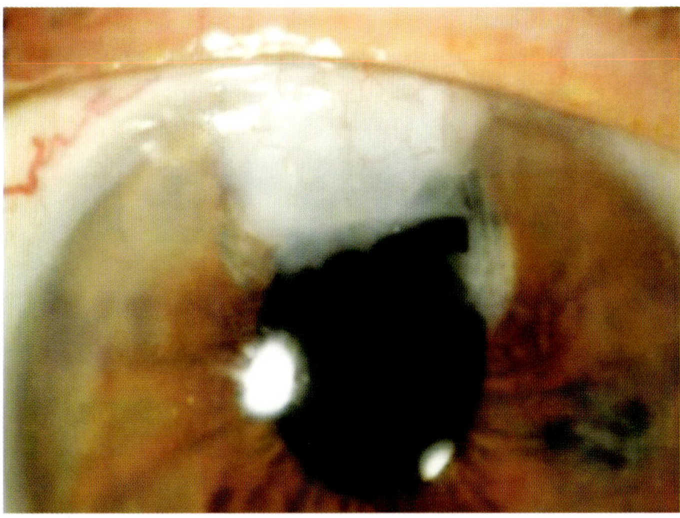

Fig. 13: Corneal burn after surgery. Personal case. This is the only one corneal burn so far in our transmission to MICS and was related to use high viscosity viscoelastics

Fig. 14: Cruise Control™ System (STAAR Surgical Company Monrovia, CA USA)

It can be easily located in the wound of the cornea. The correct profile of the hilt assures the ergonomic use and normal movements inside the eye. At the end of the forceps a pointed catch is found. This enables a controlled puncturing of the anterior bag of the lens. Pressure is applied on the bag and then with a little movement the slice in anterior bag is made. The wide gauged shoulder forceps enables a free manipulation of the torn capsular bag.

The next step is to pull the flap by tearing the bag in harmony or anticlockwise. The size of the surgical wound and the diameter of the forceps prevent the possibility of the OVD leakage and flattening of the anterior chamber, the lens and the bag are stabilized. The probability of bad tearing is decreasing. The size of the capsulorhexis should be 5-6 mm. The diameter of the anterior capsule tear should have 0.5 mm less than the diameter of the IOL. MICS Capsulorhexis Forceps allows capsulorhexis without the necessity of the help of the second tool. There is no need of more previous leading, cystotom which can considerably damage edges of the operating wound.

MICS HYDRODISSECTION, HYDRODELINEATION

The next stage of the cataract operation is the dissection of the lens from the cortex.

The hydrodissection process is important, because it separates the nucleus of the lens from the remaining motionless and delicate structure of the eye. This is important for pre-chopping as it enables the process of pre-chopping to be carried out in a safe way and does not cause complications. Hydrodissection can diminish the power of ultrasound and surgery time.

Following the process of capsulorhexis, a small amount of balance salt solution (BSS) liquid is applied directly onto the lens in order to remove the OVD from the anterior chamber. This maneuver makes a smaller power exerted on the lens from the side of the cornea. Thanks to that nucleus after BSS passing will more easily separate from the cortex and the lens will rise without problems from the bag.

In the time hydrodelineation liquid is applied under the ring of the anterior bag into the space of the lens masses. It is enables the nuclei to be elevated and separated from the cortical masses. During this maneuver it is possible to observe lines by BSS flowing in, these are called- shock waves. The maneuver should be carried out as quickly as possible and with very little amount of liquid. Pressure is then applied on the lens in order to smooth the position and BSS disposing outside of the bag into the anterior chamber. If the nuclei rotation is not possible, hydrodissection maneuver should be repeated.

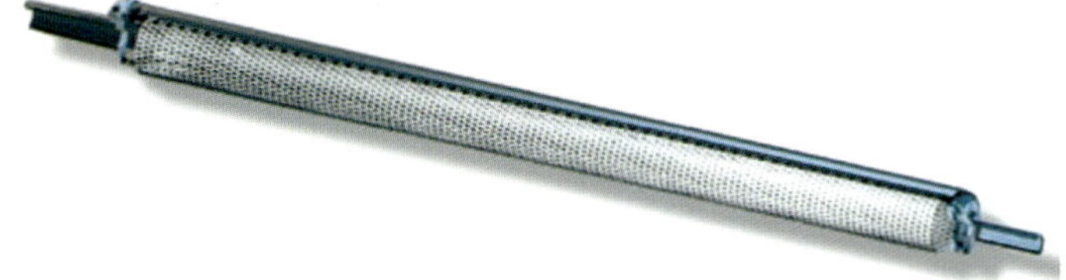

Fig. 15: Stable Chamber System (Bausch & Lomb Company Rochester, NY, USA)

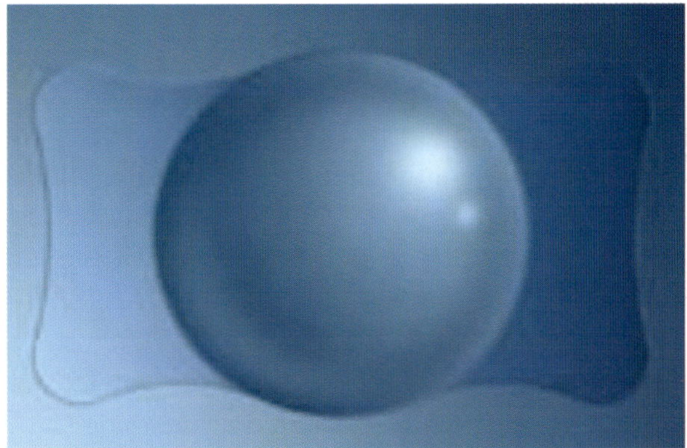

Fig. 16: Acri.Smart 46 S (Acri.Tec GmbH, Hennigsdorf, Germany)

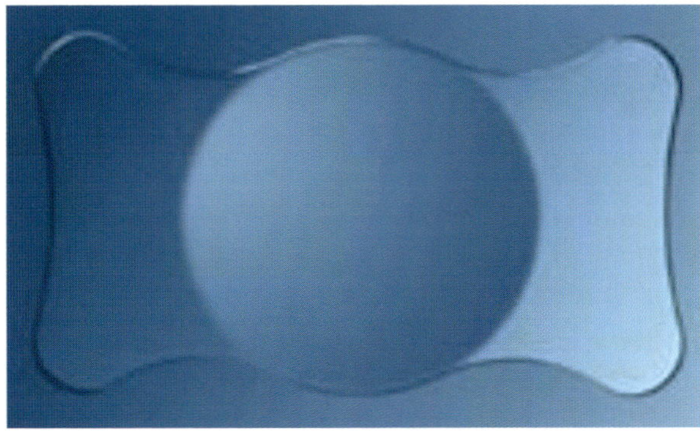

Fig. 17: Acri.Smart 48 S (Acri.Tec GmbH, Hennigsdorf, Germany)

MICS PRECHOPPING

After the hydrodissection of the lens a mechanical division is made. This activity is aimed to make four lens quadrants. Prechopping is making smaller the amount of the ultrasonic, laser or mechanical energy delivered for fragmentation into the anterior chamber. This makes manual activities smaller in the anterior chamber created by the phacoemulsification tip. There is a very important activity in the process of the energy reduction delivered to the eye. This is made with the help of two prechoppers —Alio-Rosen MICS prechoppers (Katena Inc, Denville, NJ, the USA).

Two prechoppers should be inserted into the bag under the anterior capsular rim as the first stage of the operation, so that they are opposite to each other. The hook of the chopper should be parallel to the anterior capsula bag. Next chopper should be gently rotated along the axis of the tool. The chopper should now be situated behind the masses of the lens under the bag on the perimeter.

This activity should be made symmetrically by both hands. The Choppers are crossed by, situating symmetrically opposite oneself. Next a movement of the cutting of lens masses is being made, gently crossing prechoppers. The cut will be made from the perimeter to the center nuclei. Internal edge prechoppers have a sharp edge which facilitates the incisions of the lens masses. This ambidextrous activity is important so that zonular stress does not occur. It can also be made in the case of subluxated cataracts. When the cut is made two dividing hemispheres are made. The nucleus is then rotated about 90° and then for the second time prechopping is repeated as described. After carrying out prechopping we have four lens quadrants in the bag. Fast and effective division nuclei are contributing for shortening the time of the operation.

MICS PHACOEMULSIFICATION AND REMOVAL SECTION

Having divided nuclei we can start to remove sections. We always start this stage of the operation by inserting an irrigating instrument as first tool to the anterior chamber. It assures stability of the chamber. Phacoemulsification hand piece with a tip is a basic tool which is being led through the main incision. The second incision is only carried out by the hydromanipulator. Having shared quadrants we can begin to remove phacoemulsification from the first quadrant.

We are used Alio's MICS hydromanipulator irrigating fingernail (Katena Inc, Denville, NJ, the USA). Its end is a fingernail-like shaped. This tool has 18G diameter and helps to remove rather soft cataracts. There is irrigation hole on the bottom lower side of the tool. The hole diameter is 1 mm. It has also very thin walls to increase internal diameter of instrument. This irrigation cannula is assuring infusion in borders 72 cc/min.

A large infusion directed to the bottom assures the excellent flow of liquids and also a fast and effective chilling phacoemulsification tip. An outstanding stability of the anterior chamber is assured through the function infusion and

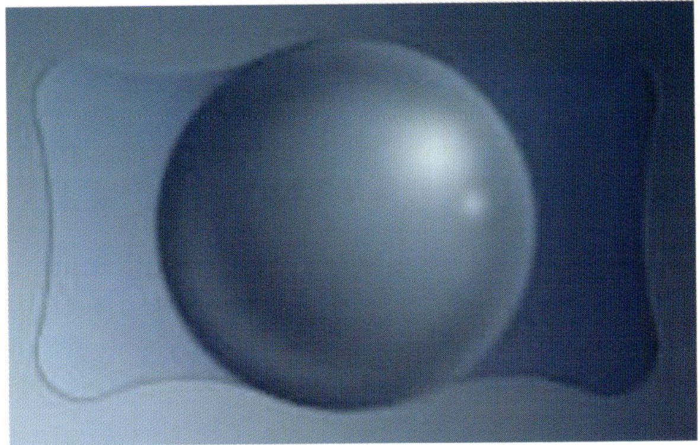

Fig.18: Acri.Smart 36 A Aberration Correcting IOL (Acri.Tec GmbH, Hennigsdorf, Germany)

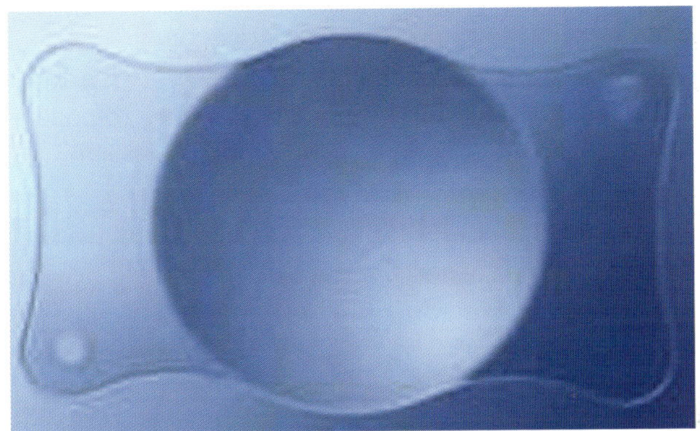

Fig. 19: Acri.LISA 366D multifocal IOL (Acri.Tec GmbH, Hennigsdorf, Germany)

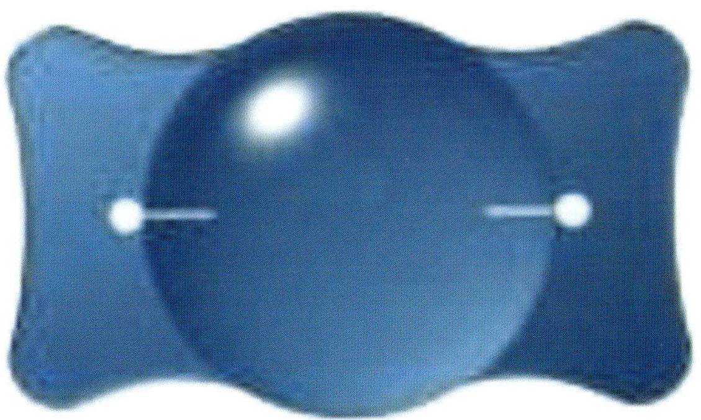

Fig. 20: Acri.Comfort 646 TLC Bitoric Aberration Corrected Aspherical Foldable One Piece Lens for Capsular Bag Fixation (Acri.Tec GmbH, Hennigsdorf, Germany)

directs the liquid to the lens masses at the bag back, independently from high vacuum sets of phacoemulsification machine.

The strength of the stream permits the bag to be held in a safe distance from the phacoemulsification tip and at the same time enables convenient manipulations of tools and lens masses. Additionally, this stream can clean the back bag from remaining cortical cells. A very fertile directed stream to the back bag is provided with the preservation of cells endothelium corneas before mechanical and thermal damage. The irrigation hole can be found situated on the side of the irrigating probe or on top and this can result in the turbulences in the anterior chamber. This effect can damage the endothelium cells and stabilities of the anterior chamber.

The tool which allows the removal of harder cataracts is Alio´s MICS Irrigating Stinger (Katena Inc, Denville, NJ, USA).

This tool has a 19G diameter and it is equipped with a tip at the end which is angled downwards. This tool is useful to chop off segments or dividing masses of the nucleus in the phacoemulsification tip.

The Stinger is also equipped with a 1 mm diameter irrigation hole directly to the underneath. This structure enables a safe distance to be kept between the back bag and the tool as well as guaranteeing the stability of the anterior chamber and a fast removal of the remaining masses.

Aspiring masses of the lens with phacoemulsification tip we can gently rise the quadrant up. In the case of soft cataracts having the placed under pressure on 500-550 using mmHg we can only use Alio's MICS hydromanipulator irrigating fingernail. This makes it possible to divide and aspirate fragment masses of the lens without using ultrasound or using ultrasound in the minimum way. In this case, a system torsional phacoemulsification can be helpful. Thanks to the oscillatory, mechanically moving tip, the need to use ultrasound is eliminated. A convenient and safe way to remove the remaining fragments from the bag is by using the hydromanipulator. The next fragment is being removed by the hydromanipulator into the phacoemulsification tip. The Kelman Tip is preferred. The Infinity System (Alcon Laboratories, Inc.) is equipped with OZil energy. The procedure of grinding down using hydromanipulator, phacoemulsification tip and high under pressure is being repeated. In the case of hard cataracts, when total occlusion tip isn't causing aspiration of masses

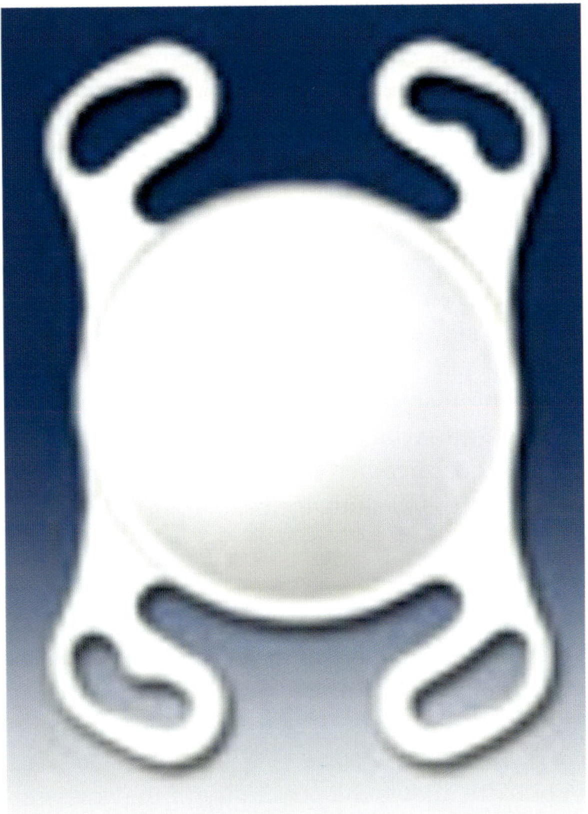

Fig. 21: Akreos AO Micro Incision (Bausch & Lomb, Rochester, New York, USA)

Stinger-Alio´s MICS Irrigating Chopper would be more useful. This headpiece has a narrow edge at the end which divides the masses and allows easy aspiration of the phacoemulsification tip. The fragmented elements of the hard cataracts are now easily aspirated using the high under pressure and in rare moments using of the ultrasound energy. Usually MICS is performed with up to 4% ultrasound power and fewer than 10 seconds of real phacoemulsification time.

For removing remains of cortical masses is serving Alio's MICS Aspiration Handpiece (Katena Inc, Denville, NJ, the USA).

There is a tool especially designed for delicate and safe manipulations within the anterior chamber. It has a diameter of 18G and the cylindrical shape allows this tool to gently manipulate within the surgical wound. At the same time the port diameter has a 0.3 mm which assures the stability of the hydrodynamic of liquid within the anterior chamber, light removing remnant masses from the bag and the full comfort of polishing the bag back.

Other Auxiliary Instrument

Useful scissors exist for complicated cataracts which may require applying the cutting within the anterior chamber of the eye. It can cut delicate membranes, adhesions, to make iridotomy, and also to cut the fibrosis of bags. In this cases you can use Alio's MICS scissors. This tool has 23 gauge curved shaft with horizontal micro blades.

The 0.6 mm breadth allows the possibility of the access into the anterior chamber without the need to widen the incision. Their shape is allows the comfort of free manipulating in the corner parts of the anterior chamber.

Basic Conditions for Fluidics in MICS

In order to use the additional tool the flow of liquids must be fulfilled with the following conditions:

1. Stabile incision with no leakage
2. Stable anterior chamber
3. High vacuum.

Together with the decreasing of the diameter of the infusion cannulas a serious problem occurred. The anterior chamber doesn't start to fill up with right amount of liquid. At the diameter infusion cannulas 21 G wasn't being able to hold stable chamber anterior at aspiration and the under pressure 500-600 mmHg. Every such an attempt would end with cave-in of the anterior chamber.

Getting the high inflow of liquids into the anterior chamber is possible thanks to a new generation for tools. Tools delivering liquid have the relatively big infusion diameter and the right profile allowing the right flow and the small internal

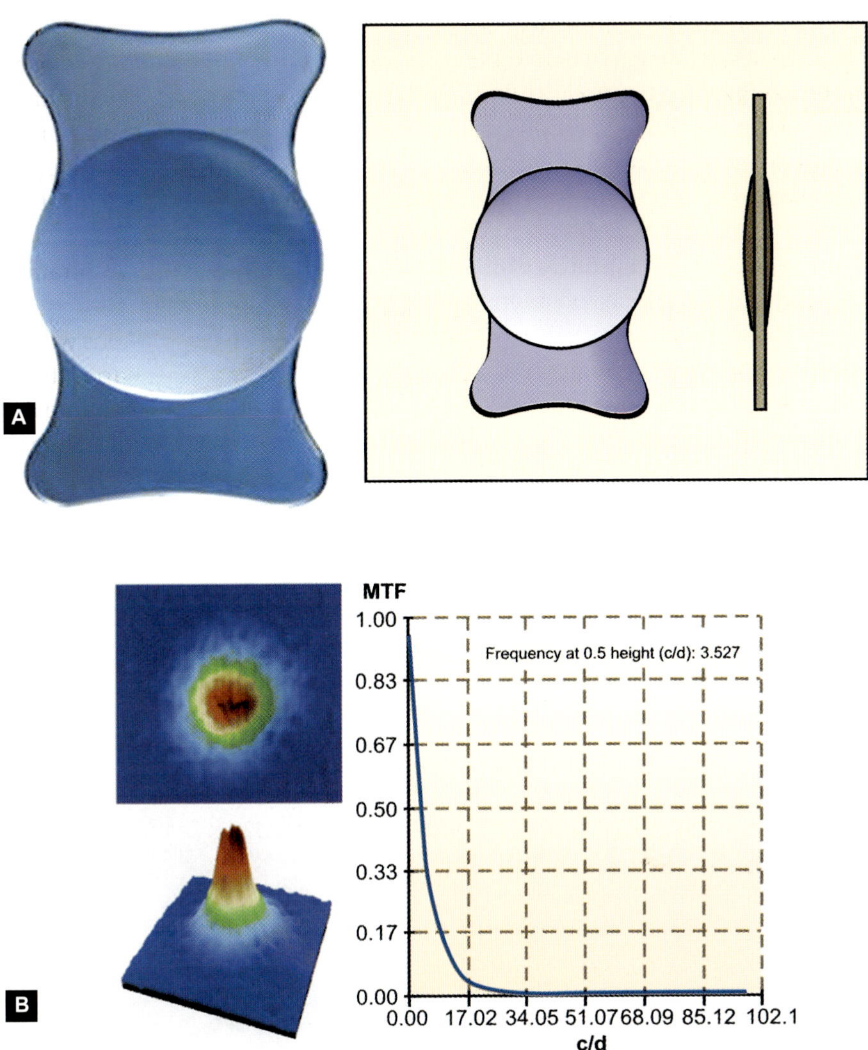

Figs 22A and B: Acri.Smart lens (A) Acri.Smart lens. (B) Optical Quality Analysis System (OQAS) image comparison with the PSF of treated and untreated Acri.Smart IOL

resistance. These conditions can prevent, making the anterior chamber shallow or rippling of back bag. An also right amount of liquid is securing for chilling phacoemulsification tip, and can cope with highly efficient aspiration pumps.

According to with laws of physics the inside diameter and tool lumen has and major influence on fluidic resistance, because resistance is proportional it the diameter. Therefore, one isn't allowed to apply standard infusion tools from the attention to the insufficiency hydrodynamic of these units. Tools assuring the flow higher up 50 cc/min are needed for MICS making. Present aspiration pumps have utility which considerably exceed flow function of standard tools. The activity of standard infusion cannulas is estimated only for 30 cc/min.

Therefore a need of creating new tools arose, they had to meet MICS needs. A Katena Inc company, Denville, NJ, the USA took on the workmanship. A tool set came into existence with very small diameter. It is answering to MICS requirements. Simultaneously the flow in instruments is high about 72 cc/min.

However, progress in the field of the efficiency of aspiration pumps rice a level of requirements for new irrigation handpiece.

Using the highly efficient pump we must allow the right inflow of liquid into the anterior chamber. In the case Accurus, Infinity type equipment we have the additional mechanism of pressurized inflow of fluidics -"gas forced infusion". It can allow controlling increase the pressure in the irrigation bottle. This mechanism pumps filtered gas into the irrigation bottle. It permits infusion to additional increase. Highly efficient irrigation cannulas and the forced help infusion give a comfort to job in stable anatomical conditions.

Anterior chamber stability we can achieve on to ways. First of them is high inflow of fluidics with proper instrument fluidics flow and forced infusion of fluidics. The second way is reduced outflow. Diminished diameter of tools and stabile chambers system, Cruse Control lead to proper outflow and they don't reduce the vacuum.

MICS can be made with different kinds of aspiration systems. However, a Venturi Pump system is most popular and recommended. It has great flexibility, fast reaction. It permit for using high value of under pressure and the flow as the additional important tool in breaking and removing masses of the lens. The flow can be adjusted, through amount of vacuum and degree of occlusion of the tip. At present venturi is the most efficient system.

MICS SETTINGS AND PHACOEMULSIFICATION PLATFORMS

Alcon Accurus 600

This device functions very well in MICS. Accurus device has the exerted inflow, high rate of the under pressure, advanced steering pump and fast efficiently in reacting. It cause that this system is very useful for the MICS surgery.
In the table we offer settings for cataract grade 3 (LOCS 3) (Table 1).

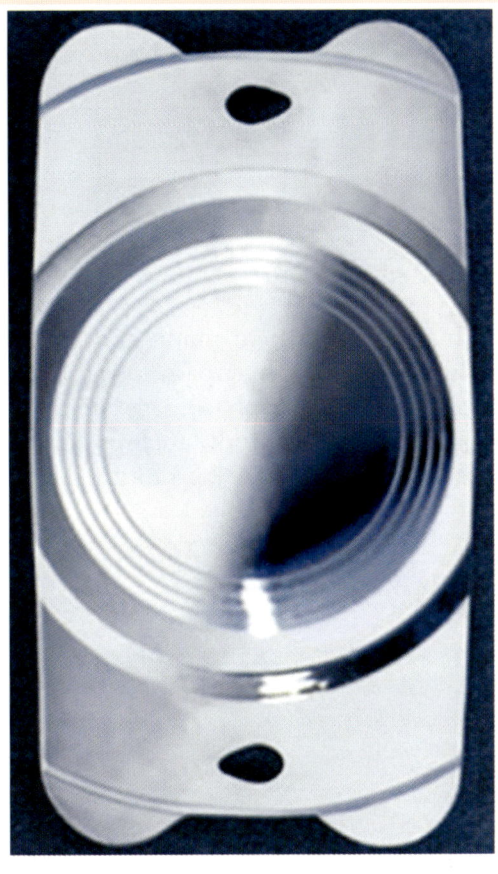

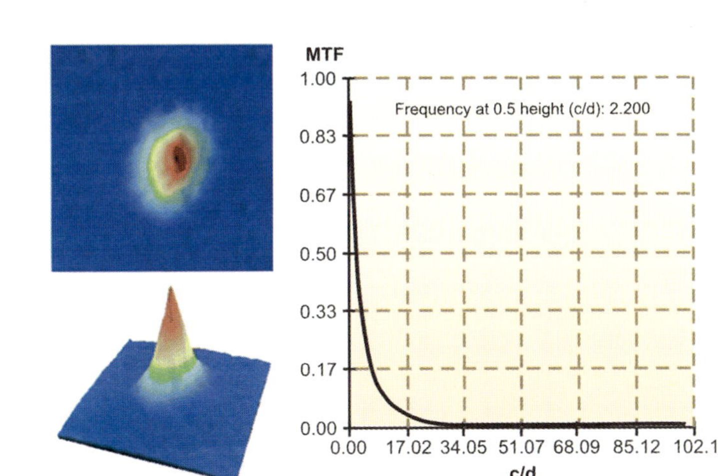

Figs 23A and B: The ThinOptX IOL (A) The ThinOptX IOL. (B) OQAS image comparison with the MTF of treated and untreated ThinOptX IOL

TABLE 1: Accurus 600 Alcon settings for 19G MICS		
Quad	*Phacoemulsification power*	*20%*
	Vacuum	300 mmHg
	Irrigation	90
	Mode burst	30 ms

Alcon Infinity

This is a device with a highly efficient pump and good software which is effective in practice. For two years the company introduced the new system for the lens emulsification it is—torsional phaco. This lateral movement system of the phacoemulsification tip lets practically total preliminaries the energy of ultrasound and risks connected with it. For infinity most useful settings are shown in Table 2.

TABLE 2: Infinity Alcon settings for 19G MICS		
Chop	*Phacoemulsification power* Dynamic rise Vacuum Irrigation Torsional amplitude Aspiration rate	*0* 0 150 110 Limit 40 On: 20 Off: 40 15
Quad	Phacoemulsification power Dynamic rise Vacuum Irrigation Torsional amplitude Aspiration rate	0 2 500 110 Limit 80 On: 20 Off: 40 30
Epi	Phacoemulsification power Vacuum Irrigation Torsional amplitude Aspiration rate	0 28 110 Limit 30 On: 20 Off: 40 28

Note: For 21 G MICS forced air infusion with air pump is necessary

Bausch and Lomb Millennium

Millennium is also adapted to leading the operation in the MICS mode. This highly efficient device has the software reducing the power of ultrasound used for a surgery. It has modes: pulse, singles burst, fixed burst, multiple burst. Millennium updated by the mode pulsed, pulse lets for creating the model of answering cycle 250 milliseconds "on-time". It is a cut at the considerable reduction of the energy. In Table 3 are shown standard settings for MICS.

TABLE 3: Millennium Bausch&Lomb settings for 19G MICS

Sculpture	Bottle height	100 cm
	Maximum bottle infusion	40 mmHg
	Fixed vacuum	200 mmHg
	Fixed U/S	10%
	Duration	20 ms
	Duty cycle	60%
Quadrant	Bottle height	100 cm
	Maximum bottle infusion	40 mmHg
	Fixed vacuum	470 mmHg
	Fixed U/S	10%
	Duration	20 ms
	Duty cycle	60%
I/A	Bottle height	80 cm
	Maximum bottle infusion	40 mmHg
	Maximum vacuum	550 mmHg

Note: For 21 G MICS forced air infusion with air pump is necessary

AMO Sovereign WhiteStar

The WhiteStar device is working well in mode of ultrapulse around 6 milliseconds on and 12 milliseconds off. For this device a height of the bottle is 90 cm, aspiration flow rate 26 ml/min, vacuum for nuclear emulsification 400 mmHg, and for epinucleus 200 mmHg.

AVOIDING CORNEAL BURN

Present biaxial applying microincision clear cornea phacoemulsification is gives the possibility to make the treatment practically with no temperature elevation. However, a development of high temperatures and incidence of corneal burns are possible in several cases . For example, it may appear in the case of the occlusion of the phacoemulsification tip with lens masses or the part of nuclei or in the coincidence of the highly OVD material is used.

It doesn't take place when the normal flow of liquids as long as the infusion liquid is circulated adequately. Irrigation-aspiration imbalance still remains a problem. When using a high value of the aspiration, the surgeon's attention is required to insure the stability of the anterior chamber. The amount of attention towards the flow seems to be one of basic conditions of the entire procedure.

Irrigation and Aspiration: Creating a Balanced Fluidics Environment

A cortical remains removing is a part of surgery where the flow is very important for correct cortical cleanup and cleaning the back bag and the ring of the anterior bag. Tools should to be adapted for the operating wound. On the present stage the internal incision 1.2 allows to correct situating 21G tools. The aspiration cannula has the smaller internal diameter than irrigation one. This will cause disproportion in the resistance of the flow between infusion and aspiration, additionally will guarantee the anterior chamber stability. Therefore, aspirating cannula Alio's MICS Aspiration Handpiece has the irrigation hole about the 0.3 mm diameter. However, increasing the depth of the anterior chamber cause lens diaphragms movement. It can effect of lens masses getting into the space behind the iris. Masses can be placed between the iris and the anterior bag in the sulcus surrounding space, this doesn't allow the masses to be seen. However, it does allow the masses to be seen in the anterior chamber some ours after the operation. Rinsing out and cleaning this space is extremely important.

After accurate cleansing the bag, OVD is placed in the anterior chamber. The eye is prepared for MICS lens injecting.

The stability of the anterior chamber in case of MICS is indisputably higher than in coaxial phacoemulsification. MICS doesn't cause frequent and considerable changes in proportion anatomical of the eyeball and traction do not effect during the operation. From capsulorhexis to on filling up OVD before lens injection it is possible to hold the anterior chamber stable.

STABLE CHAMBER SYSTEM

Cruise Control™ of the STAAR Surgical Company is additional system streamlining works of the irrigating-aspirating system. There is device specially designed for making cataracts in the bimanual microincisional phacoemulsification mode at the high vacuum settings. Cruise Control has disposable flow restrictor with and 0.3 mm internal diameter. It is being fixed between phacoemulsification handpiece and the aspiration tubing. It prevent surge during occlusion breaks at higher vacuum level. It has mesh filter which arrangement is safeguarding against blocking. On the filter lens masses are staying. Restrictor is limiting the flow. At the underpressure of 500 mmHg anterior chamber does not become shallow.

The similar device is being offered by the Bausch and Lomb Company. Stable Chamber differs in size restrictor, however the principle of act remains similar.

MICS's Intraocular Lenses

MICS cataract surgery develops post operative astigmatism in the minimal way. Up to 80% of MICS patients the corneal astygmatism is less than 0,5D. Only the 25% of coaxial cataract surgery patients have astigmatism less than 0.5D. MICS is the useful method to do a cataract surgery with refractive surgery. The developing of MICS caused develops of foldable lenses, which can be implanted through 1.5 mm incision or less. Since Sir Harold Ridley invented and implanted first IOL in 1949, lenses became in one if most advanced scientific tool in ophthalmology. The lenses should fulfill the high technology. Most of them are made of hydrophilic acrylic biomaterial. But only some of them can be used to MICS incision. Compression during injecting can damage the lens. The lens ruptures can occur. Decompression can also be a matter of damage of the lens. For MICS IOL, it should fulfill the following requirements. The IOL should be implantable through a sub-2.0 mm incision. After unfolding the IOL shouldn't have any structural, mechanical changes or optical alteration or deformation. Haptics of the lens should defend from decantation. The structure of the lens should protect from posterior capsule opacifications (PCO). Lenses shouldn't induce halos, glare, night-vision phenomenon, aberrations or scattering.

MICROINCISION IOL

Microincision IOL in practice we use:

Acri.Tec IOL's (Acri.Tec GmbH, Hennigsdorf, Germany)

ThinOptX UltraChoice (ThinOptX, Abingdon, Virginia, USA)

Akreos AO Micro Incision (Bausch & Lomb, Rochester, New York, USA)

Acri.Tec MICS's lenses: You can use 36A Acri.LISA for multifocals implantation. For toric implants, and for cases with more than 3.00 D of astigmatism, you can use the toric Acri.Tec IOL, marking the axis of the implantation at the slit-lamp prior to surgery. Acri.Smart 48S and Acri.Smart 46S are the lenses with the optical diameter 5.5 mm i 6 mm. It is biconvex, equiconvex, nonangled lenses with hydrophobic surface. They can be implanted on both sides. Acri.Smart 48S IOLs water content of 25% in its fully hydrated state Acri.Smart lenses are designed with square truncated edges. The edge thickness corresponds to standard designed IOLs and is in the range 0.25-0.27 mm. The lens is made from acrylic material, a copolymer of hydroxyethylmethacrylate and ethoxymethacrylate with an ultraviolet absorber. The optic power of this lens range from 0.00 D to 32.00 D. Acri.Smart Glide system with Acri.Glide cartridge is used to implant lens. Acri.Smart 48S are the lenses can be injected through 1.5 mm incision or smaller. They are very easy to apply. After injection the lens unfold very quick and with the control. It has no tendency to decentration or to tilt. The adhesion between posterior capsule and lens is perfect.

Clinical results: 45 eyes with cataract grade 2, 3, 4 (LOCS III) were operated by MICS. The incision size was 1.46 mm (1.4-1.9). After 6 months after operation 98.9% of the patients had BCDVA 20/25 (0.7 decimal value) or better and 71.3% of the patients had distance UCDVA 20/32 (0.6 decimal value) or better. The safety index for distance vision of the procedure was 2.5 and the efficacy index of the procedure was 1.8.

Ninety percent of the patients had a near BCNVA of 20/25 (0.8 decimal value). 60% of the patients had a near UCNVA of 20/32 (0.6 decimal value) or better. The mean add for near was + 1,5 D or less in 70% of cases and was + 2,0 D in 26% of cases. The safety index for near vision of the procedure was 1.4 and the efficacy index of the procedure was 0.9. It can indicate that Acri.Smart has a pseudoaccommodative ability. In this study none of the lenses shoved any change in position, decentration, tilt, PCO.

UltraChoice 1.0 ThinOptX is a hydrophilic acrylic IOL. The optic is 350 um thin. It has optical power range from 15.0D to 35.0D. The diameter of the lens is 11.2 mm. The diameter of the optic is 5.5 mm. Implantation technique base on injector or on rolling by surgeon in the gloved hands. ThinOptX UltraChoice is a refractive-diffractive lens design. The ultra thin ThinOptX lens was manufactured by lathe cutting one surface to retain continuous curvature, whereas the second surface was created to be within micrometers of the opposite surface with a series of 50 μm steps keeping the lens thin. Each step could, therefore, be focused on a single point, with the goal of eliminating spherical aberration. The posterior surface of the lens has a central portion which is surrounded by a series of concentric, planar, annular rings of increasing diameter. The ThinOptX is not a Fresnel lens because in its design the second surface of the lens was designed to assist the front surface in focusing light at a single focal point, which makes ThinOptX a refractive, not a diffractive, design IOL. Each stepped ring provides the same optical information to the same focal point on the retina and MTF and visual acuity are therefore excellent.

In the study ThinOptX lenses were implanted through mean 1.56 mm incision. The results were shown 12 months after surgery. UCDVA improved from 20/125 (0.16 ± 0.09) before surgery to 20/32 (0.72 ± 0.17) at the end of the study. BCDVA improved from 20/40 (0.5 ± 0.19) to 20/25 (1.0 ± 0.21) UCNVA showed that seven out of 10 patients reported ability to see J3 or better without near correction and the BCNVA was J2 (0.7 ± 0.14). The mean add diopters for near vision had decreased from +2.95 D before surgery to 1.75 D at 12 months after surgery with a mean reduction of near vision addition of 40.6%.

A change in the IOL position and significant decentration were observed in four out of 50 eyes. Tilt after implantation was observed in three of 50 eyes. PCO developed in two out of 50 eyes. The final incision size was 1.56±0.19 mm. Other studies confirm perfect contrast attributes, flexibility and ability to retain its original memory of this lens.

Akreos AO MI60 Micro Incision is a hydrophilic acrylic with 26% hydration rate. Optic measures 6 mm and has a 360° posterior ridge—barrier to prevent PCO. Haptics geometry consists of 4 point support system, haptics angled at about 10°. Akreos has an aspherical optic. Akreos MI-60 is an aspheric lens, reduce the aberrations and improves contrast sensitivity.

Akreos AO MI60 can be implanted with a 1.8 Viscoglide cartridge and Viscoject Lens Injection System (Medicel AG, Widnau, Switzerland). This type of lenses has no tendency to decentration or PCO.

Astigmatism Control with MICS

Among the major advantages of MICS is the reduction of surgical trauma resulting in reduction of surgically induced astigmatism (SIA), aberrations and improvement of the optical quality of the cornea after surgery. Thus leading to improvement of visual outcome and high patient satisfaction.

Degraded optical quality of thecornea after incisional cataract surgery would limit the performance of the pseudophakic eye. Thus, it is important not to increase or to induce astigmatism and/or corneal aberrations after cataract surgery. Even with MICS, we could achieve reduction of the astigmatism and higer order corneal aberrations.

The optical quality of the cornea plays an important role in recovery of visual function after cataract surgery, and this is determined by combination of corneal and internal aberrations generated by the IOL and those induced by the surgery. These corneal refractive changes are attributed to the location and size of the corneal incision. The smaller the incision, the lower the aberrations, the better the optical quality.

We have described the improved control on corneal surgically induced astigmatism with MICS when compared to conventional 3 mm phaco-emulsification. A great advantage of MICS is the reduction of SIA and that the microincisions do not produce an increase in astigmatism.

The shorter the incision, the less the corneal astigmatism, as it was estimated that the magnitude of the SIA studied by vector analysis is around 0.44 and 0.88 diopters, rising as the size of the incision increases. This is considered important because cataract surgery today is considered more and more a refractive procedure.

Also, Small-incision surgery (3.5-mm incision without suture) does not systematically degrade the optical quality of the anterior corneal surface. However, it introduces changes in some aberrations, especially in nonrotationally symmetric terms such as astigmatism, coma, and trefoil. Therefore, one has to expect better results and lesser changes with sub 2 mm incision (MICS).

This is supported by the finding that the corneal incision of < 2 mm had no impact on corneal curvature. Going hand in hand with the modern concept of making cataract surgery a refractive procedure, by controlling and even decreasing astigmatism and HOA by using MICS, which is the state of the art.

We can say that MICS sub 2 mm incision effectively decreases the induction or changes in corneal (HOA) during cataract surgery.

Corneal Aberration with MICS

Nowadays cataract surgery is not only a removal of a opaque lens, but also it is a part of refractive surgery. The technical progress generated high standard of ophthalmic machines, tools. We can obtain precisely IOL power calculation, we can reduce residual astigmatism and do surgery without surgically induced astigmatism (SIA). Corneal refractive surgery becomes more popular and more excellent. That's why the lens we are using should be perfect.

The quality of vision can also be measured in objective way. The Optical Quality Analysis System (QQAS, Visiometrics SL) is the tool which analyze the reflex of the eye reflexed from retina. The system calculates the modulation transfer factor (MTF) and point spread function (PSF). The study shows that UltraChoice 1.0 ThinOptX and Acri.Smart 48S MICS lenses have excellent MTF performance. In study there was no difference between this lenses and AcrySof MA60BM in the study. This indicates that there is no difference between MICS lenses and conventional cataract lens. Small incision, folding and unfolding didn't cause structural and functional defects.

End of the Surgery

The procedure is finished by injecting into anterior chamber 0.1-0.2 cc of cefuroxime. Next corneal wound hydratation should be done to close the wound and 2-3 drops of povidone-iodine is administrated to the conjunctival sac.

Future of MICS

Unfortunately new ideas in the field of the operation of cataract are limited by technical possibilities. Making the incision smaller is natural tendency of the development of the surgeon's technique. Today is possible removing the lens through sub-1.0 mm incisions by the MICS. However a problem remains in the possibility of lens compression. The foldable intraocular lens are of 1.5 mm, it is necessary to make a larger incision to implant the lens.

MICS makes the wound smaller and this results in the shorter healing time, the convalescence of the patient therefore is also reduced. Surgically Induced astigmatism practically isn't appearing or it is minimal. The quality of the post-operative vision is considerably higher in comparison to the classic method. Therefore, the satisfaction of postoperative MICS patients is higher. A new operating method MICS will be evolving in direction of more incision reduction of the energy reduction and the reduction of eye injury. Incisions of the cornea isn't fulfilling expected hopes in spite of so for many attempts. Incision still remains one of the greatest risks of the postoperative infection and large incision results in the astigmatism development. This element of the operation passed one of the biggest transformation. Wound size decrease, incision place change, the different shape were the main courses of evolution. The future belongs to the miniaturization of the tools and the wound size. New materials should be used to construct new incision knives which increase the opportunity to make the incision.

Viscoelastics will change their chemical and physical properties. They should preserve endothelial corneas cells, with the excellent stability of the anterior chamber. Setting them will be widened for the greater possibility of suppressing the energy in the anterior chamber. The application and removal of theses should not create the problem.

Fragmentation nuclei of the lenses are the most important element of this operation. Shortening the time breaking and removing the lens must come but at the same time it must be safe. A minimization of the energy and minimalization of manual activities must come into the anterior chamber. A reduction of zonular stress is important from capsulorhexis till the lens implantation.

The problem of energy still remains a problem for explain. Phacoemulsification which at present is most often used still free the high quantity of wave energy which is occurs as the thermal energy. Cells, endothelium corneas are most sensitive to damage. In the MICS cataract surgery we can use minimum amount of necessary ultrasound energy. Using the system torsional phacoemulsification we can additional decrease energy during emulsification the medium or hard cataract. The evolution of this part of the treatment is just coming. The next step could be the subsonic oscillation and lasers.

In the future the laser will supply the ultrasound and may become standard technology of breaking nuclei lenses. However at the present stage of technology it isn't possible to remove hard cataract with the help of new types laser. Laser doesn't give off the mechanical, thermal energy, it will be perhaps the golden mean for fragmenting masses of the lens in the future. YAG laser could be the solution. Also connecting the ultrasound energy and laser energy can bring the desired effect in the future. Laser energy will make possible to remove cataract with smaller than 0.7 mm incision.

Managing the flow of liquids also will change together with the development of infusion and aspirating pumps. A minimization of the wound is connected with minimization of tools. The problem with providing by irrigation tool the large amounts of liquids is still occurs. The development of highly efficient fluid injectors and new liquid substances with the different viscosity will be the perfect solution.

A minimization of lenses is still coming. The development of new materials perhaps will permit for creating new injected lenses through 0.7 incisions mm which will not be multifocal or accommodative but different much better. Polymers filling the bag of the lens up in the future can substitute for traditional IOL. In the future the MICS development will be a necessity. Polymers should be apply for filling the bag of the lens after removing cataract by the micro cut. But now foldable IOL should be improved to make the further minimalization of the incision.

MICS is a first between standard technique cataract surgery and with future. It is assuring minimizations of the operating wound, minimizations of the used energy, shortening the time of the operation, reduce in the possibility of complications allows the good quality of the vision and gives simultaneous satisfaction of the patient from the first days after operation.

13

Truly Endocapsular MICS (TECMICS)

Armando Capote, Marcelino Río,
Eneida de la C Pérez (Cuba)

Introduction

Cataract surgery has experienced a vertiginous advance in the last decades. Many ophthalmic Surgeons still active have been part of these changes by beginning their careers doing Intracapsular Extraction of the crystalline lens with incisions of 11mm or more; shifting to Extracapsular Cataract Extraction through large sutured incisions either on the cornea or on the limbus; later to surgery through self-sealing scleral tunnels like the Mini-nuc Technique or several alternatives of phacosection. Also have seen the initially slow, but constant and successful development of Phacoemulsification since the late sixties to become established in the last decades as the method of election for the surgery of the cataractous lens, in the countries with more development in the specialty. In 1998 the first cataract surgery through incisions of approximately 1mm was carried out. The technology to decrease the generation of heat with Phacoemulsification has been improved in order to perform cold Phaco and nowadays MICS, Phakonit, Bimanual Phaco or Microphaco among other denominations finds itself in a stage of expansion and generalization worldwide, mostly in highly developed centers.

Eye Surgeons have been involved in two quests in the field of cataract surgery, the first is to achieve the least invasive possible surgery, that facilitates a prompt recovery of the patient and a quick and high visual quality by reducing incision size. This search has been highly successful.

The second, is the search for an accommodative effect that permit the patients to reach good sight at all distances. This is a much more distant and difficult frontier because there are multiple complex barriers that have to be broken in order to achieve it.

There are several current surgical alternatives to treat Presbyopia. One of the more extended options is Monovision either with intraocular surgery in cataract patients or with Corneal Refractive Surgery with Excimer Laser, this has the inconvenient of anisometropia and decreased quality of binocular vision. Multifocal Intraocular Lenses, as well as the carving of multifocal corneas with laser are controversial and can cause adverse effects as the loss of contrast sensitivity, glare and vision of haloes. The patient is placed in a not physiologic situation of multiple images focussed in the retina, requiring sensorial adaptation to this phenomenon.

Conductive Keratoplasty and the techniques in the sclera either with the use of implants or relaxing incisions, result equally controversial.

An interesting option is the Accommodative IOLs, however their efficacy is questioned due to the fibrosis and capsular shrinkage that may affect their long-term effect.

According to our criterion the most anatomic and physiologic alternative would be to replace the opaque hardened lens material for a gel or lens of comparable characteristics to those of the natural crystalline lens with regard

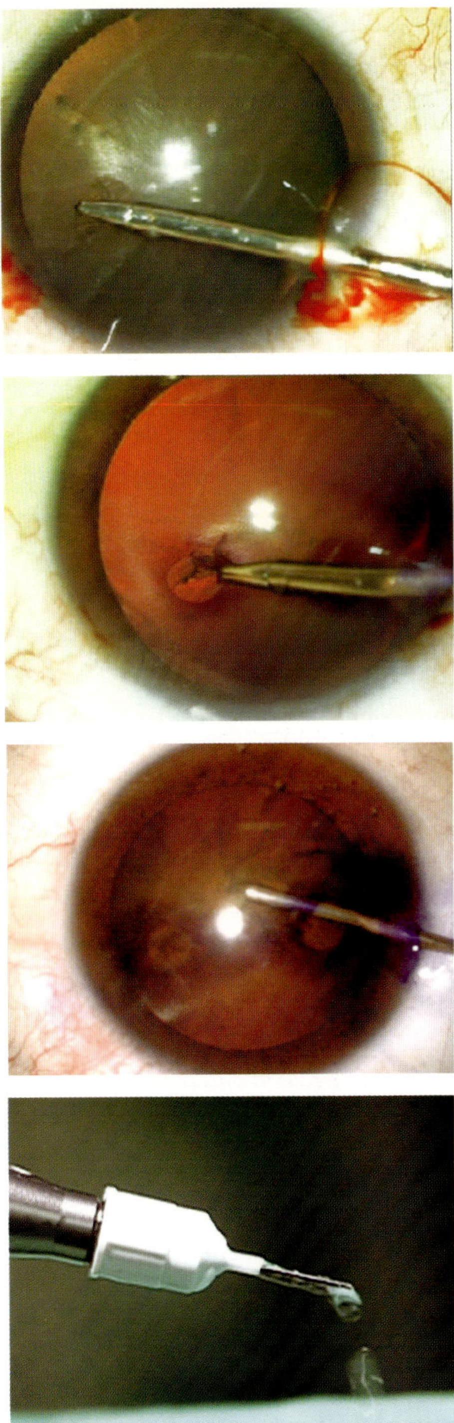

Figs 1 to 4: Various Surgical Steps of TECMICS

to its optical properties, elasticity and biocompatibility. This has been researched in the last decades; already in 1964 Kessler introduced the idea to fill the crystalline lens with a synthetic material after removing the cataract. Parel (1986) in the Bascom Palmer Eye Institute with the Phaco-Ersatz Study began experimental works by using a gel of polymer of silicone after cataract surgery by preserving the capsule and zonules in monkeys. Hettlich (1992) used an acrylic copolymer and a photosensitive catalyst system. Nishi has also been a pioneer in these researches in animals. At present there are several groups working in this search of accommodation, some with very promising results.

Various difficulties still have to be solved in order to make this dream come true.

There is still doubt regarding the true theory of accommodation, the most accepted is the Helmholtz Theory, but there are others proposed by authors as Schachar, Fukasaku, among others that are opposed and that have supported the development of some surgical techniques. It is clear today that the ciliary muscle and the suspensory apparatus are capable of reacting still in presbyopic patients.

Capsular opacification and retraction is a significant problem. Different physical, chemical and mechanical alternatives have been investigated, but still there is not a definitive solution.

Infrared refractors could be combined with the surgical microscope to control refraction during the surgery and decide the quantity of polymer to inject. Nishi and other authors have designed plugs to avoid leaks outside of the capsular sac, this still needs to be perfected.

The polymer with the necessary characteristics could be available in a relatively short-term.

Can the lens material be removed through microincisions and microcapsulotomies preserving as intact as possible the capsular sac?

The extraction of the crystalline lens through a minicapsulotomy has been reported in animal and cadaver eyes by multiple authors as part of studies to inject accommodative materials in the capsular sac. Dr Hara T. reported his technique of Endocapsular Phacoemulsification through one anterior capsular opening of 1.5 to 2.5 mm in 1989 and also developed Electric Vacuum microtrephine to facilitate the creation of very small tear free holes in the lens capsule.

This work describes a surgical technique that has the goal to perform a Truly Endocapsular Microincision Cataract Surgery (TECMICS), keeping as much as possible, the integrity of the capsular bag.

Corneal incisions of 1.4 mm, and two minicapsulorhexis of 1 to 1.5 mm of diameter are done in the peripheral area of the capsular sac lined up with the microincisions, which can be placed according to the preference of the surgeon, as they are astigmatically neutral. We perform them with a Diamond Knife for MICS and are located in hours 2 and 10.

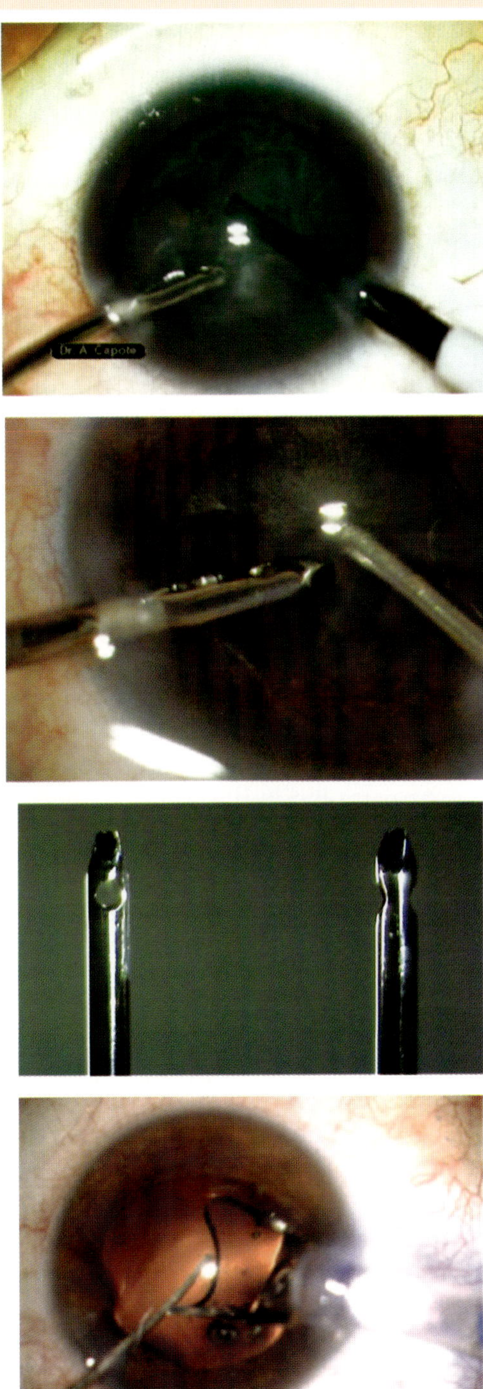

Figs 5 to 8: Various Surgical Steps of TECMICS

The minirhexis are started making a tiny capsular tear with a needle cystotome and with a 23G Capsulorhexis Forceps for MICS manufactured by Janach complete them in a very gentle and careful way. These forceps allow an excellent control of the maneuvers required through the small clear corneal incisions. The Anterior Chamber remains filled with a sufficient, but not excessive quantity of viscoelastic, to avoid positive pressure on the capsular sac that could cause its collapse and rupture during Phacoemulsification.

There must exist a perfect view of the capsule to avoid enlargement or peripheral tears, if there is not good visibility, a capsular stain should be used.

Hydrodissection must be carried out in a very careful way, because the BSS is injected in a closed capsular sac and it can explode. We recommend the use of a small syringe of 1cc or 2cc and to push the piston slowly, watching the wave of fluid and interrupting the injection when this is completed.

Phacoemulsification has been performed with the machine Pulsar 2 of Optikon, using the Phaco Tip for MICS with an external diameter of 0.9 mm. As Phacoemulsification is done inside the capsular bag and the technique is of recent introduction, conservative parameters have been used by programming relatively low values of ultrasound, vacuum and flow. The irrigation cannula or chopper used have two holes of 0.5 mm.

During Endocapsular Phacoemulsification the Anterior Chamber remains full of viscoelastic and the wound is less irrigated by BSS, so we have used a cut silicone sleeve to provide external irrigation and cooling as an extraprotection against corneal burns. An extra-BSS bottle is used for the irrigation cannula or chopper.

The Phaco tip is introduced creating a central tunnel and not a groove and then the irrigation cannula is entered, or in harder nucleus an irrigating chopper, and begin to sculpt the nucleus by varying the strategy according to its hardness, in the harder ones after creating the tunnel the chopper is used to cut the nucleus pushing forward and laterally against the Phaco tip. This instrument was particularly designed to chop inside the sac and is manufactured by Janach, has edges to cut forward and laterally, two models are available, one with lateral holes and a second with holes superior and inferior to the frontal edge in order to separate the posterior and anterior capsules by means of the fluid pressure. Soft lenses are emulsified without any strategy of fracture.

It is important to be sure that both, the Irrigating cannula and the Phaco tip remain inside the sac during the procedure, if the first one goes outside, the bag may collapse and rupture, if the phaco tip is not well inserted through the minirhexis it may cause capsular tears.

We have performed surgeries in cataracts of hardness from + to ++++, even in hypermature lenses. The used ultrasonic powers have varied depending on the hardness of the nucleus from 10 to 40%, in Continuous Burst Mode to create the tunnel and in Pulse Mode to emulsify the fragments. The vacuum has been

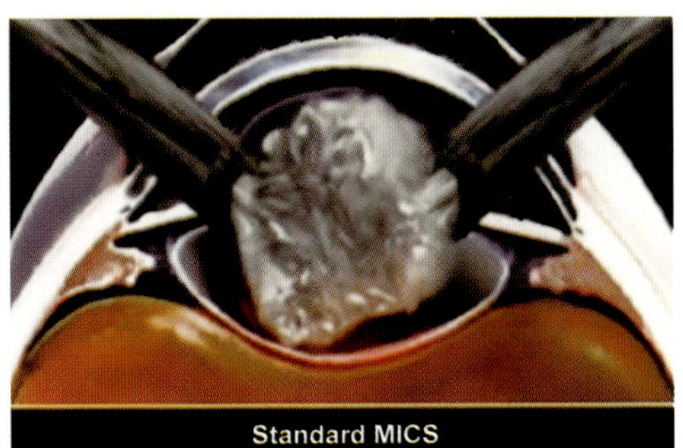

Fig. 9

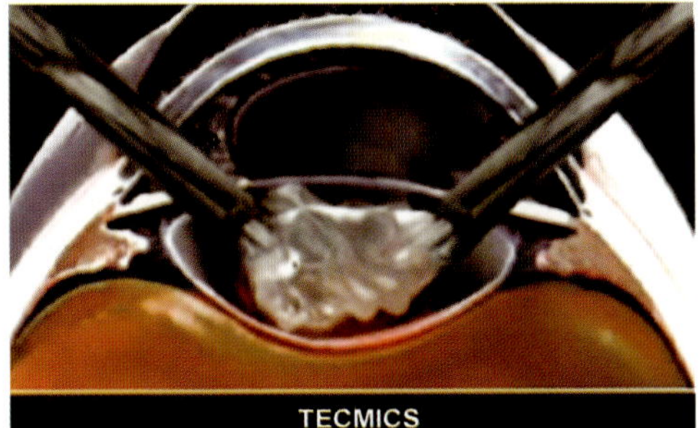

Fig. 10

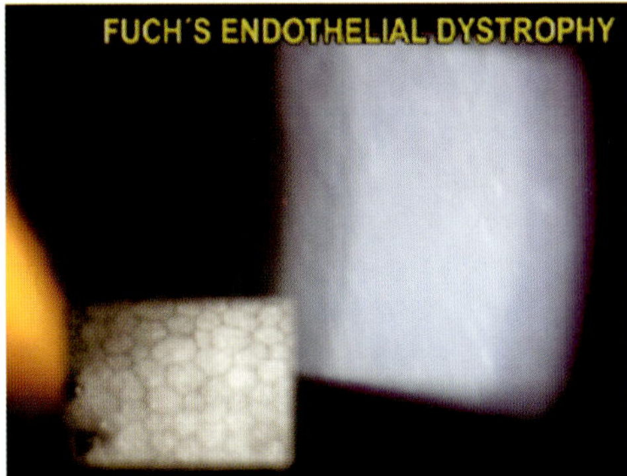

Fig. 11

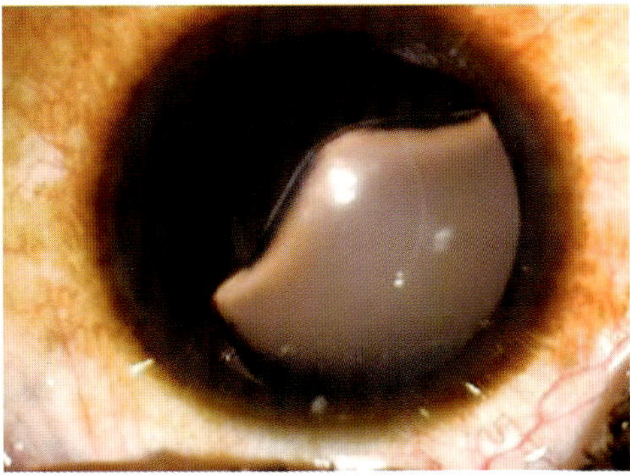

Fig. 12

raised as maximum to 180 mm Hg with a fixed flow of 30 cc/min, always working with the peristaltic pump.

Up to now we haven't had the case of Posterior capsule rupture; our strategy in this case would be to unite the 2 minirhexis with microscissors and forceps completing removal of lens and vitrectomy if necessary. In this case the anterior capsule should provide an excellent support for Lens implantation in the sulcus.

Aspiration of cortical remnants is done bimanually, and a careful polishing of the subcapsular epithelium is made. This is a step that is necessary to perfect, by means of the use of larger zoom in the surgical microscope and the dedication of more time and care, because the future success of accommodative IOLs and injectable materials will depend in great part on the possibility to maintain the transparency and elasticity of the capsular sac.

The small rhexis may facilitate in the future the placing of epithelium growth inhibitors in the sac with the Anterior Chamber filled of viscoelastic to protect the other structures of the Anterior Segment.

The minicapsulorhexis are enlarged to one of 5 to 6 mm with forceps, after doing two relaxing incisions with microscissors or with needle cystotome.

The incision is enlarged to 1.8 mm and a MICS IOL is implanted. We have experience with the Acrismart 46S-5 with very satisfactory results regarding stability.

TECMICS requires refinement and has more technical complexity than the traditional techniques of coaxial phaco and MICS due to the need of performing two microcapsulotomies and mostly because the crystalline lens is emulsified inside the capsular sac, working near the anterior and posterior capsules. Being so, we can ask ourselves why doing this technique?

In first place because this could be a surgical alternative for the future if the adequate IOLs or injectable polymer is developed. But this technique also has characteristics that make very interesting its use in the present.

In coaxial phaco and in Standard MICS turbulence is produced in the whole Anterior Chamber damaging the cells of the Corneal endothelium and inducing inflammation of the iris and other intraocular tissues. In TECMICS the dynamic of fluidics is generated inside the capsular bag, protecting therefore the Corneal Endothelium and other structures of the Anterior Segment.

A study with Specular Microscopy to determine the effect of the technique on the corneal endothelium shows that it could be of usefulness for patients with damaged endothelium, as in Fuch´s dystrophy.

In 57 eyes operated with TECMICS a low endothelial cell loss of 2. 8% endothelial cells per square mm has been observed. Very clear corneas and reactive pupils are regularly seen the day after the surgery.

Other current indication may be subluxated lenses. During Phaco or extracapsular extraction of the crystalline lens, zonular dialysis may be enlarged

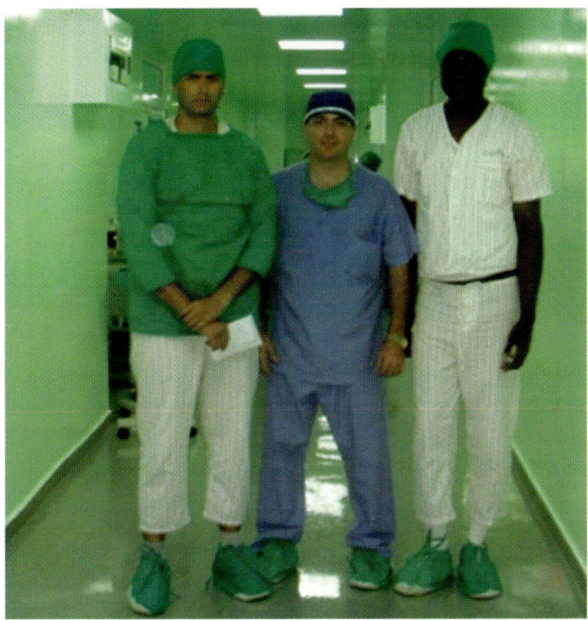

Fig. 13: Two Marfan's syndrome patients operated by TECMICS and artificial zonules

due to capsular bag collapses. In TECMICS the bag remains expanded by the endocapsular irrigation. Moreover a curved irrigation cannula can be used to hold the sac by the minirhexis or also Grieshaver iris retraction hooks.

TECMICS in Subluxated Lenses: "Ring in the Loop Technique"

Ectopia Lentis or Lens subluxation means a challenge to the Eye Surgeons due to the instability and abnormal position of the lens caused by weakness or absence of zonular fibers. Its etiology can be congenital or acquired and its severity can vary from very mild, manifested only by phacodonesis, to severe dislocation.

In patients with Ectopia Lentis without history of trauma, a careful ophthalmological and systemic examination must be performed due to its frequent association with ocular and systemic diseases.

Surgery may not be necessary unless the patient has decreased quality of vision secondary to cataract or lens malposition causing Diplopia or optical aberrations. It is indicated in presence of secondary ocular hypertension and must be considered a surgical urgency if the lens is luxated to the Anterior Chamber.

Dozens of surgical alternatives have been proposed to treat subluxated lenses. A number of variables should be considered to plan the right strategy, like the cause of the ectopia, its severity, its stability (It may be progressive in some cases like Pseudoexfoliation), the extension and direction of the dislocation, the existence of other ocular conditions like the presence of vitreous in the Anterior Chamber, iris dialysis, etc. systemic diseases (Ex. General Anesthesia complications may occur in patients with Homocystinuria); and the nucleus hardness among others.

Factors related to the surgeon like experience and skills, as well as availability of required resources at the moment of the surgery are also important.

With so many variables involved every patient should be seen individually. This is not routine surgery, every aspect should be carefully planned. Surgical steps like the location of the main and side port incisions, size of the rhexis, etc. , that we perform mechanically in standard lens surgery, here should be customized to each particular patient.

Depending on the magnitude and cause of the subluxation it may be enough in mild cases just to perform a careful surgery to avoid extradamage and implant the lens in the bag where sometimes it is convenient to place the lens haptic in the dialysis area to expand the bag. If the zonular rupture is bigger, it may be necessary to insert a Capsular Tension Ring either before or after doing the phaco. This maneuver can be done with injector or with forceps, I personally prefer the latest as they allow more control, and cause less zonular stress.

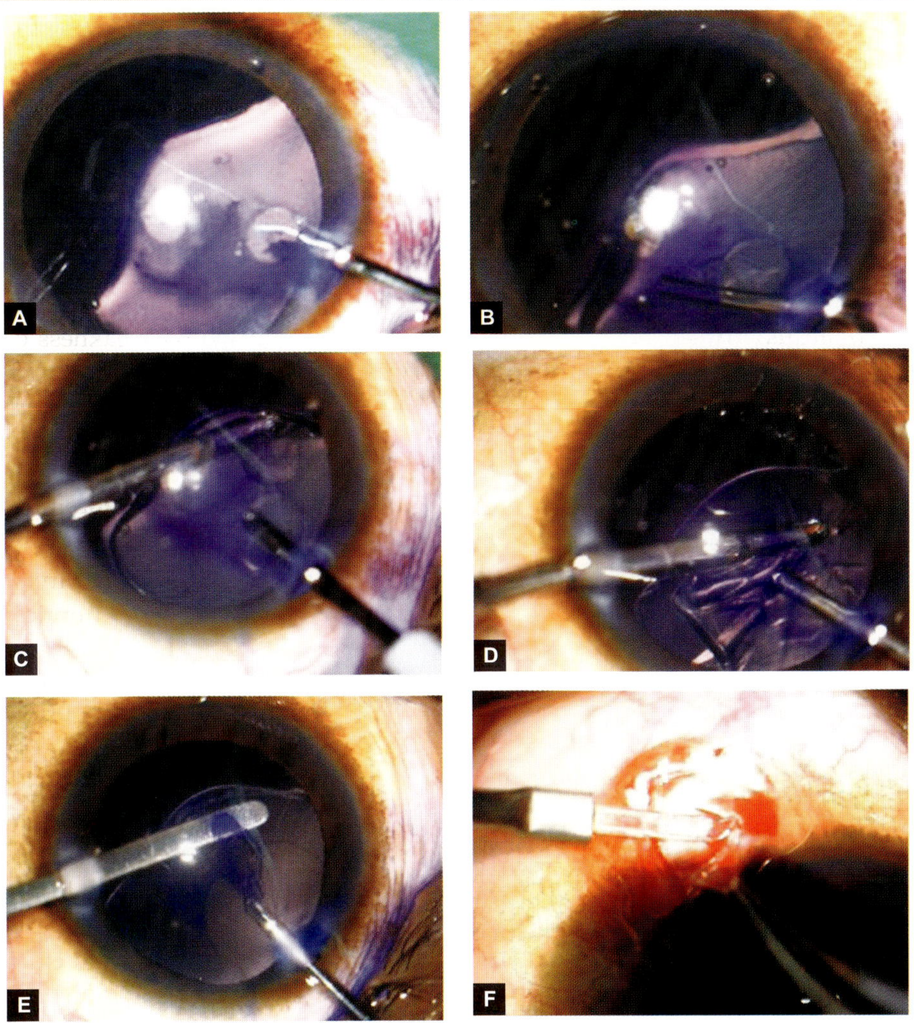

Figs 14A to F: Surgical Steps of TECMICS Technique

These cases are usually very complicated to manage and the solution alternatives offered to the patients are to perform an ICCE or Lensectomy and implanting an AC IOL or a PC IOL sutured to the Sclera or Iris with the possible complications related with each option like glaucoma and corneal decompensation in AC IOLs and tilting or descentration with sutured lenses. The situation is even more complex in larger subluxations with more than 180° dialysis, because the Capsular Tension Rings may not be enough to provide appropriate centration and stability to the bag.

Phacoemulsification can be attempted and a capsular tension ring designed to be sutured to the sclera can be implanted. These are not always available and need particular care in the position where the fixating arm is located. There are several designs like the Cionni Ring, or the Endo-Exo-Capsular Ring of Villar-Kuri, etc. most of them have an arm to be sutured to the ciliary sulcus and sclera.

TECMICS has been very useful in subluxated lenses, first of all as the phacoemulfication is performed in a closed bag, this will remain expanded without the collapses that are frequently produced when performing a standard Phaco or Extracapsular, that contribute to brake more zonules and enlarge the dialysis area. While doing TECMICS most of the BSS doesn´t escape from the bag which is advantageous in such patients.

Before I started doing TECMICS I sutured some standard rings to the sclera by passing one needle below and one above the ring already inside the bag, through the capsular equator, but this may cause capsular tears either when passing the needle or when pulling the ring to the desired place with the polypropylene suture. If the ring is sutured before implantation and brought out of the capsule anteriorly through the rhexis, the 10-0 polypropylene may tear the capsulotomy edge.

The surgical technique described below was developed by us for patients with subluxated lenses with more than 180 degrees dialysis in which TECMICS is combined with artificial zonules in order to achieve an adequate fixation and stability of the IOL-bag complex.

One clear corneal incision of 1.4 mm is placed 180° away from the center of the subluxated area, the second one is located to provide comfortable access to the capsular sac in the loosen area.

The two mini-capsulorhexis of 1 to 1.5 mm diameter are lined up with the incisions, the one in the middle of the subluxated area should be as peripheral as possible, this will not harm zonules as they are not present in these cases. Zonular stress has to be avoided during the entire procedure.

Hydrodissection is important, to release all the contents within the bag to facilitate the Phacoemulsification and cortex aspiration.

Bimanual Endocapsular Phaco must be done very smoothly, the blunt irrigation cannula can be used to hold the sac and even to pull it according to the surgeon's needs. The instruments can change hands facilitating the access to all areas, even the part of the bag hidden under the iris. Bimanual Irrigation-Aspiration is done as in Phaco with a fully distended bag.

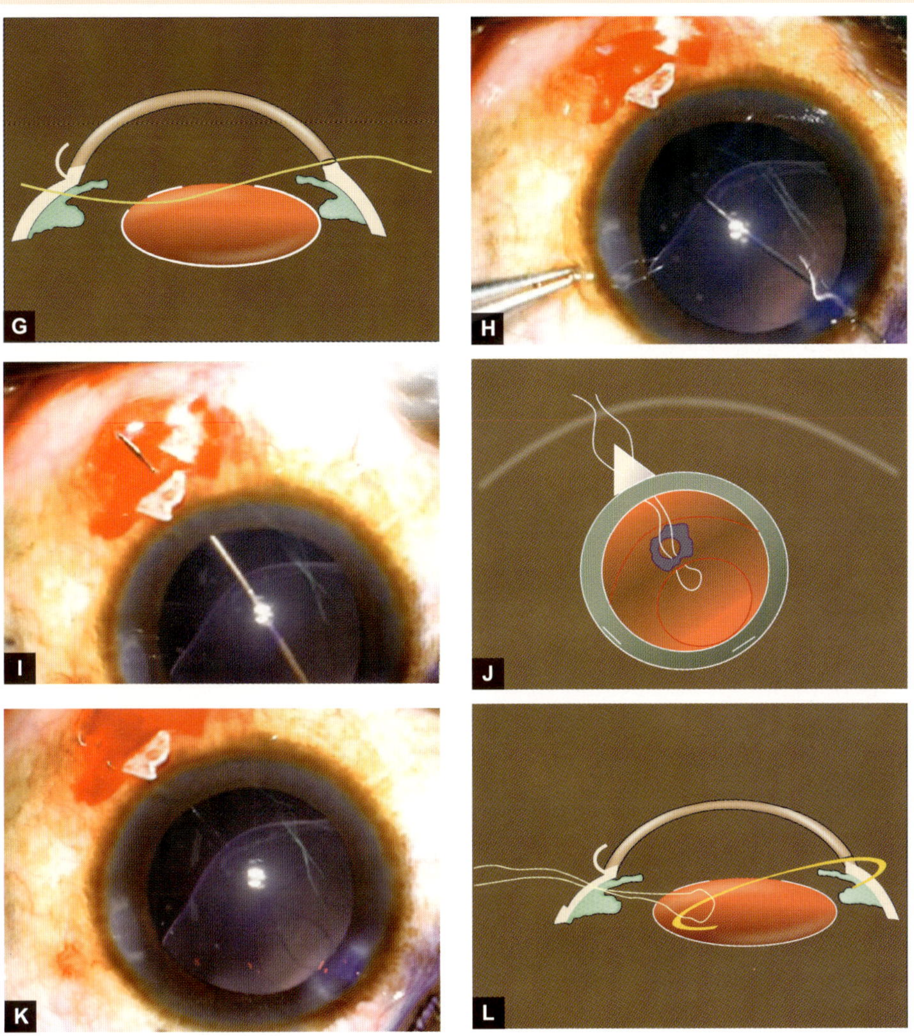

Figs 14G to L: Surgical Steps of Tecmics Technique

After filling the bag and Anterior Chamber with viscoelastic, the rhexis is enlarged to 5 or 5.5 mm, it should not be large, to permit the Capsular Tension Ring to remain inside the sac.

A blunt instrument like an iris spatula can be used to pull the capsular bag to the pupillary area to permit the completion of the capsulotomy and then a partial thickness scleral flap is aligned with the incision and peripheral minirhexis.

A Polypropylene 10-0 suture with 2 long needles (16 mm) is passed through the incision opposite to the flap, enters inside the bag through the large rhexis and goes out all the way through the minirhexis.

It perforates the sclera on the ciliary sulcus and exits the globe at approximately 1.5 mm from the limbus under the scleral flap.

The same maneuver is repeated with the second needle and once they are both out of the eye, they are pulled away until a loop of Prolene suture forms inside the capsular bag. The loop is conveniently positioned in a vertical situation in the middle of the sac to ease the insertion of the Capsular Tension Ring (CTR) all the way through it, inside the bag.

The ring expands the sac very widely while it is gently inserted with forceps and Sinskey Hook, but as consequence of the great extension of the subluxation it is not enough and a mild upwards displacement of the sac remains as predicted.

The two ends of the prolene suture are pulled using tying forceps and the ring and capsular bag are moved to the desired central position and then the suture is tied leaving the knot under the flap.

A Foldable three pieces IOL is implanted inside the bag achieving an excellent centretion and after suturing the scleral flap and conjunctiva and aspirating the viscoelastic material, the surgery is completed.

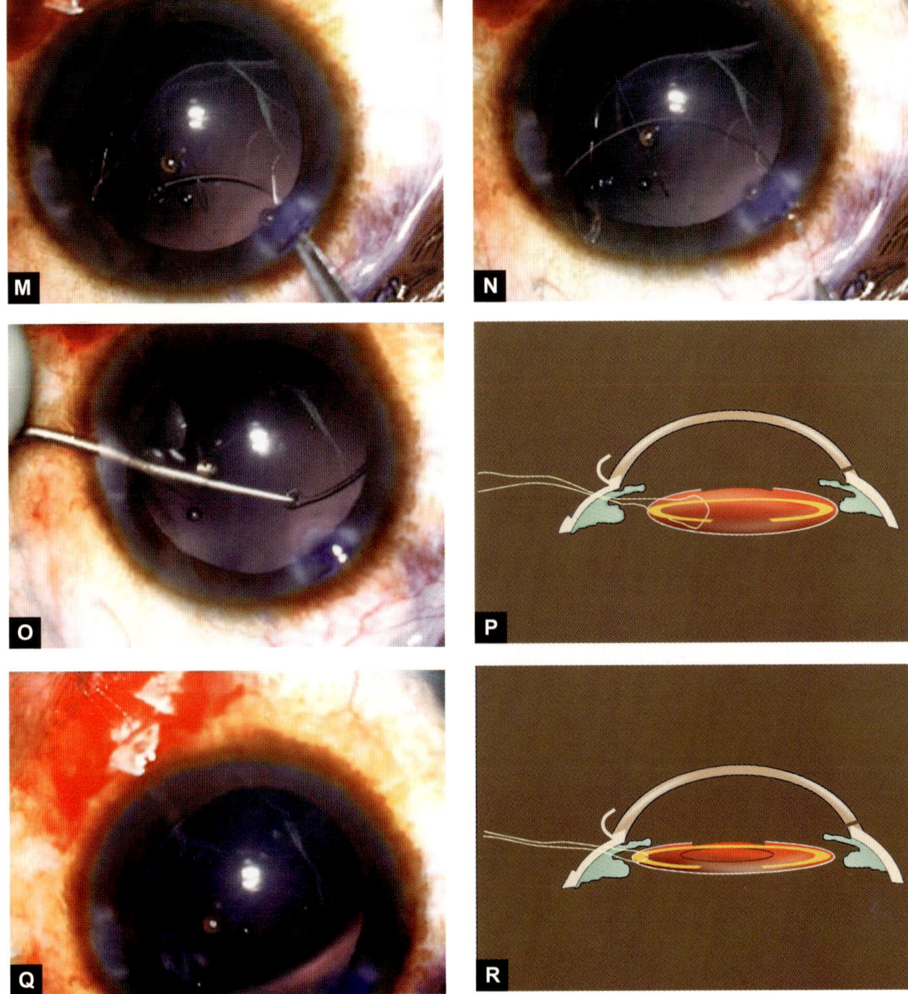

Figs 14M to R: Surgical Steps of Tecmics Technique

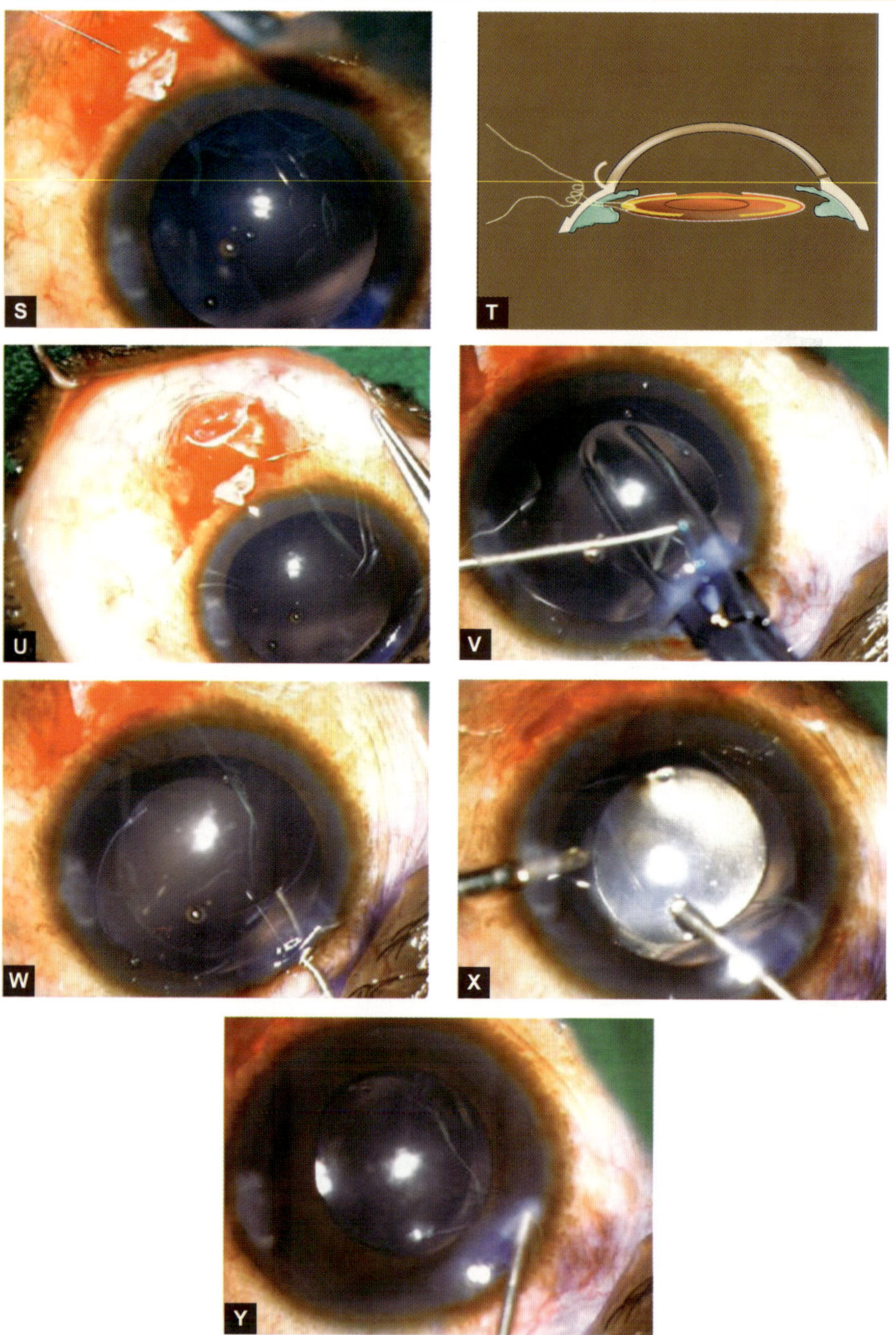

Figs14S to Y: Surgical Steps of Tecmics Technique

14

Advances in Cataract Removal Technology

Cyres K Mehta, Keiki Mehta (India)

Introduction

Ever since the advent of phacoemulsification, cataract surgery has shifted to automated modalities

Newer modalities for cataract removal have arrived on the scene like Vortex Phacoemulsification,Yag Lasers, subsonic oscillation in the form of Neo-SoniX and the Staar Sonic Wave, Pulses of warmed water(AquaLase) and Oscillatory phaco (Ozil), just to enumerate a few.

In addition conventional phaco machines have evolved further to include micro or "hyper" pulse power delivery, vacuum settings can go as high as 700 mmHg and flow rates have touched 100 cc/min, all with relatively stable chambers.

The ability to micropulse has led to new terminologies like "Cold Phaco" and is responsible for the proliferation of unsleeved "Microphaco" techniques.

In this chapter, lets examine these new developments for their effectiveness and application.

Catarex: Endocapsular Vortex Phacoemulsification

This was first demo'ed to ophthalmologists by Richard Kratz MD at the 1998 ASCRS meeting and evoked great interest. It has certain great advantages over normal existing phacoemulsifiers.

After a small 1 mm capsular opening, nucleus and cortex are emulsified by the probe tip in a one handed, single step procedure that obviates the need for chopping cracking and other maneuvers.

The center piece of this technology is the single use hand piece which is a 1. 37 mm diamond tipped impeller probe. This tip is contained in a translucent protective sleeve and can be withdrawn or advanced. Similar to dental drills a turbine spins the impeller between 20,000 and 100,000 rpm. Inflow, aspiration and air lines attach to the main unit on the Millennium (Bausch & Lomb) console.

The tip has 3 struts. Each strut has a vertical and a horizontal component. The horizontal component looks like a propeller and generates the vortex flow that brings the nucleus and cortex to the impeller where the vertical component essentially emulsifies it.

Technique

A clear corneal tunnel is created after which a decentered 1 mm capsulotomy is fashioned in the anterior capsule with SW dithermy. After hydrodissection with a specially designed cannula the tip is inserted 1 mm into the bag and the device started. Inflow pressurizes the bag and the propellers generate a fluid vortex which draws the lens contents to the tip which emulsifies them. This process took 1 to 3 minutes in eye bank eyes with grade 1 to 3 cataracts.

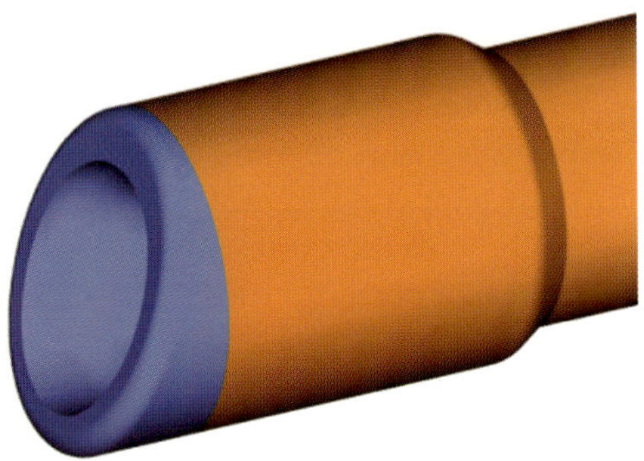

Fig. 1: Smooth bevelled silicone tip of the aqualase handpiece

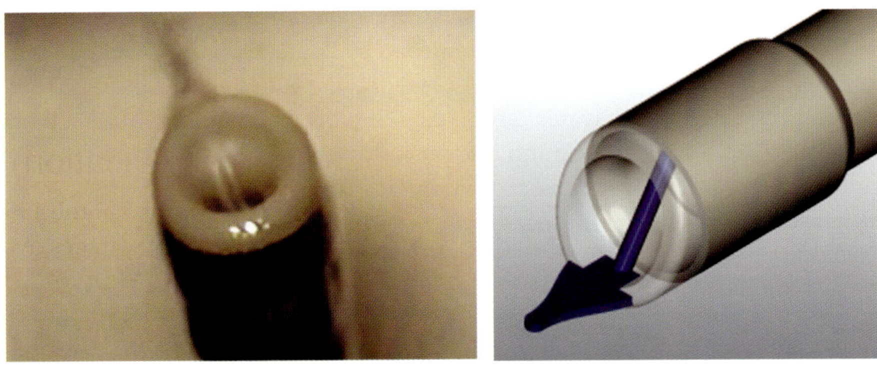

Fig. 2: Fluid exiting the aqualase tip as a spray

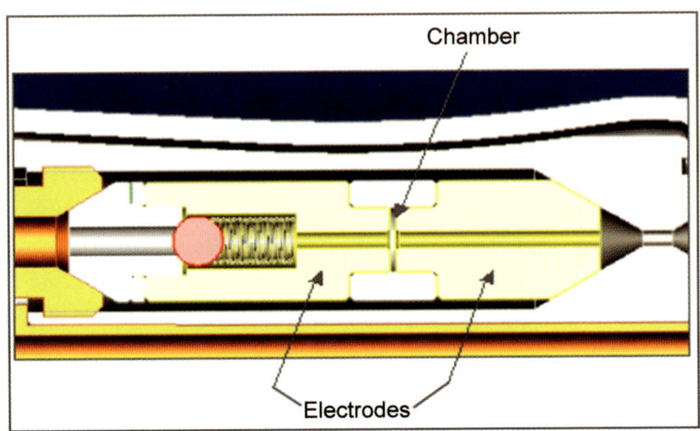

Fig. 3: Chamber where pulses of fluid are generated

The great advantage is that no nuclear manipulation is required and the process is quick and reproducible. Further studies are being carried out and this new technology may soon appear in our operating rooms. The ability to remove a cataract through a 1 mm opening is highly appealing as this will allow the injection of a room temperature vulcanizing polymer which will restore accommodation. Naturally with the vortex most lens epithelial cells will be stripped away so the chance of posterior capsular opacification developing is remote.

Laser Technology in Cataract Removal

The idea of a single handpiece which would vaporize the lens material leading to rapid cataract removal through a microincision is not a new discovery.

The Erbium YAG laser was first researched by Peyman and Tsubota 2 decades ago. This laser produces a wavelength of 2. 94 micrometer. This is an infrared laser highly absorbed by water. This is how it works. In the first micron ahead of the laser tip a cavitation bubble forms allowing the beam to traverse that bubble. In front of the first bubble another bubble forms and so forth. In the nuclear matter of the lens a succession of bubbles form due to the cavitation effect causing a shock wave to generate. This disrupts lens material forming an emulsate that can be aspirated from the eye. This laser came to market in 1997 brought by Asclepion-Meditec (Jena,Germany),and was called the MCL-29. The handpiece of this unit had irrigation and aspiration and the fiber that delivered laser energy was made of zirconium fluoride.

Acceptance of this laser led to the development into the Phacolase system which is coupled to Geuder's Megatron unit which has a dual peristaltic-venturi pump.

The next entrant was the Paradigm medicals Photon laser PhacoLysis system. This uses an Nd:Yag 1064 nM laser to provide a photo-acoustic ablation of cataract material under aspiration. The tip design is such that aspirated nuclear fragments are trapped in the tip and the laser fiber is aimed at this so called "photon" trap. This laser is coupled to the Mentor SIStem peristaltic I&A unit.

The next unit on the scene was the Dodick Photolysis Q-Switched Nd:Yag Laser system(ARC Corporation) introduced in 2000.

This unit has the following features.

Q switched Nd:Yag laser shots are focused on a titanium plate. This results in shock waves generating that can emulsify the nucleus. Laser and aspiration are on the same probe which is inserted through a 1. 4 mm clear corneal tunnel. In the other hand, an irrigation cannula enters the eye through 0. 9 mm. The laser shots impact on a titanium target resulting in shock waves at 200 to 400 nanoseconds intervals.

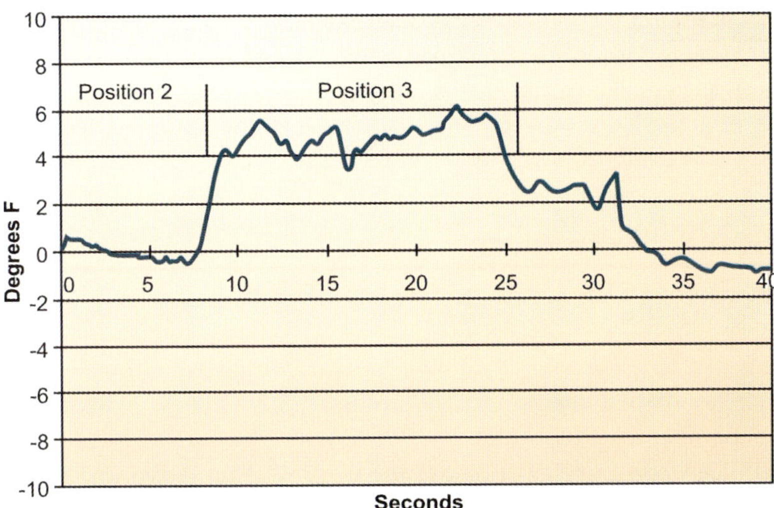

Fig. 4: Intraocular Response – Temperature-Note that in the eye the temperature never rises more than 3°C

Conditions:

Fast responding thermocouple
Aspiration flow rate: 12 cc/min
AquaLase™ power: 100 %

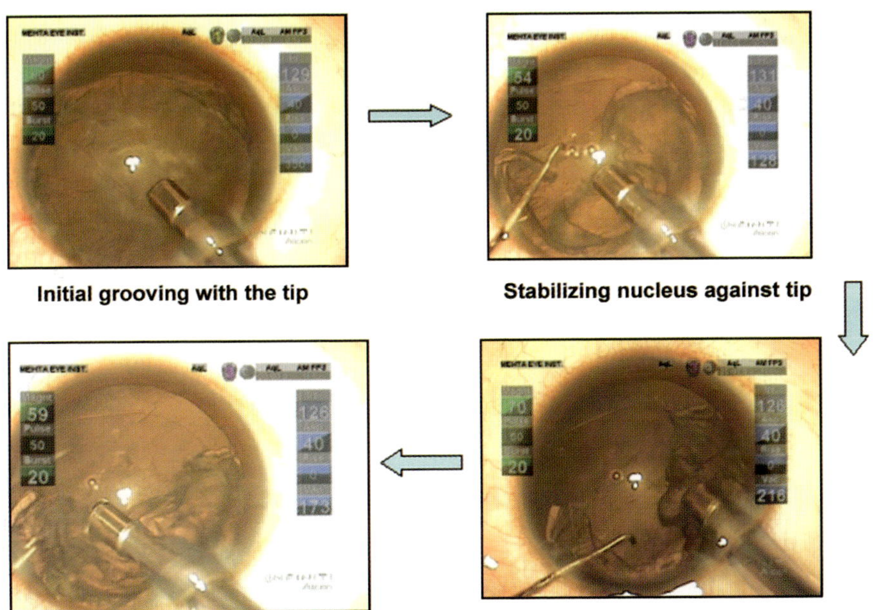

Fig. 5: Aqualasing the nucleus

The machine uses a venturi pump and has a regular phaco-ultrasound handpiece for cataracts which are too dense for the laser. The laser method works to about grade 2 cataracts beyond which the regular handpiece is much quicker. The obvious advantage here is that we can easily perform bimanual cataract surgery as there is no heat generation by the unsleeved laser-aspiration probe.

NeoSoniX Technology

Since the dawn of Phacoemulsification its known that ultrasound has certain undesirable effects on ocular tissue. Endothelial cell loss continues to occur for sometime after the surgery as demonstrated in long term studies. Our effort today is to reduce to the minimum the amount of ultrasound energy used in the anterior chamber to a minimum.

In 2001, Alcon Surgical (Texas) incorporated its Advantec NeoSoniX technology into the Legacy 20000 series phacoemulsifier.

NeoSoniX is a hardware upgrade consisting of a handpiece which incorporates a motor . This produces a 100Hz oscillation of the tip from side to side of upto 2 degrees from neutral. This oscillation is programmable for power level in foot position 3, starting time, and percentage of 2 degrees of oscillation. This has the effect of continuously repositioning the nuclear matter at the tip thereby allowing the surgeon to use less ultrasound power for a comparable grade of cataract. When the motor in the handpiece is on a distinct vibration is felt as the tip rotates from side to side. Its possible to remove grade 1-2 cataracts using zero ultrasound power and NeoSoniX alone to embed the tip for chopping techniques. This side to side oscillation effectively repositions nuclear material at the tip. Its greatest use in my opinion is in grade 4 and 5 hard brown or black cataracts where it reduces by nearly 30-40% the amount of phaco power needed to emulsify the nucleus. In Dr. Fine's studies comparing the Legacy with and without NeoSonix, effective phaco time with NeoSonix dropped from 11.5 to 1.5 seconds, and average power dropped from 15 to 6.5%. The percentage of clear corneas rose from 90 to 98%, and the percentage of patients with postoperative uncorrected vision of 20/40 or better (at two to 24 hours postop) rose from 70 to 96%.

Aqualase

Aqualase is a new technology from Alcon. It has been incorporated into its Infiniti platform as a separate handpiece.

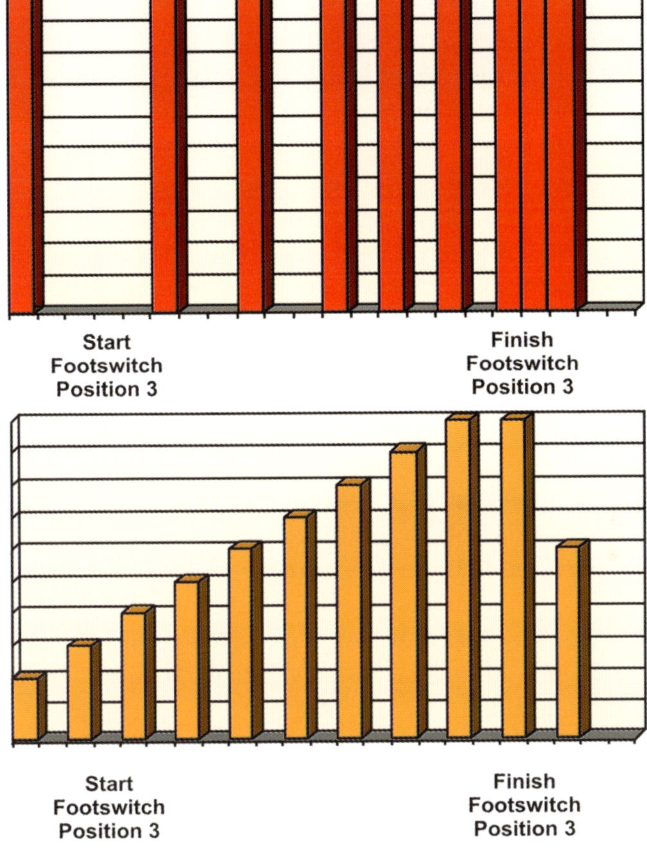

Fig. 6: Fixed burst mode vs pulse mode

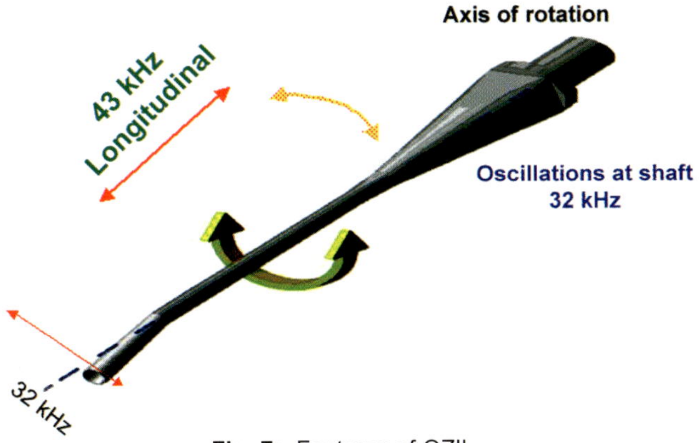

Fig. 7: Features of OZIL

HOW DOES THIS WORK?

The handpiece has electrodes in its body. When the salt containing BSS is in the handpiece and a current is applied to it, this warmed fluid pulses at the volume of 4 microliters per pulse, propelled upto 50 times a second (50pps).

This impact of warmed pulses rapidly strains the cataract causing liquefaction.

There is no high frequency mechanical motion of the tip and thus no heat generation at the incision. Magnitude of aqualase can be increased, i.e. pulse length increases from 3 to 9 microseconds.

This aqualase handpiece has both irrigation and aspiration and a smooth disposable silicone tip. Basically the cataract is emulsified using a sculpting technique. Stop and chop is difficult with this handpiece until a large part of the cataract has been emulsified by sculpting as the tip does not embed. A great advantage of this tip is that its absolutely atraumatic and even cortical cleanup can be done with it. This shows us that its not the shape of the phacotip or the fact that its port size is large that leads to capsular breakage on occlusion, rather that the edge should be smooth and pliable.

This lends itself well to refractive lens exchange and to pediatric cataracts. The only problem with this technology is that cataracts harder than grade 2 need an inordinate amount of time and are faster managed with conventional pulsed ultrasound.

OZIL

Another new technology from Alcon is the Ozil upgrade to the Infiniti platform. OZiL™ is Alcon's brand name for a torsional phaco handpiece.

HOW DOES THIS WORK?

- Oscillatory torsional amplitude creates lateral tip movement that cuts more efficiently due to less repulsion, and results in decreased thermal energy at the incision. Thus torsional phaco cuts the lens by shearing as against regular phaco which employs a jackhammer effect.
- When a conventional phaco tip encounters a nuclear fragment part of the forward stroke of the tip actually pushes the fragment away until vacuum pulls the fragment back to the tip. This decreases cutting efficacy. The harder the cataract the greater the repulsion. This is totally avoided in OZIL as here there is no forward repulsion and thus greater followabilty.
- This torsional oscillation with a Kelman tip generates the same stroke *at the tip end* as phaco but in transverse direction
- Oscillations of the OZIL handpiece are 32 kHz (32,000 times per second)

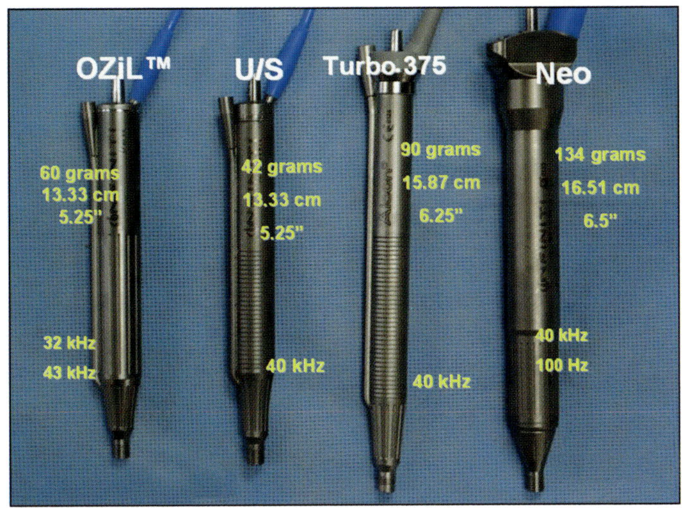

Fig. 8:

Comparison	*Phaco*	*Torsional*
Frequency	40 kHz	32 kHz
Max. Stroke	85 μm	85 μm
Stroke direction	Longitudinal	Side to Side
Preferred Mode	Pulse or Burst	Continuous
Cutting Action	During forward stroke only	During both left and right directions
Vacuum Needs	Benefits from high vacuum to reduce repulsion	Medium vacuum is sufficient to pull material through
Repulsion	Mitigated by vacuum and pulse/burst	Reduced or not present
Heat	Proportional to power	Proportional to amplitude but 2/3 less than in phaco
Best Phaco Tip	1.1 Flared	0.9 mm Tapered

Fig. 9: Physical Dimension Phaco Vs Torsional

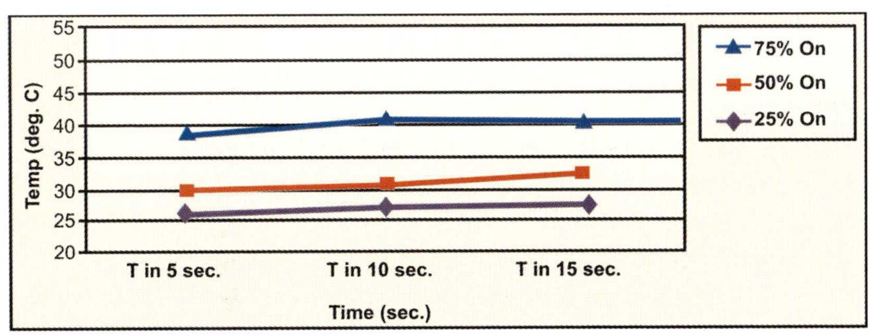

Fig. 10: Temperature rise with variation due to pulse duty cycle (Cadaver Eye; 12 cc/min Asp; 0.9 mm tip through 1.2 mm incision; 50 pps pulse at 100%).

This is much faster than 100 Hz for NeoSoniX, so oscillations alone have enough energy to cut. It's, however, lower than the 40 kHz of regular phaco which results in a 20% energy saving and much less heat generation at the incision.

Overall there is about 2/3 less heat at wound site according to studies.

The company maintains that torsional is most efficient when applied continuously – pauses will slow down removal and may induce clogging on the 4+ lenses. However in my experience it works great in pulse mode and corneas are much clearer the next day than if continuous power is used.

In contrast as it has repulsion, regular phaco is best in pulse or burst mode to minimize repulsion by using high vacuum.

Sonic Phaco with the Staar Sonic Wave

Staar has produced a machine called the Sonic Wave that on the same handpiece can give both sonic and ultrasound. The Sonic WAVE™ blends low frequency pulses (40-400 Hz) with new ultra vacuum technology to produce a cataract removal system which is more efficient than ultrasound.

The company claims that there are no thermal burns as sonic vibrations produce no heat . Indeed at 100% sonic power you can hold the bare tip in your fingers without feeling any heat. In similar circumstances a ultrasound tip would rapidly cross 100 degrees centigrade.

A special feature of the Staar machine is its coiled ***supervac*** tubing. This tubing is attached in the aspiration line and greatly decrease or eliminates surge on occlusion break. It generates turbulence in the line and forces the aspirated fluid to slow down on occlusion break. Its the sudden speeding up of the fluid in the aspiration line on occlusion break that's responsible for surge The SuperVac tubing increases vacuum capability up to 650 mm Hg. The key to chamber maintenance is a positive fluid balance between infusion flow and aspiration flow. When occlusion is broken, vacuum previously built in the aspiration line generates a high aspiration flow that can be higher than the infusion flow. This results in anterior chamber instability. The coiled SuperVac tubing limits surge flow resulting from occlusion breakage in a dynamic way. The continuous change in direction of flow through the coiled tubing increases resistance through the tubing at high flow rates such as on clearance of occlusion of the tip. This effect of generating turbulence only takes place at higher flow rates (more than 50 cc/min). The fluid resistance of the SuperVac tubing increases as a function of flow, and most importantly unoccluded flow is not restricted.

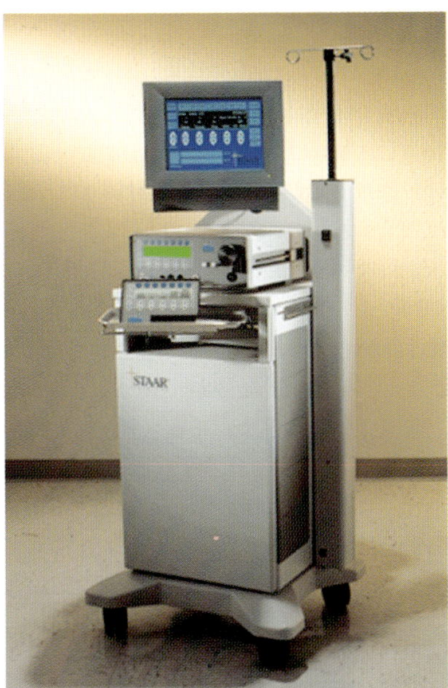

Fig. 11: Staars sonic wave machine

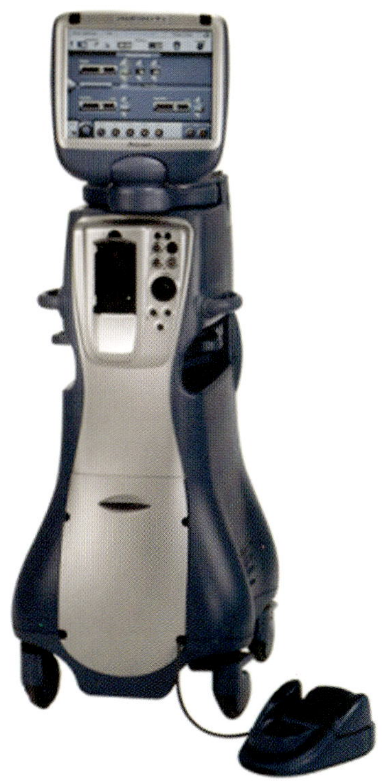

Fig. 12: Alcons infiniti platform

RESULTS

Comparing the sonic to the ultrasonic machine, using the same parameters, Dr Fine found an increased effective phaco time, as expected. The power was approximately the same at around 7. 5% phaco power. The percentage of clear corneas was exactly the same at 96%, and the patients' uncorrected visual acuity 20/40 or better remained the same at 79%.

"It still is a spectacular system," Dr Fine said. With the foot pedal, one can move back and forth between ultrasound and sonic energy, thus covering all grades of cataract. "With harder grades, the tip tends to become occluded, so we kick over to ultrasound for a second, clear the tip and then move back into the sonic mode," he said.

The Staar Wave also has a unique tightly coiled aspiration vacuum tubing. The continuously changing direction of fluid leaving the eye is associated with a dramatic increase in the resistance of flow at high flow rates. "This is fabulous for chamber stability and as an antisurge device," Dr Fine said.

Pulsatome (Visijet Inc. and Ponte Nossa Acquisition Corp.)

This new device uses a lower pressure, pulsed waterjet for the fragmentation, irrigation, hydrodissection and aspiration of cataracts. The Pulsatome hand piece goes through a 2. 9 mm incision, and it uses short pulses of 20 mL of BSS under a pressure of 1,000 psi to break the nucleus into smaller fragments that are aspirated through the aspiration port on the hand piece.

The advantages of this system are its potentially high safety profile, no wound heat and easy learning curve, noted Richard L. Lindstrom, MD. However, it is likely good only for soft cataracts and may be slower than ultrasound, he said, but the technology is still in the lab.

Hyperpulse Microburst and Whitestar Ice Technology

This is a proprietary technology of AMO on its flagship Soverign phaco machine. Designed to reduce heat build up at the phacotip and minimize the US power needed thus enhancing purchase on the fragment the Soverign pioneered this technology 5 years ago.

These pulses of ultrasound energy are as short as 1/100 of a millisecond. This is shorter than the thermal relaxation time of the tissue, thus there is no heat build up.

This basically means that we can have hyperpulses of even 5 millisec with a offtime of 995 millisec at every pulse cycle. AMO was the first to launch this technology in the Soverign with its ICE upgrade. Now however the capability to simply generate hyperpulses can be found in much cheaper machines and

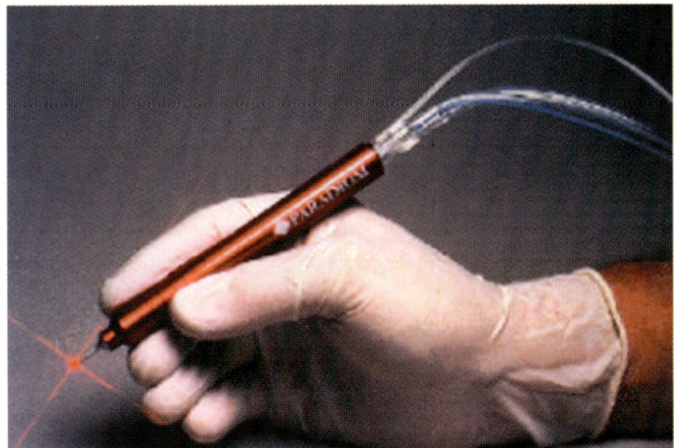

Fig. 13: Paradigm laser phaco handpiece

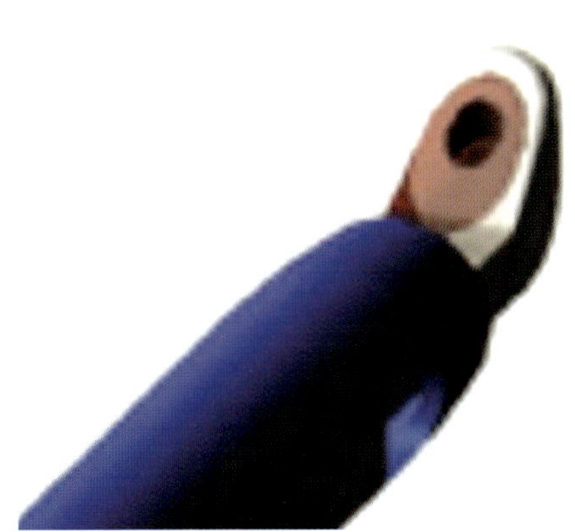

Fig. 14: The ski-shaped tip of paradigm laser system which acts as a photon trap

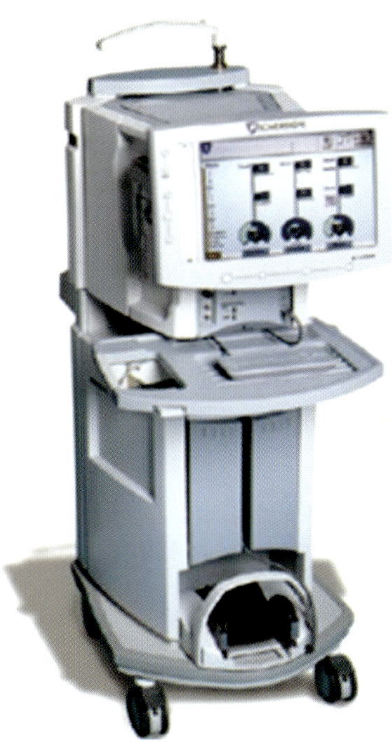

Fig. 15: Soverign system from AMO

basic models as well. Another feature of the Soverign is that once the tip is embedded the vacuum can be lowered automatically to a previously preset value thus reducing surge on occlusion break. This is a worthwhile feature and is termed CASE (Chamber Stabilisation Environment) by the company.

To take it one step further the ICE upgrade added to this the concept of shaped pulses . This means that in the first millisecond of the pulse the power automatically steps up and then decreases for he rest of the pulse. This reduces cavitation and increases followability of the fragment which the company refers to as magnetic followability.

Conclusion

Endocapsular phaco technology will combine well with refillable lenses. Hyper and customized pulses will further reduce ultrasound expended in the anterior chamber. Alternative modalities like aqualase and NeoSoniX will continue to appear. The further development of laser technology will indeed allow true cold bimanual phaco as a procedure of choice.

15

Persistent Hyaloid Artery: Surgical Solution and Postoperative Management

Simonetta Morselli, Roberto Bellucci (Italy)

Introduction

The persistency of Hyaloid Artery is not a common disease but it could be confused with a retinoblastoma. The primary vitreous is the embryonic vasculature of the eye and supplies nutrients to the developing lens and retina during early gestation. The hyaloid artery is the main arterial supply within this network. Abnormal persistence of the primary vitreous and tunica vasculosa lentis and concurrent hyperplasia of the embryonic connective tissue produce the basic lesion. Persistent hyperplastic primary vitreous has been described in association with fetal alcohol syndrome, fetal hydantoin syndrome, and midline congenital cranial defects. Most cases (90%) are unilateral; bilateral cases can be associated with trisomy syndromes 13, 15, 18, and 21. Normally a retrolental membrane is present in the eye. Children with persistent hyperplastic primary vitreous usually present in the perinatal period with leukokonia and microphthalmos and are examined for possible retinoblastoma. Only the use B-mode sonography for orbital evaluation could be helpful to distinguish the two diseases.

Surgical Solution

The young patient must be operated under general anesthesia. It is very difficult to have the exact idea of the problem that the eye present. If it is possible the axial length is measured preoperative, if not, the axial length is measured before surgery under general anesthesia . The calculation of the IOLs is in every case performed before starting the surgery even if the IOL could not be implanted, due to the anatomical reason. Most of the time the K-reading values could not be obtained before or during the surgery; therefore the power of IOL implanted is based on axial length. We normally follow the rules of Dr Dahan for babies less than one year. If the axial length is about 20 mm we use 25 D IOL if it is about 19 mm we implant 26 D, if the length is about 18 mm we implant 28 D IOL. If the axial length is between 21 and 23 mm the power of the IOL will be: axial length value + 1D per mm more than 21. If the axial length is more than 24 mm the power implated will be: axial length value –1D per mm more than 24. We are able to use 5.5 mm three piece optical IOL with 12.5 mm of length.

Our goal is to obtain emmetropia or slight hyperopia to give to that eye the option to develop a visual acuity. After the surgery the hyperopia and the pseudophakic presbyopia must be corrected with contact lens or with glasses considering the age of the patient. The pre-operative mydriasis is obtained with 1cc of phenylephrine 10% and tropicamide 0.5% + 1 cc of cyclopentolate diluted in the same syringe with 8 cc of distilled water. This solution is applied in the eye two hours before surgery until the pupil will be mydriatic.

The incision is placed al 12 o'clock under conjunctival flap to protect the incision as soon as possible.

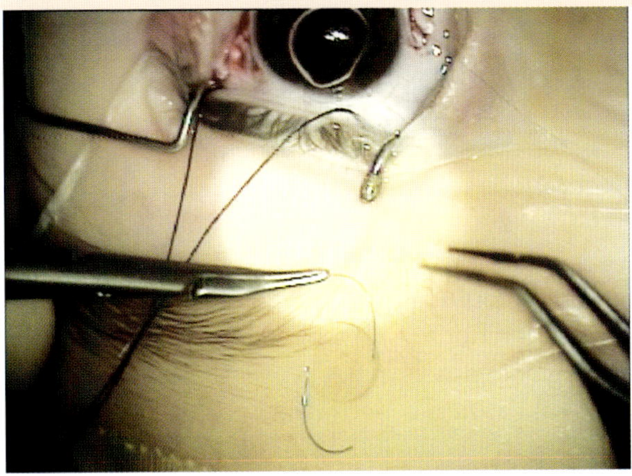

Fig. 1: IOL used for congenital cataract surgery

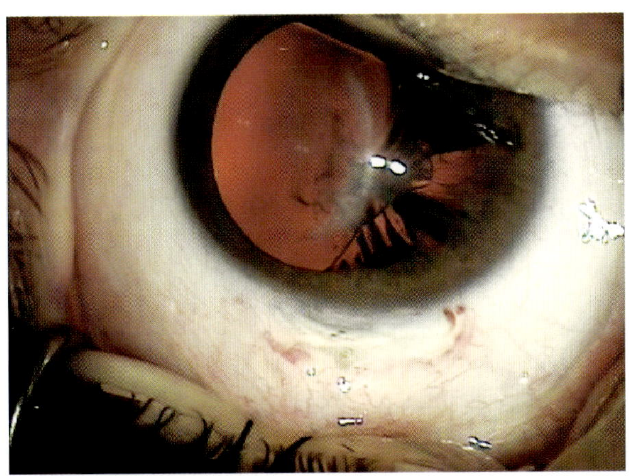

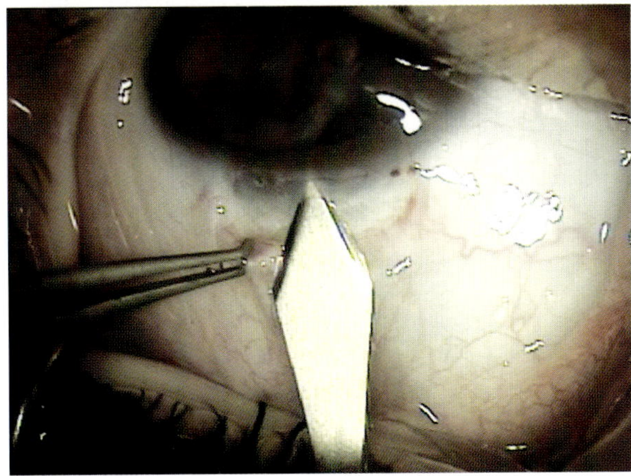

Figs 2 and 3: The incision is placed at 12 o'clock under conjunctival flap

Then the high molecular weight viscoelastic substances is used to protect the tissues and to maintain the spaces into the eye. A capsulorhexis is performed to aspirate the intracapsular material.

Then in most of the cases the retrolental membrane must be cut with a microscissor. The membrane is removed after cauterizing the hyaloid artery with endodiathermy retinal system, increasing the value until the artery is visible closed and cut.

Then the membrane could be removed together with the anterior vitrectomy to avoid vitreoretinal tractions.

The capsular bag sometimes is not present and a scleral fixation of IOL is necessary. The scleral fixation is performed with ab externo technique with a three pieces acrylic hydrophobic IOL.

This type of IOL could follow the growing of the eye due to the elasticity of the loops. The incision is closed with a 10/0 vicryl. The scleral flaps and the conjunctiva is also closed with a 10/0 vicryl.

Postoperative Management

The postoperative therapy is the association with antibiotics plus corticosteroids, quad per day, for a three weeks period and omatropine drops, bid per day, for a five-six weeks. The contralateral eye is immediately patch after the surgery. We normally used to prescribe the amount of the hours,that the healty eye is patched, depending on the age of the patient. For example, if the patient is 3 months old, we prescribe three hours per day (at that age the baby is woke up not more), that means a permanent patching. At one year old we prescribed half a day of patching following the potential visual recovery of the operated eye. The postoperative examination of the operated eye is conducted under general sedation after one, three, six postoperative months. Sometimes inflammatory membrane could be occluded the visual axis. This membrane must be excised with posterior or anterior vitrectomy, depending on the position of the membrane. Every eye is different, but we had a great experience of 5 cases in 4 years and thus technique was generally applied in every of that cases successfully.

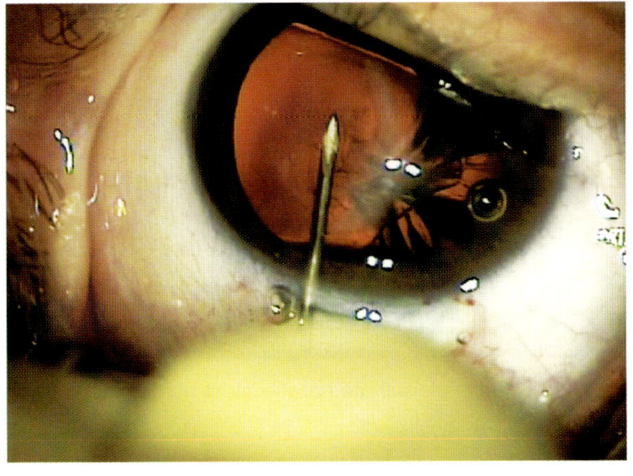

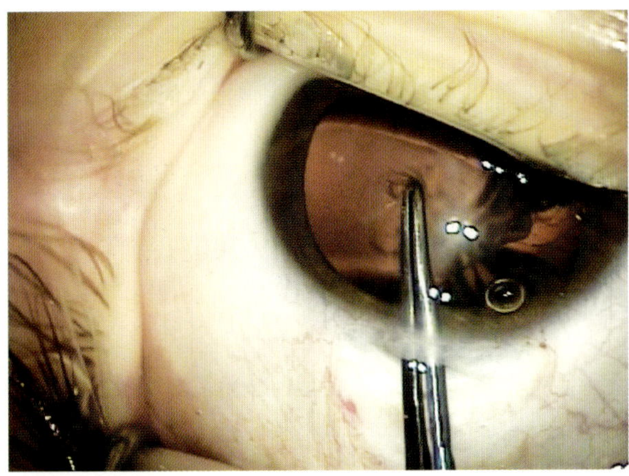

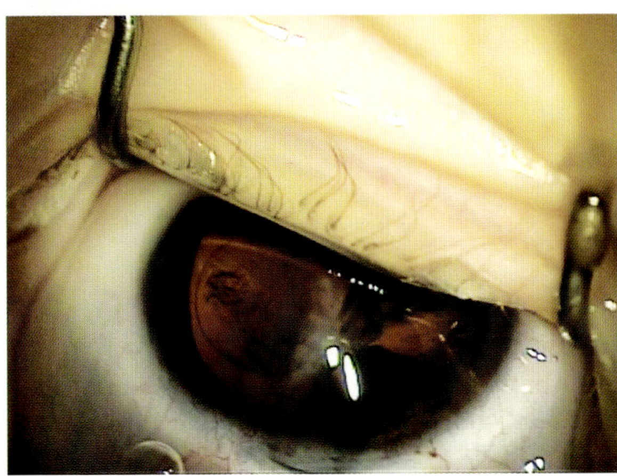

Fig. 4 to 6: The capsulorhexis is performed

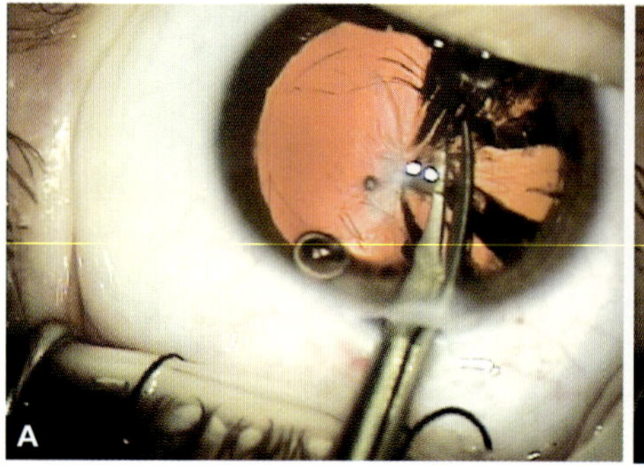

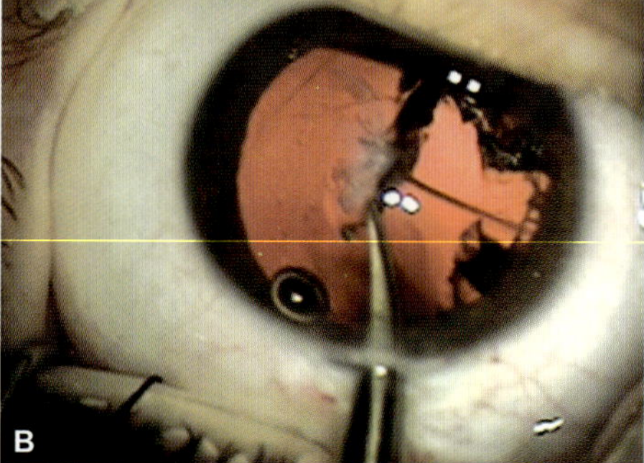

Figs 7A and B: The retrolental membrane must be cut with a microscissor

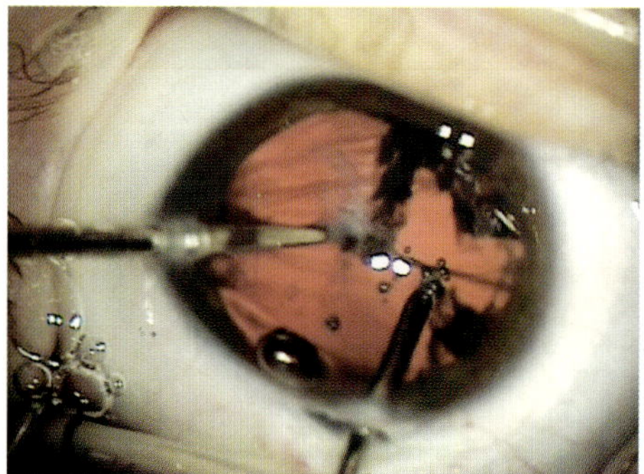

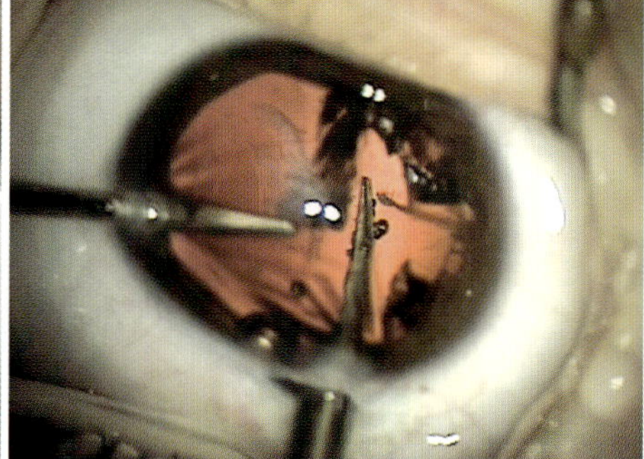

Figs 8 and 9: The membrane is removed after cauterizing the hyaloid artery with endodiathermy retinal system, increasing the value until the artery is visible closed and cut

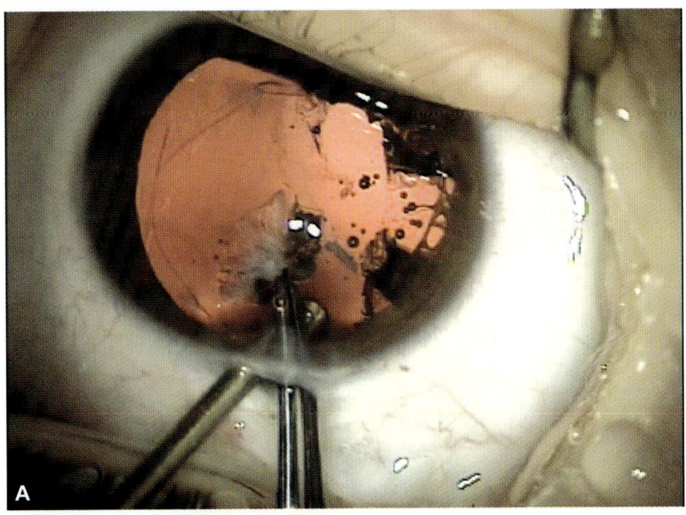

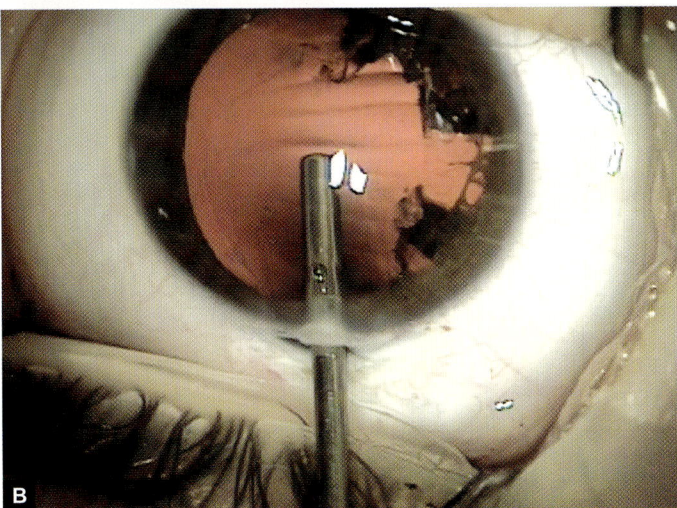

Figs 10A and B: Then the membrane could be removed together with the anterior vitrectomy to avoid vitreoretinal tractions

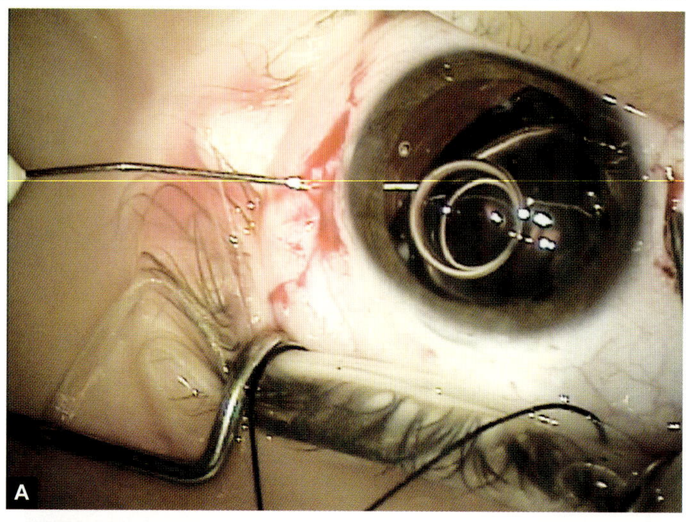

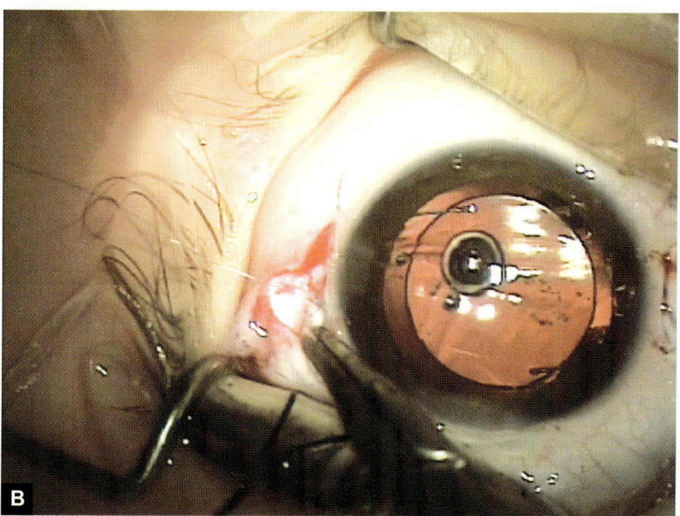

Figs 11A and B: The scleral fixation is performed with ab externo technique with a three pieces acrylic hydrophobic IOL

16

High Definition 3D Visualization for Cataract Surgery

Robert J Weinstock, Stephen M Weinstock,
Forrest Fleming (USA)

Introduction

The human body is a clearly a three dimensional system. Some of the most complex geometric shapes in nature are expressed within both the macro (i.e. specific organs, bone, vascular, nerve, tumor etc) and micro (cell structure, protein shapes etc) systems of the body. Because there is an ongoing need to better understand human anatomy within the real-time context of surgery, one can reasonably expect 3D visualization technology to advance. This chapter will provide a brief review of imaging technology used in medicine today and also a specific example of a new 3D visualization technology for microsurgery applied in cataract removal and artificial lens replacement.

Visualization in Medicine

The original visualization system for medical procedures was the physician's eyes. Subsequent innovation (i.e. X-ray, Ultrasound, CT, MRI, loupes, microscopes, endoscopes, etc.) attempted to either enhance natural vision or enable the physician to see through opaque tissue. Many of these technologies provided 2D views of 3D objects. This has proved very helpful in diagnostics and preoperative surgical planning. However, for most surgeries, a 3D view is desired and provided by the inherent nature of the human 2-eye system. The right eye and left eye triangulate with the target to create stereoscopic vision providing a perception of depth in the z-axis. Loupes and stereomicroscopes with separate right-eye/left-eye optical paths provide a magnified 3D view for procedures on small structures (Eyes, Ear, Nose, Throat, Brain, Spine, Vascular, Hand, etc.). Presently, this magnification is accomplished with optical science and the resulting image is an optical image. Increasingly this optical image technology is being replaced with digital imaging technologies.

With the advent of endoscopes in the 1980s, new minimally invasive procedures were developed for internal large organ surgeries (gynecology, urology, gastrointestinal, orthopedic, etc.). Most of the endoscopes used 2D cameras as their vision system and required surgeons to rely on a tactical feel to compensate for a lack of 3D vision. Most likely these vision systems will evolve to include a 3D capability.

Using a Digital Hi-Definition 3D Vision System for Cataract Surgery

BACKGROUND

Advances in computing and digital imaging are making it possible, and soon perhaps desirable, to perform many microsurgical procedures by viewing and

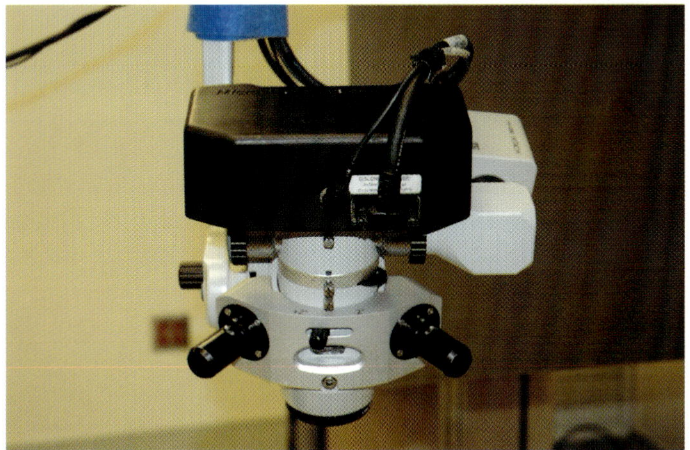

Fig. 1: Image capture module connected to Zeiss microscope

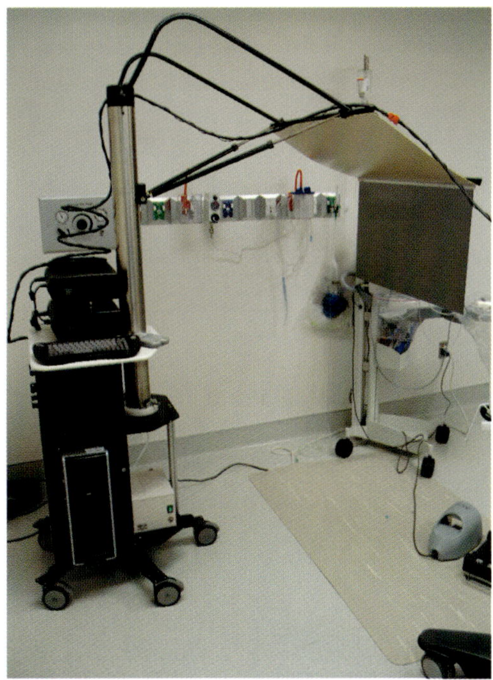

Fig. 2: Image processing unit located on bottom half of stand

manipulating tissue in the surgical field by looking directly at a high definition 3D digital display rather than optically through the microscope eyepieces. This paper documents the use of such a system from TrueVision Systems of Santa Barbara CA (www.truevisionsys.com) to perform cataract surgery.

True Vision Systems (TVS) has developed a patent pending digital 3D vision system that can be retrofitted to most standard Leica and Zeiss surgical microscopes. The novel nature of the TVS imaging system lies in that TrueVision is both 3D and high definition; suggesting ophthalmic and other microsurgeries can be performed without looking through the microscopes eyepieces. Currently 2D video cameras and displays are used as secondary viewing systems in microscopy or even the primary viewing system in endoscopy. This system provides a vastly improved view in high definition which not only allows observers to view the surgical field in 3D, but also can be used by the surgeon in lieu of the conventional view through the oculars of the microscope. The TVS system has three primary components.

The Image Capture System (ICM)

The ICM is a compact, ergonomic module which replaces the eyepieces of any surgical microscope. This procedure involves loosening and tightening one set screw and literally takes less than 15 seconds. The ICM contains two high definition (1280 × 1024p) sensors (one for the right eye and one for the left) that emulates the human two eye system thus providing visual depth perception as one sees through the eyepieces in real time. The ICM sends an integrated, encrypted, data stream at 2.5 Gbits/sec along a special hi-bandwidth cable to the information processing unit. The ICM works naturally with all of the other controls of the microscope, such as zoom and focus.

Image Processing Unit (IPU)

The IPU is a high powered, customized, Windows/Intel based, workstation. It receives and processes the ICM data and formats it for a variety of display technologies, which in this case was a dual projection system. Within the IPU there are a variety of image enhancement functions such as brightness, gamma, contrast etc. The IPU outputs DVI formatted data at up to 350 MB/sec to the projectors.

Image Display System (IDS)

The IDS consists of a fold up 4′ × 3′ specialized screen and two 1280 × 720p, 60 hz projectors that generate real time images simultaneousely for the right eye and left eye on screen. By wearing polarized glasses the right or left eye only sees the right eye/left eye image captured by ICM and delivered by the IPU. This creates the stereo effect to see in 3D. The IPU and IDS are housed together in an ergonomic, OR friendly cart that is compact, mobile, and FDA class 1 compliant.

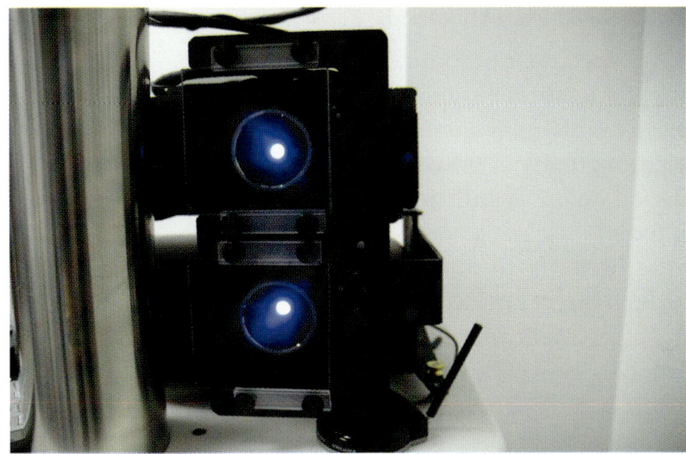

Fig. 3: 3D High definition digital projectors

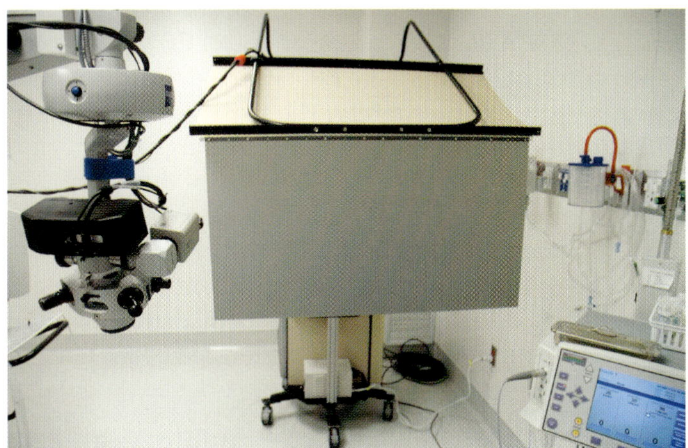

Fig. 4: High definition view in screen

OBJECTIVES AND METHODS

This was a prospective randomized evaluation of the safety and efficacy of performing cataract surgery with a 3D high definition indirect viewing system. Further objectives of our evaluation were to explore several questions:

1. Is the picture quality of the digital image equal to the optical image?
2. Is the digital image of sufficient quality to safely perform eye surgery on a routine basis?
3. Are there benefits to an indirect digital 3D vision system over the conventional direct optical view?
4. Are there other applications and advantages with a digital 3D vision system?

Established in 1974, The Eye Institute of West Florida is a multi-specialty ophthalmic practice. The current facility is over 30,000 sq ft with an integrated Ambulatory Surgery Center with 4 modern operating rooms. All ORs have Zeiss OPMI-view microscopes and networked 2D video systems with a macro and surgical view capability. With the help of TrueVision personnel a TVS system was installed in March 2007 after we became aware of the product at AAO in Las Vegas Nov 2006. We configured one of the OR's to accommodate the device. Two different layouts were established depending on whether we were doing a right eye or left eye surgery. The TVS screen was simply rotated to a position that provided optimum viewing for the surgeon.

To initially test the visual quality and viability of the system, a superficial conjunctival lesion biopsy and a pterygium resection were completed without complication. 300 patients scheduled for routine cataract surgery were then randomized to one of three operating rooms. Room 1 had the TVS indirect viewing system attached to the microscope. Room 2 and 3 had conventional ocular microscope viewing. All cases were performed by the authors.

RESULTS

Over the course of 10 operating room sessions, all 300 cataract cases were performed successfully. 100 cataract surgeries were completed using TrueVision as the primary viewing and manipulation system. The additional 200 cases were performed with the conventional system. There were no surgical or postoperative complications in either group. The average case time was slightly longer in patients who had the TrueVision system.

OBSERVATIONS

Both surgeons noted that the brightness and detail clarity were slightly better in the optical image while the depth of field was superior in the digital image. The resolution was also noted to be marginally better in the optical view. Both surgeons preferred the room lights out with the TrueVision cases to aid in visualization, while normally they operate with the room lights on. Remarkably,

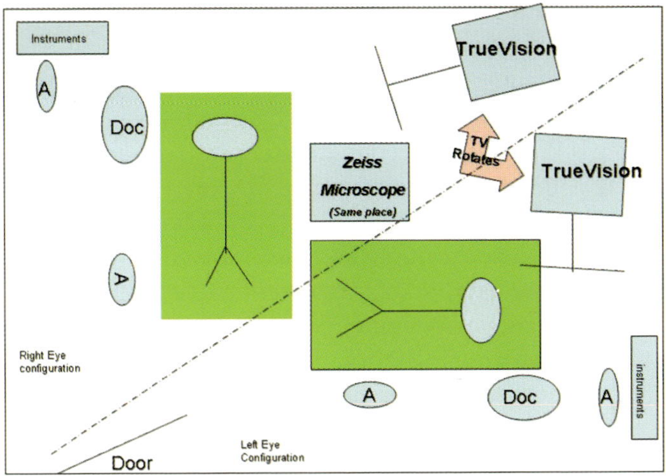

Fig. 5: Schematic of operating room setup for the Truevision system for left and right and eye

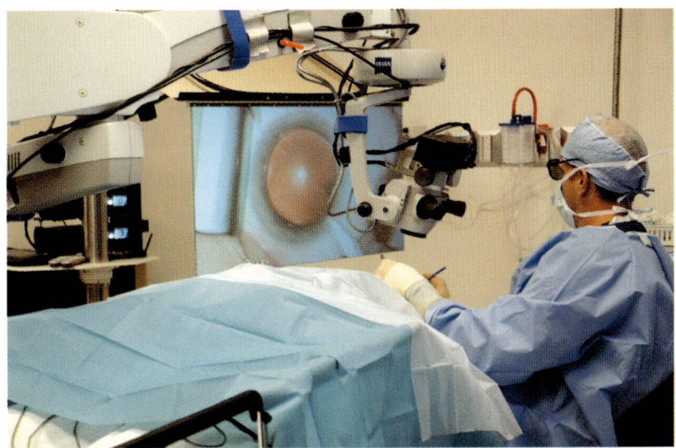

Fig. 6: Dr Robert Weinstock using the Truevision system for cataract surgery

both surgeons felt comfortable with the slightly different hand-eye orientation of the TrueVision system after one day of use. Both surgeons also noted that the depth of field was greater in the TrueVision and was very helpful in nucleus removal. Magnification was also found to be an advantage of the TrueVision system. Dr. Robert Weinstock noted that the large screen and the magnification it provides along with the improved depth of field made him remove the nucleus more slowly and methodically. This may account for the slightly longer case times seen in the TrueVision group. The TrueVision system, because of the large screen format, suggested amplified instrument movement on the screen which in effect gave the surgeon a feeling of better instrument control. The surgical scrub, who also was viewing in 3D noted that the improved view enhanced her ability to identify the stages of the procedure and increased her efficiency in passing the correct instrument to the surgeon.

Discussion

The TrueVision 3D viewing system is truly a revolutionary product that is in its infancy regarding its potential applications throughout the microsurgical field of medicine. Within ophthalmology there are many immediate applications including the possibility of negating the need for a surgeon to view the eye through the microscope oculars and improving the surgical view.

Residency and teaching institutions can find an immediate benefit from the system. By attaching the 3D camera to a binocular observers scope, a 3D view of the operating field is available to everyone watching in or out of the OR. The surgeon can still maintain a direct view of the eye through the primary oculars if desired. Future capabilities include applications in telemedicine, given the near perfect 3D view of the surgical subject from remote locations. This could also translate into 3D virtual surgery and training applications. Once 3D recording capability is added to the system, it is possible for educational forums and meetings to offer educational video clips in 3D. This may be a tremendous aid in education to microsurgeons translating into improved patient outcomes and a more meaningful learning experience for the doctor.

Aside from an immediate benefit in teaching, perhaps the greatest justification for a digital vision system is other potential applications that can be added once the operative visualization occurs in the digital realm. The applications may include:

1. Measurement overlays to assist with incision placement and size. For example, location, length, and axis of limbal relaxing incision and size can be overlayed on the screen to aid in placement.
2. Using annotation and colored shadings to establish boundary zones for safety and guidance. An example of this would be shading the

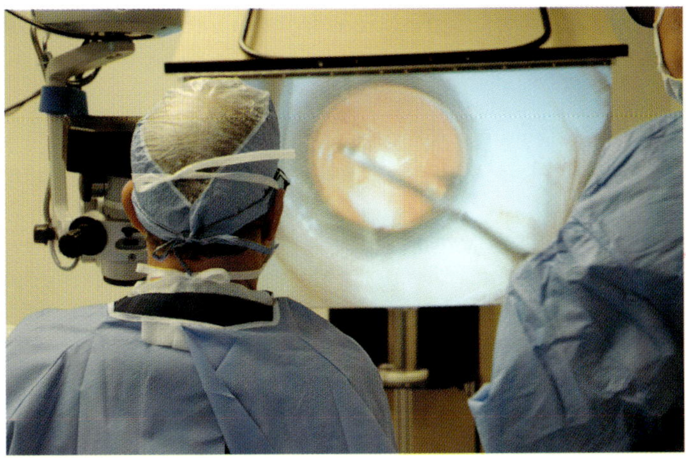

Fig. 7: Dr Weinstock and surgical assistant Jay both viewing the eye in 3D during a cataract case

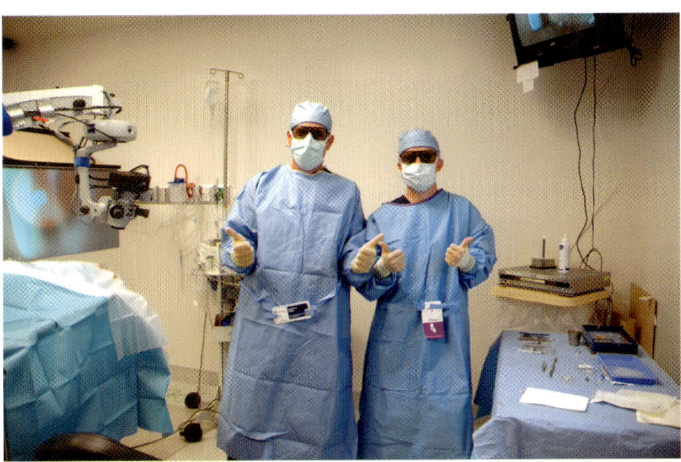

Fig. 8: Dr Weinstock and assistant Jay after a successful day using the Truevision system

cataract green, yellow and red from front to back to allow the surgeon to have an added visual signal of how deep the phaco needle is in the capsular bag.

3. Integration of other data into one heads up display (i.e. phaco machine parameters, patient data, measurement scales, overlay drawing with mouse and keyboard, etc.).

These added features are not available with current optical views through the microscope. As they become available on the Truevision digital system it may prove to be a significant advantage.

Conclusion

The advancement in 3D digital technology has produced an image quality that now approaches the optical image seen through the microscope oculars. The case for a 3D digital vision system in surgical microscopy is increasingly compelling. Digital images can be recorded, replayed, transmitted, integrated, and enhanced in ways never before possible with optical images. For similar reasons, digital cameras are quickly replacing film as the world's primary image capture medium. As this technology improves with better clarity, brightness, and resolution coupled with digital overlays and adjunctive data display on the heads up screen, this technology will significantly improve the way we operate, educate and communicate with patients in the future.

17

Torsional Phacoemulsification

Rohit Om Parkash (India)

Introduction

Phacoemulsification has seen a constant evolution in the techniques, surgical parameters, power modulations and fluidic management since 1968. The only thing, which has not changed, has been the forward-backward motion of the phaco tip in a linear direction along the axis of the shaft.

Longitudinal Phaco has innate problems like (1) repulsion (2) heat production (3) chamber instability. It is around these three issues that Phacoemulsification has evolved.

Issues Associated with Longitudinal Phacoemulsification

REPULSION

The main problem associated with longitudinal phaco is repulsion. High vacuum with high flow rate are used to take care of repulsion. In addition, we have been employing methods of Intermittent Energy delivery like Pulse, Hyper Pulse, and Burst etc. This strategy of using intermittent energy allows for fluidics to attract the chattering nuclear matter to the tip and aspirate it. Repulsion for pulsed-mode axial phaco was reduced to 40% of the total stroke at the start of each pulse.

HEAT PRODUCTION

The other basic problem is wastage of energy in half the period when the tip is coming back. Subsequently, excessive heat is produced. Intermittent energy in the form of Pulse, burst and hyperpulse with numerous variations are used to take care of excessive heat. However, there is no denying that the wastage of energy is still there and problems related with excessive heat are still far from ideal.

CHAMBER STABILITY

Modern Phacoemulsification procedures are involved with high fluidics parameters to counter the repulsion aspect and to increase the efficiency of cataract removal procedure. The fluid management system of the machines plays a decisive role in preventing surge. The problem of chamber instability becomes all the more important in difficult situations like Hard Cataracts, Posterior Polar Cataracts, Subluxated cataracts and cataracts with small pupils.

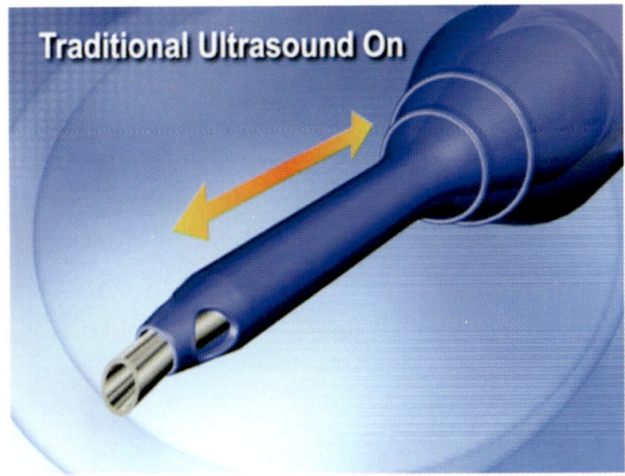

Fig. 1: Forward and backward movement in traditional ultrasound

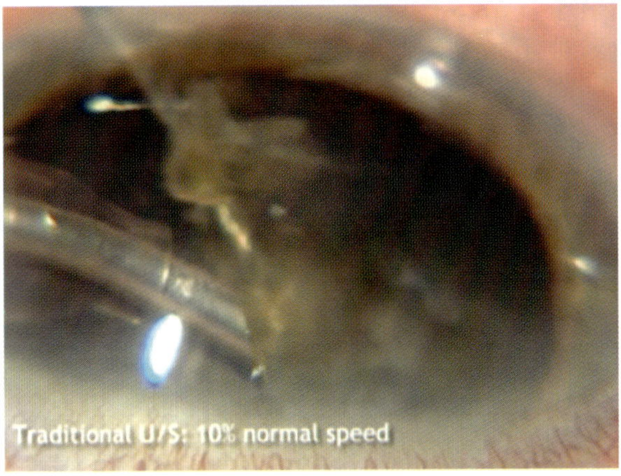

Fig. 2: Traditional ultrasound at 10% normal speed showing chatter at sweet spot

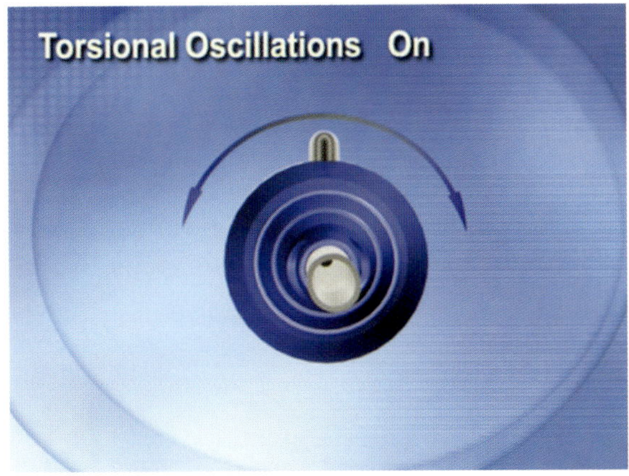

Fig. 3: Torsional ultrasound with side to side cutting

OZil™—TORSIONAL EMULSIFICATION

OZil™, a new cataract removal modality on the Infiniti® Vision System was introduced during the AAO meeting in 2005. Torsional phaco utilizes ultrasonic oscillations of an angulated or bent phaco tip, which dramatically changes both the energy profile of the tip and the surgical efficiency.

OZil™ stands for the torsional ultrasound handpiece, offered with the Infiniti Vision System®. It has a torsional motion of the tip i.e. side to side cutting. This is quite contrary to the longitudinal ultrasound which has a forward and backward traditional motion.

TORSIONAL HANDPIECE AND PHACO TIP

The torsional handpiece weighs only 1.5 ounces. It is one of the lightest handpieces available. Its tip is similar to other handpieces. It is angled and tapered which makes the distal end wider than the shaft. Different-sized infusion sleeves can be used with the handpiece which enables functioning through a small incision of 2 to 2.2 mm.

Key Features of Kelman Tips

- The 0.9 mm Kelman tip works the best. This provides the greatest displacement and shearing action.
- The Kelman ABS tips have an aspiration bypass system in the form of 0.22 micron hole in the side near the distal end. This provides an alternative part for fluid to pass when the tip is occluded. Whenever there is an occlusion break less fluid is needed for replacement from the chamber. This provides better chamber stability.
- A 45-degree tip works a bit easier than the 30-degree tip because it makes the quadrants tumble more easily than a 30-degree one due to more surface area on the lumen at the bevel.
- The energy created within the incision by the rapidly oscillating Kelman tip is significantly less than at the distal end.

REPULSION AND OZIL

In Torsional Phaco, the cutting of the lens matter is by shearing action instead of the jackhammer effect of Traditional Phaco. It rubs and does not push. There is a continuous contact between the tip and the nucleus. In other words, in OZil there is no repulsion.

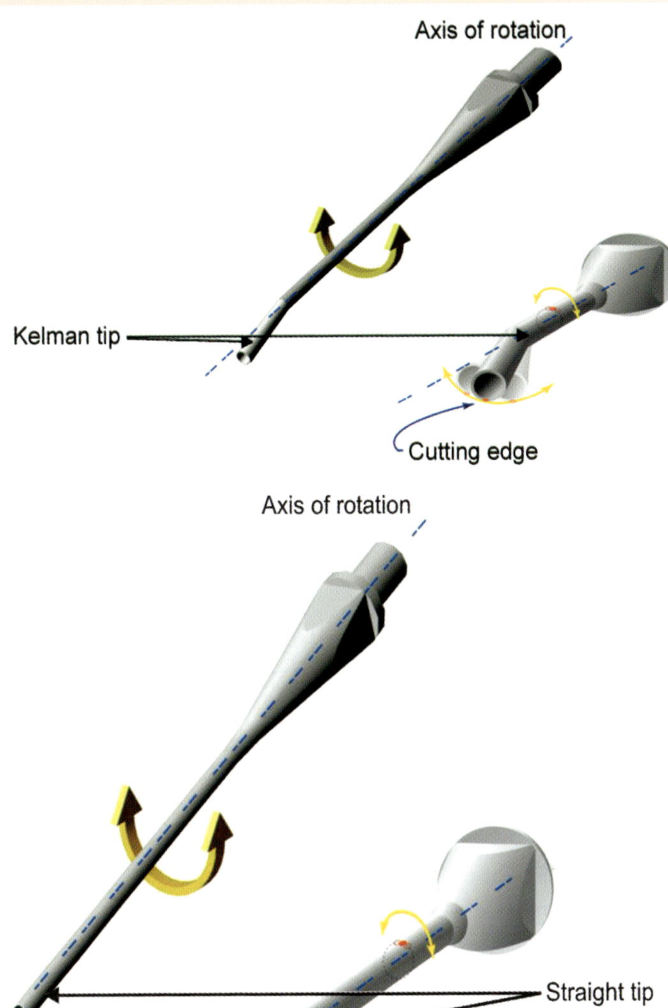

Fig. 4: Kelman tip

The zero repulsion in Torsional emulsification of one of the major problems associated with Longitudinal Phaco. This repulsion rate dropped to almost zero using torsional phaco the nucleus appears to evaporate. It just disappears into the tip quickly because it doesn't just sit on the tip and microscopically there is no chatter during removal.

The absence of repulsion has resulted in another dimension in Nucleus Emulsification. The Nucleus pieces just come to the tip and stay at the tip. There is no need to reach or fish for them in the periphery. The whole procedure takes place by just staying in the middle of the eye.

The zero repulsion has helped in protecting the Corneal Endothelial Cells in Torsional Emulsification. There is continuous contact between the tip and the Nucleus. This causes reduced flow and turbulence in the anterior chamber which keeps endothelial cells in much better shape. In addition to this, the reduced turbulence keeps the protective viscoelastic in the anterior chamber much better than if we use traditional ultrasound.

The decreased chatter and decreased turbulence is quite evident from the decreased number of loose nuclear pieces at the side port incision as compared to traditional ultrasound. The only time there are occasional loose particles in the side port incision is when the paracentesis is a little too large.

In Traditional emulsification we require to attain the sweet spot for the best use of Energy delivery and fluidics. This involves some dexterity in foot switch handling. A heavy footed surgeon is not able to have a perfect energy and fluidics usage.

In Torsional emulsification, we use continuous delivery. Torsional is most efficient when applied continuously because pauses slow down removal and induce clogging on the 4+ lenses

In Torsional Emulsification, there is no need to be dexterous in using the foot switch. The nucleus piece just starts clinging on to the tip of the needle at foot position two. The occlusion of the nucleus piece gets to the maximum at the top of foot position two. The Torsional ultrasound is activated. There is no repulsive effect and nucleus piece is removed. Torsional emulsification by its simplicity is able to help the surgeon raise his surgical skill.

HEAT AND OZIL

Heat energy produced is not an issue with Torsional Emulsification. There are obvious reasons why heat is no issue with OZiL

1. The Operating frequency of the OZil™ is 32 kHz as compared to traditional 40 kHz. The operating frequency of 32 kHz is good enough for OZil™ as it is a bidirectional cutting.

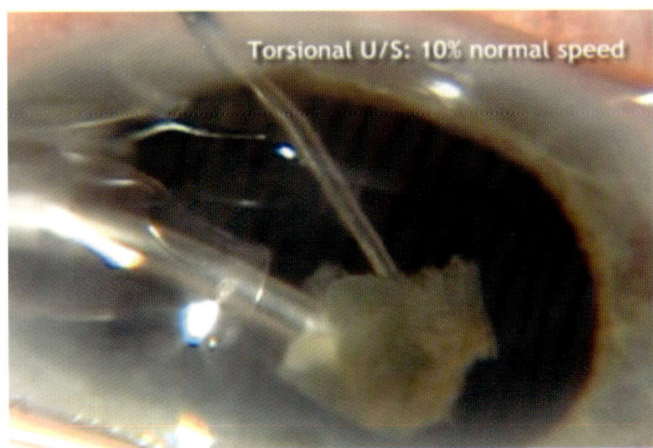

Fig. 5: Torsional ultrasound at 10% of normal speed showing zero repulsion

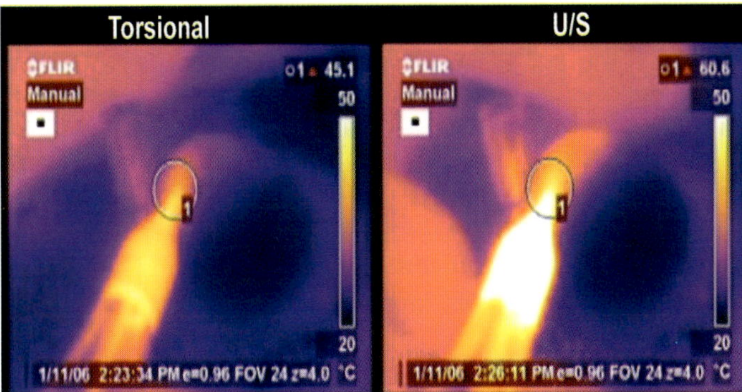

Fig. 6: Comparative evaluation of heat generated by torsional ultrasound and traditional ultrasound with no irrigation and total occlusion

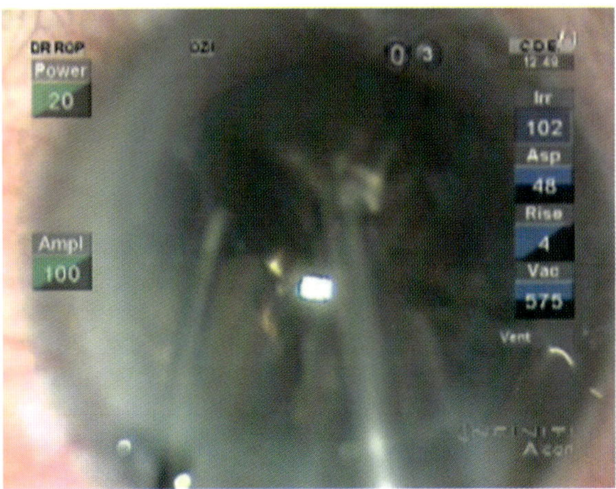

Fig. 7: A programmed torsional handpiece with combination of traditional and Torsional oscillations used in very hard cataracts

A 32 kHz OZiL is as effective as 64 kHz of Traditional ultrasound. In Traditional Ultrasound the tip cuts only in the forward motion. The reverse motion does not contribute to the cutting of the lens matter. In Torsional emulsification there is no wastage of half the cycle. In other words, in Torsional Emulsification, every complete stroke of the tip, one side to another and back, is like two strokes making it effectively 64 kilohertz.

There is non wastage of energy in one half of the cycle in Torsional emulsification. This has helped in decreasing the time period for which the Torsional ultrasound has to be kept on for effectively removing the same nucleus as would be required for Longitudinal Phacoemulsification. Subsequently, there is less heat produced.

2. The Kelman tip has further combined with the OZiL to decrease the Energy produced at the incision site. With each oscillatory cycle, the distance traveled by the tip is approximately is 5.5° which translates into 90 microns of stroke at the cutting edge. At the incision the stroke is approximately half of it, 40 microns. The reason is that the velocity of the angled tip of the torsional handpiece is about three times greater than the velocity of its shaft. Consequently, there is more delivery of energy by the tip to lens than by the shaft to the incision site and surrounding collagen. The decreased velocity of the shaft and the dramatically reduced friction within the incision reduces the incidence of thermal injury to the incision. The energy created within the incision by the rapidly oscillating tip is significantly less than at the distal end.

   Cionni also found that its lower stroke movement required 10% less ultrasound energy.

3. There is another striking reason why less of energy is used in Torsional Emulsification. While chopping or in any other nucleus removal methodology because of the absence of repulsion there is lesser amount of ultrasonic play required in position three to embed in the nucleus.

In short, the Wound site thermal injury is no issue with OZiL in continuous mode even with the hardest of cataracts. It is a much better option to use torsional ultrasound in cataract training centers (Dr Tjia).

Dr Boukhny and colleagues purposely occluded the aspiration line and created a leak-tight incision to eliminate cooling. The research showed that the temperature increase as a result of 80% ultrasound power application was approximately two times as fast as the temperature increase due to 100% Torsional amplitude.

STABLE CHAMBER AND OZIL

The cold incision site permits the surgeon to create a smaller incision because leakage of infusion fluid alongside the instrument is not required to lower its temperature.

Nucleus Removal Time

The other major advantage of Bi directional cutting is in improving the over all efficiency of the procedure. Subsequently, using the same flow and vacuum settings that the cataract surgeon might normally set for traditional ultrasound, the nucleus is removed more quickly with torsional ultrasound. In other words, Torsional phaco emulsification had a significantly shorter nuclear removal time as compared to longitudinal phacoemulsification.

TORSIONAL EMULSIFICATION AND LOWER PARAMETERS

The absence of such repulsive dynamics helps in having better fluidics at lower parameters of flow rate and vacuum. During traditional phaco surgery, nuclear fragments may be repelled from the tip with the forward stroke of the phaco tip, forcing the surgeon to use power modulations or increased fluidics to recapture nuclear fragments to the vibrating tip. There is no such repulsion in Torsional Emulsification and lower parameters work much better.

Fluid dynamic settings can be adjusted to lower levels without compromising on efficiency resulting in an increased safety margin level. The efficiency of torsional ultrasound with low fluid dynamic settings is still extremely good.

TORSIONAL EMULSIFICATION AND LOWER FLUID USAGE

Torsional Technology has one more clinically significant advantage. There is significantly lesser amount of fluid consumed during the procedure than that with longitudinal phacoemulsification. This observation may be attributed to the following reasons:

- Torsional phaco has virtually no repulsion so the lens matter stays at the tip throughout so the amount of fluid transfer through the eye is less.
- Torsional emulsification does not require very aggressive fluidic parameters.
- The overall efficiency and efficacy of the procedure is much better with the Torsional ultrasound. The time the tip remains in the eye is less which helps in lowering the consumption of fluid.

PLANE OF EMULSIFICATION WITH OZIL

There is another fine change in the technique. One is able to stay more at the level of or below the level of the iris plane in the central zone of safety. The tissue is not repelled to the extent that it is with standard longitudinal phaco. There is less fluid flow through the eye and increased efficiency.

MISCELLANEOUS POINTS

- Sculpting is easier, faster and more efficient with torsional ultrasound because with a greatly reduced repulsion the occlusion is maintained at all the time.
- The CDE is less than half when the Phaco tip is driven deep into the Nucleus from the peripheral side as compared with the approach from the center.

CLEARER CORNEAS AND OZIL

The OZiL provides a perfect blend of factors which contribute to clearer corneas.

1. Minimal repulsion
2. Remarkable chamber stability
3. Vastly improved followability
4. Thermal injury free profile
5. Efficient settings
6. Reduced BSS consumption
7. Decreased turbulence
8. Deeper plane of emulsification

OZIL IN COMPLICATED CATARACTS

OZiL is a revealation in complicated cataracts like:

1. Hard cataracts
2. Subluxated cataracts
3. Small pupils
4. Floppy iris syndrome
5. Posterior polar cataracts
6. Posterior capsule rupture
7. Corneal endothelial dystrophy
8. Posterior vitreous pressure

HARD CATARACTS

In harder cataracts, the Torsional Emulsification finds special usage because the wound site thermal injury (WSTI) is minimal. Tighter incisions are not a problem because of minimal WSTI. Consequently, one can work in harder cataracts with stable anterior chamber settings. The advantages of stable chamber settings make it easier to work in such harder cataracts. We need not worry about turbulence as stated earlier. This results in clearer corneas.

In Rocky Hard lenses (4+), the first change is the fluid parameters which should be increased and titrated according to the surgeon's convenience. The Non Tapered ABS Kelman tip should be used to avoid clogging. A 45 degree tip facilitates nucleus emulsification better than 30 degrees because it makes the quadrants tumble more easily.

In rocky hard cataracts, one can use the option of pressing the foot pedal fully in position 3. If one feels that the emulsification is still difficult then a combination of torsional and traditional longitudinal is used to avoid occlusion of the handpiece tip. The problem may be caused by a large sheared-off piece obstructing the tip. The short repulsive effect of longitudinal ultrasound helps reposition the quadrant and facilitate the quadrant to be tumbled and emulsified without being lollipopped.

A programmed Torsional handpiece with a combination of 80% torsional oscillation and 20% traditional ultrasound is used for such hard cataracts. In other words, 80 msec is used for torsional and 20 msec for traditional.

SOFT CATARACTS

The absence of repulsion and efficient working at lower parameters has a double edged advantage in Soft Cataracts. In Torsional Emulsification, holding of a soft and thin plate of Nucleus can be efficiently managed.

In soft cataracts, there is a need to hold the soft nuclear piece with accurate fluidics and energy delivery. This becomes possible with OZiL while using lower machine parameters. The absence of repulsion makes the embedding and holding of a thin and softer plate of Nucleus piece easily possible.

In contrast in longitudinal Phaco, the delivery of energy associated with repulsion requires a somewhat thicker and harder nucleus plate to fully embed and hold the nucleus piece.

Posterior Polar Cataracts, Small Pupils, Floppy Iris Syndrome and Subluxated Cataracts

These difficult cataracts require low fluid dynamics settings which is mandatory for a successful outcome. A low aspiration flow of 20 ml/min or less and a low bottle height help to prevent vitreous or iris being caught by the phaco tip. A low vacuum setting of 250 mmHg with the low compliant FMS cassette of the Infiniti machine produces no significant surge flow on occlusion break. In other words, there is a stable chamber setting which is mandatory for such difficult cataracts.

These low parameters are not without problems. These settings do not provide sufficient holding power with traditional longitudinal ultrasound during quadrant removal. The settings would lead to repulsion and scattering of nuclear pieces in the anterior chamber. Therefore, a great deal of manipulation would be required which may result in increased risk of complications. With torsional ultrasound, however, followability and holding power, even with very low parameters, is still excellent. The level of control of the procedure is remarkable, enabling the surgeon to feel much more confident when handling such difficult cases.

Torsional Phaco is a truly revolutionary and futuristic technology. It is all set to replace traditional longitudinal phaco completely in the coming years. It qualifies the very essence of the term advancement. It is simple. It takes care of the shortcomings of the earlier longitudinal phacoemulsification. Torsional Phacoemulsification takes surgical skills to a different plane, increasing efficiency and safety while allowing the surgeon to remove a larger segment of cataract varieties with ease and confidence.

18

Pearls of Supracapsular Surgery Using the Tilt and Tumble Technique

Elizabeth A Davis , Richard L Lindstrom (USA)

Introduction

The technique of tilt and tumble is a modified form of supracapsular phacoemulsification. It uses a bimanual technique to tilt one pole of the nucleus above the anterior capsule. Phacoemulsification is then performed while supporting the lens in the iris plane with a nucleus rotator.

In the following paragraphs we will describe and illustrate this technique in enough detail to allow an ophthalmologist to perform it on his own.

Indications

The indications for the tilt and tumble phacoemulsification technique are quite broad. It can be utilized in either a large or small pupil situation. Some surgeons favor the technique with small pupils where the nucleus can be tilted up such that the equator is resting in the center of the pupil and is then carefully emulsified. It does require a larger continuous tear anterior capsulectomy of at least 5.0 mm. If a small anterior capsulectomy is created, the hydrodissection step of tilting the nucleus can be dangerous, and it is possible to rupture the posterior capsule during the hydrodissection step. If, inadvertently, a small anterior capsulectomy is created, it is probably safest to convert to an endocapsular phacoemulsification technique or enlarge the capsulorhexis. If it is not possible to tilt the nucleus with either hydrodissection or a manual technique, the surgeon should also convert to an endocapsular approach. Occasionally the entire nucleus will subluxate into the anterior chamber. In this setting if the cornea is healthy, the anterior chamber deep, and the nucleus soft, then the phacoemulsification can be completed in the anterior chamber supporting the nucleus away from the corneal endothelium. The nucleus can also be pushed back inferiorly over the capsular bag to allow the iris plane tilt and tumble technique to be completed.

In patients with severely compromised endothelium, such as Fuchs' dystrophy or previous keratoplasty patients with a low endothelial cell count, endocapsular phacoemulsification is preferred to reduce endothelial cell loss. In a normal eye, corneal clarity on the first day postoperatively is excellent. Nevertheless, the tilting and tumbling maneuvers do increase the chance of endothelial cell contact of lens material compared to an endocapsular phacoemulsification. Therefore, the endocapsular technique should not be employed in eyes with borderline corneas or shallow anterior chambers.

Preoperative Preparation

The patient enters the anesthesia induction or preoperative area and Tetracaine drops are placed in both eyes. The placement of these drops increases the patient

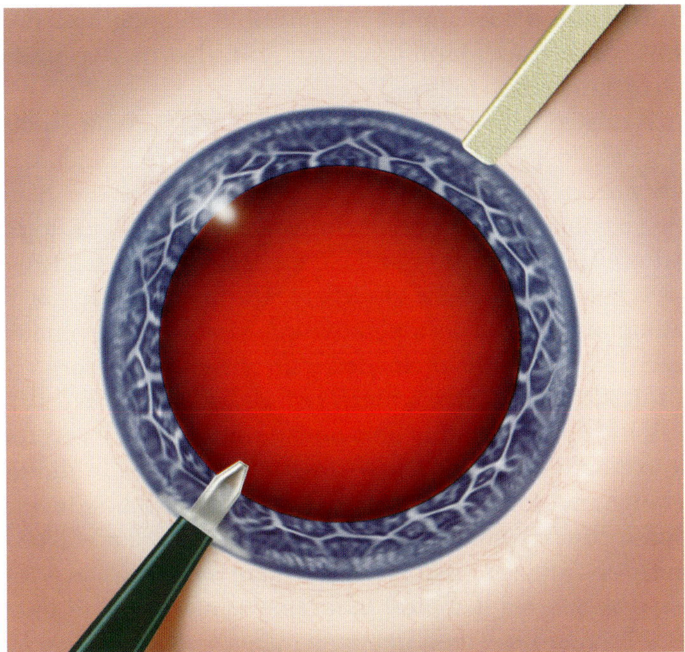

Fig. 1: Counterpuncture site of 1.0 mm is made with a diamond stab knife

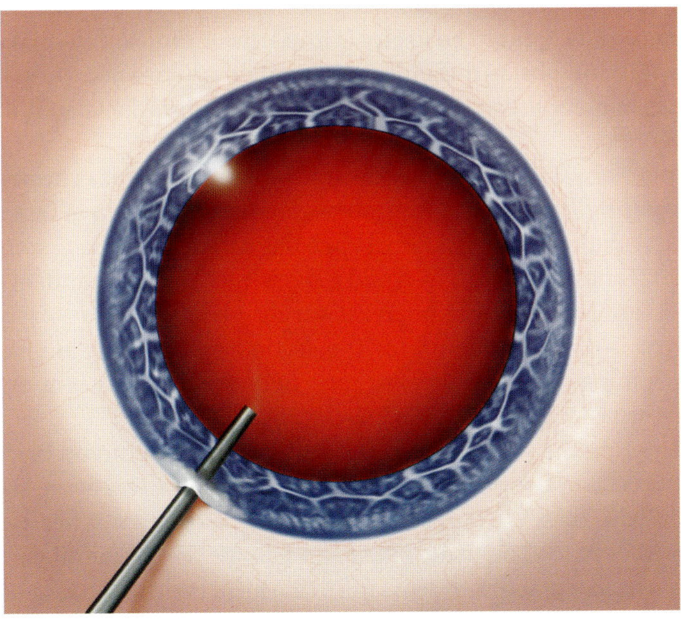

Fig. 2: Preservative-free xylocaine is injected intracamerally

comfort during the placement of the multiple dilating and preoperative medications, decreases blepharospasm and also increases the corneal penetration of the drops to follow.

The eye is dilated with 2.5% neosynephrine and 1% cyclopentolate every 5 minutes for three doses. Additionally, preoperative topical antibiotic and anti-inflammatory drops are administered at the same time as the dilating drops. We favor the combination of a preoperative topical antibiotic, topical steroid and topical nonsteroidal. The rationale for this is to preload the eye with antibiotic and nonsteroidal prior to surgery. The pharmacology of these drugs and the pathophysiology of postoperative infection and inflammation support this approach. An eye that is preloaded with anti-inflammatories prior to the surgical insult is likely to have a much reduced postoperative inflammatory response. Both topical steroids and nonsteroidals have been found to be synergistic in the reduction of postoperative inflammation. In addition, the use of perioperative antibiotics is supported in the literature as reducing the small chance of postoperative endophthalmitis. Since the patient will be sent home on the same drops utilized preoperatively, there is no additional cost.

Our usual anesthesia is topical tetracaine reinforced with intraoperative intracameral 1% non-preserved (methylparaben free) xylocaine. For patients with blepharospasm a "miniblock" O'Brien facial nerve anesthesia, utilizing 2% xylocaine with 150 units of hyaluronidase per 5 cc of xylocaine, can be quite helpful in reducing squeezing. This block lasts thirty to forty-five minutes and makes surgery easier for the patient and the surgeon. Patients are sedated prior to the block to eliminate any memory of discomfort. One way to determine when this facial nerve block might be useful is to ask the technicians to make a note in the chart when they have difficulty performing applanation pressures or A-scan because of blepharospasm. In these patients a mini-facial nerve block can be quite helpful.

In younger anxious patients and in those with difficulty cooperating, we perform a peribulbar block. Naturally, general anesthesia is used for very uncooperative patients and children. While this is controversial, in some patients where general anesthesia is chosen and a significant bilateral cataract is present, we will perform consecutive bilateral surgery completely re-prepping and starting with fresh instruments for the second eye. Again, this is a clinical decision weighing the risk to benefit ratio of operating both eyes on the same day versus the risk of two general anesthetics.

Upon entering the surgical suite the patient table is centered on pre-placed marks so that it is appropriately placed for microscope, surgeon, scrub nurse and anesthetist access. We favor a wrist rest, and the patient's head is adjusted such that a ruler placed on the forehead and cheek will be parallel to the floor. The patient's head is stabilized with tape to the head board to reduce unexpected movements, particularly if the patient falls asleep during the procedure and

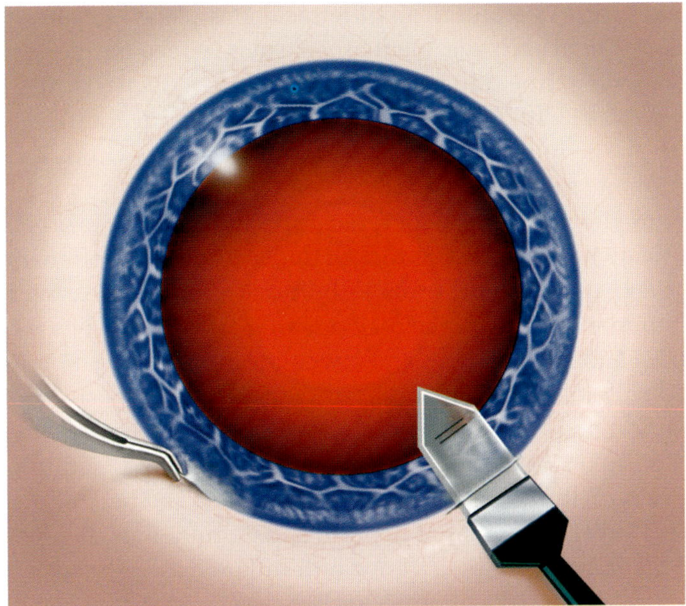

Fig. 3: A clear corneal incision is made temporally in right eyes and nasally in left eyes

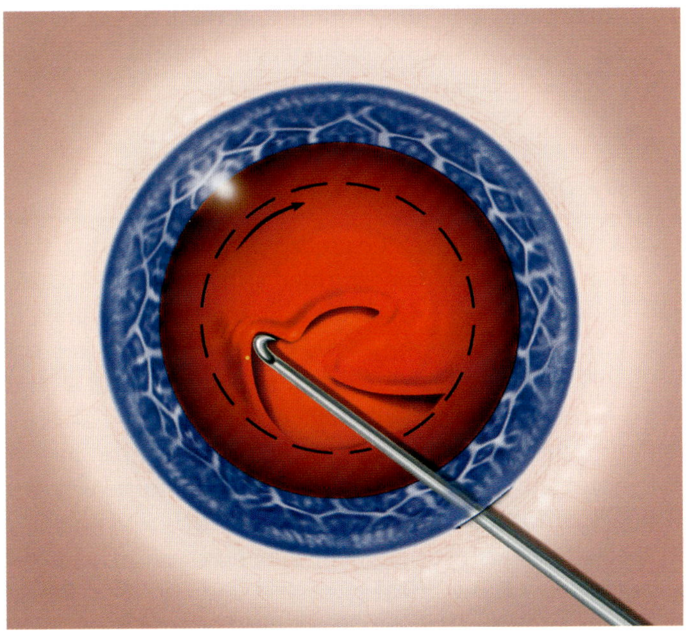

Fig. 4: A continuous curvilinear capsulotomy is made with a cystatome

suddenly awakens. A second drop of tetracaine is placed in each eye. If the tetracaine is placed in each eye, blepharospasm is reduced. A periocular prep with 5% povidone-iodine solution is completed. We do not irrigate the ocular surface and fornices with povidone-iodine. Under topical anesthesia we have found that the patients note a significant burning. If a few drops leak into the eye this is certainly acceptable.

An aperture drape is helpful for topical anesthesia to increase comfort. We have noted that when the drape is tucked under the lids this often irritates the patient's eye and also reduces the malleability of the lids, decreasing exposure. Since it is important to isolate the meibomian glands and lashes a Tegaderm adhesive cut in half for the upper and lower lids may be used.

Balanced salt solution is used in all cases. For the short duration of a phacoemulsification case, BSS plus does not provide any clinically meaningful benefit. We place 0.5 cc of the intracardiac non-preserved (sodium bisulfate free) epinephrine in the bottle for assistance in dilation and perhaps hemostasis. We also add 1 ml (1,000 units) of heparin sulfate to reduce the possibility of postoperative fibrin. This is also a good anti-inflammatory and coating agent. At this dose there is no risk of enhancing bleeding or reducing hemostasis.

The lids are separated with a Lindstrom/Chu aspirating speculum (Rhein Medical). A final drop of tetracaine is placed in the operative eye or the surface is irrigated with the non-preserved xylocaine. We do not like to utilize more than three drops of tetracaine or other topical anesthetic as excess softening of the epithelium can occur, resulting in punctate epithelial keratitis, corneal erosion and delayed postoperative rehabilitation.

Operative Procedure

The patient is asked to look down. The globe is supported with a dry Merocel sponge, and a counter puncture is performed superiorly at 12 o'clock with a diamond stab knife. (Osher/Storz) The incision is about 1 mm in length. Approximately 0.25 ml of 1% non-preserved methylparaben free xylocaine is injected into the eye. We advise the patient that they will feel a "tingling" or "burning" for a second, and then "the eye will go numb". This provides a psychological support for the patient that they will now have a totally anesthetized eye and should not anticipate any discomfort. We tell them that while they will feel some touch and fluid on the eye, they will not feel anything sharp, and if they do, we can supplement the anesthesia. This injection also firms up the eye for the clear corneal incision. We do not find it necessary to inject viscoelastic prior to constructing the corneal wound.

We perform a temporal or nasal anterior limbal or posterior clear corneal incision. Care is taken not to incise the conjunctiva as this can result in ballooning during phacoemulsification and irrigation aspiration. Some surgeons define

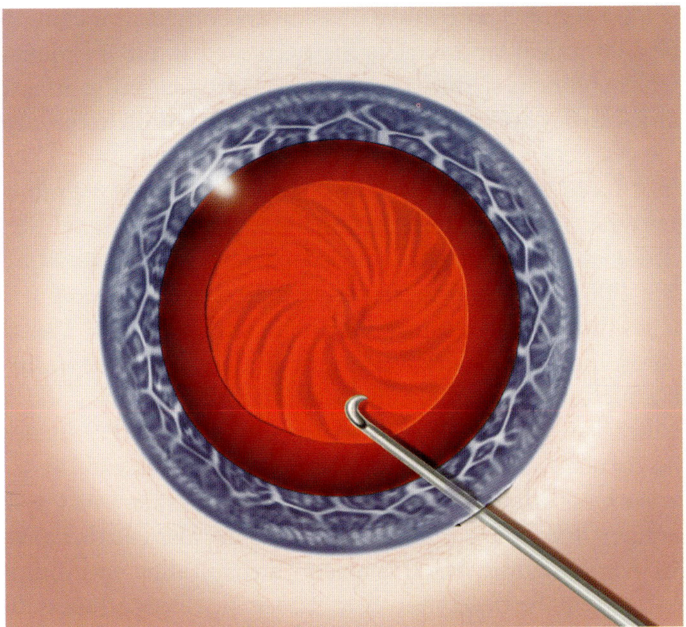

Fig. 5: The capsulotomy is optimally 5.0 to 6.0 mm in diameter

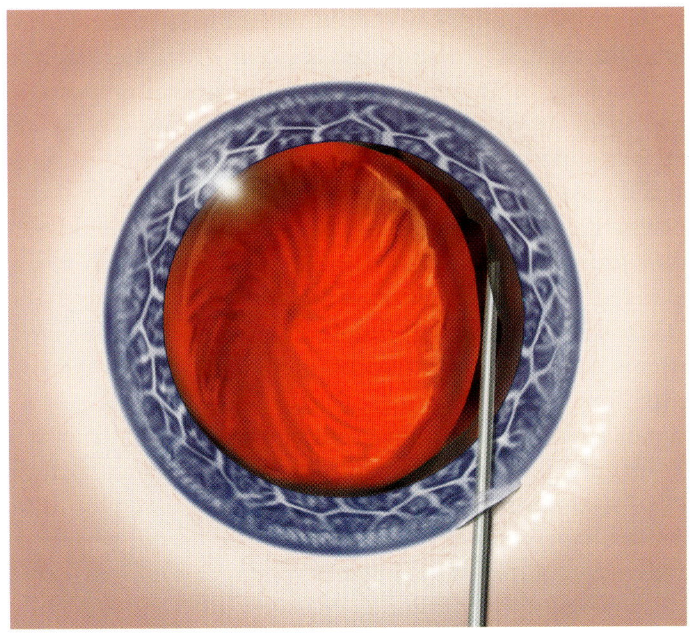

Fig. 6: Continuous slow hydrodissection leads to tilting of the nucleus out of the bag

this as being a posterior clear corneal incision and others as an anterior limbal incision. The anatomical landmark is the perilimbal capillary plexus and the insertion of the conjunctiva. Since the incision is into a vascular area, long-term wound healing can be expected to be stronger than it is with a true clear corneal incision. True clear corneal incisions, such as performed in radial keratotomy, clearly do not have the wound healing capabilities that a limbal incision demonstrates where there are functioning blood vessels present.

The anterior chamber is then entered parallel to the iris at a depth of approximately 300 microns. This creates a hinge type of incision.

In right eyes the incision is temporal, and in left eyes, nasal. This allows the surgeon to sit in the same position for right and left eyes. The nasal cornea is thicker, has a higher endothelial cell count and allows very good access for phacoemulsification. The nasal limbus is approximately 0.3 mm closer to the center of the cornea than the temporal limbus, and this can, in some cases where there is excess edema, reduce first day postoperative vision more than one might anticipate with a temporal incision. There also can, in some patients, be pooling of irrigating fluid. For this reason, an aspirating speculum is useful. It is also helpful to tip the head slightly to the left side. Nonetheless, in left eyes a nasal clear corneal approach is an excellent option, particularly for surgeons who find the left temporal position uncomfortable.

In some patients it may be safest to create a corneal scleral incision. Examples of these include patients who have had a previous radial keratotomy or demonstrate findings of peripheral corneal ulcerative keratitis, in some patients with very low endothelial cell counts, and any case where there is any significant peripheral pathology or thinning. The anterior limbal or posterior corneal incision described above can be made temporally, nasally, in the oblique meridian or even superiorly without induction of significant corneal edema or endothelial cell loss.

The incision, if 3 mm in length, tends to cause an induction of 0.25 ± 0.25 diopters of astigmatism. If it is placed on the steeper meridian, it can therefore be expected to reduce the astigmatism somewhere between 0 and 0.50 diopters. An incision in the 3 mm range will almost always be self sealing. With modern injector systems most foldable intraocular lenses can be implanted through a 3 mm anterior limbal incision.

In select patients an intraoperative astigmatic keratotomy can be performed at the 7 to 8 mm optical zone. This can be done at the beginning of the operation. The patient's astigmatism axis is marked carefully using an intraoperative surgical keratometer which allows one to delineate the steeper and flatter meridian and not be concerned about globe rotation. One 2 mm incision at a 7 to 8 mm optical zone will correct 1 diopter of astigmatism and two 2 mm incisions will correct 2 diopters of astigmatism in a cataract age patient. One 3 mm incision will correct 2 diopters, and two 3 mm incision 4 diopters. One can combine a

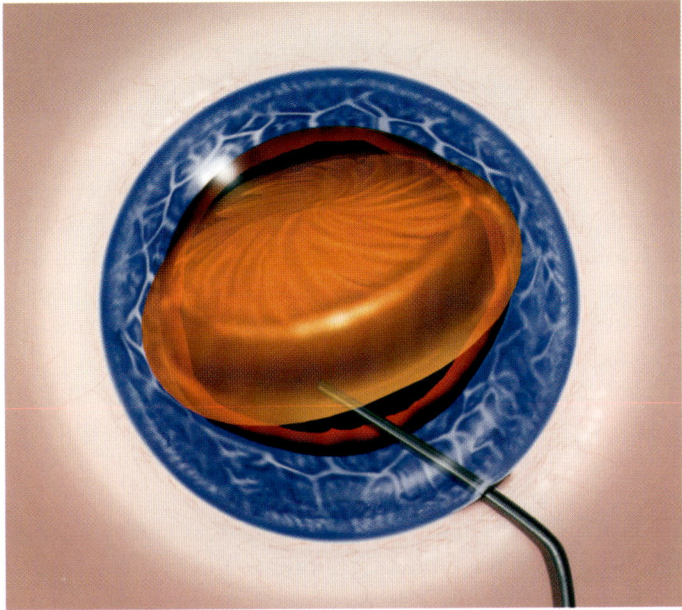

Fig. 7: The nucleus is rotated to face the incision

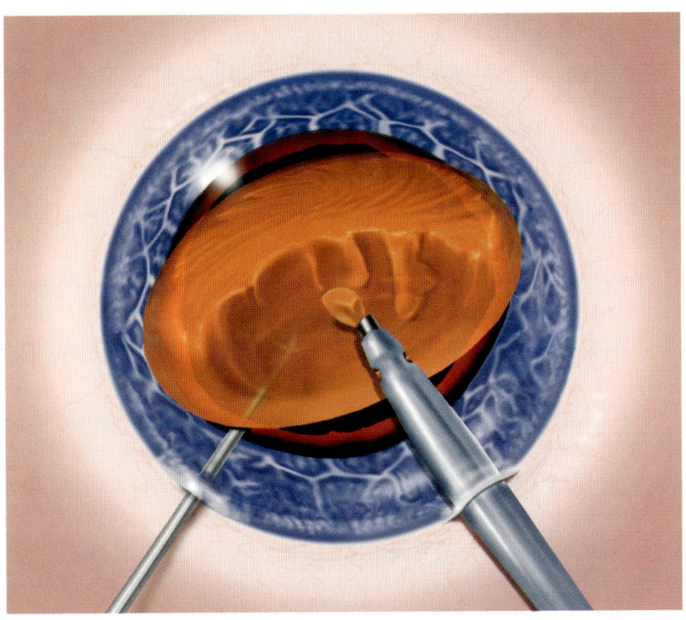

Fig. 8: The nucleus is supported during phacoemulsification with a second instrument

3 mm and 2 mm correcting 3 diopters. Larger amounts of astigmatism can also be corrected utilizing the Arc-T nomogram. Depending on the age of the patient one can correct up to 8 diopters of astigmatism with two 90° arcs. Many surgeons have moved to a more peripheral corneal limbal arcuate incision, but we favor the 7 - 8 mm optical zone because of years of experience with this approach. There certainly is a variation in response, but there have not been any significant induced complications with this approach. The outcome goal is 1 diopter or less of astigmatism in the preoperative axis. It is preferable to under-correct rather than over-correct. The key in astigmatism surgery is "axis, axis, axis". If one is not careful in preoperative planning and the incision are placed more than 15° off axis, one is better avoiding this approach.

The anterior chamber is constituted with a viscoelastic. Our studies have not found any significant difference between one viscoelastic or another in regards to postoperative endothelial cell counts. Amvisc Plus works well and we can obtain 0.8 cc of it at a very fair price.

Next a relatively large diameter continuous tear anterior capsulectomy is fashioned. This can be made with a cystatome or forceps. The optimal size is 5.0 to 6.0 mm in diameter and inside the insertion of the zonules (usually at 7 millimeters). Larger is better than smaller, as there is less subcapsular epithelium and thus lower risk of capsular opacification. Additionally, a larger capsulorhexis makes for an easier cataract operation. With this technique there has not been any change in the incidence of intraocular lens decentration. With some intraocular lenses the capsule will seal down to the posterior capsule around the loops rather than be symmetrically placed over the anterior surface of the intraocular lens. These eyes do extremely well and this might be preferable to having the capsule anterior to the optic. This is also certainly a controversial position.

Hydrodissection is then performed utilizing a Pearce hydrodissection cannula on a 3 cc syringe filled with BSS. Slow continuous hydrodissection is performed gently lifting the anterior capsular rim until a fluid wave is seen. At this point irrigation is continued until the nucleus tilts on one side, up and out of the capsular bag. If one retracts the capsule at approximately the 7:30 O'clock position with the hydrodissection cannula, usually the nucleus will tilt superiorly. If it tilts in another position, it is simply rotated until it is facing the incision.

Once the nucleus it tilted some additional viscoelastic can be injected under the nucleus pushing the iris and capsule back. Also, additional viscoelastic can be placed over the nuclear edge to protect the endothelium. The nucleus is emulsified from outside-in while supporting the nucleus in the iris plane with a second instrument, such as a Rhein Medical or Storz Lindstrom Star or Lindstrom Trident nucleus rotator. Once half the nucleus is removed, the remaining one half is tumbled upside-down and approached from the opposite

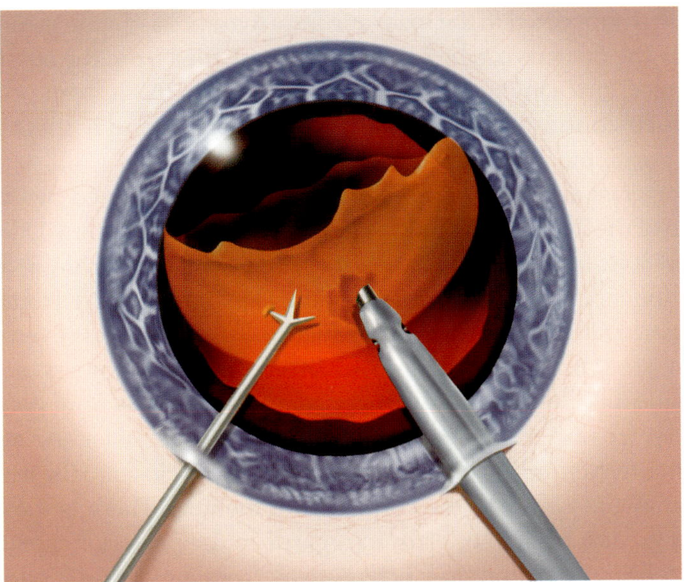

Fig. 9: The second half of the nucleus is tumbled upside down

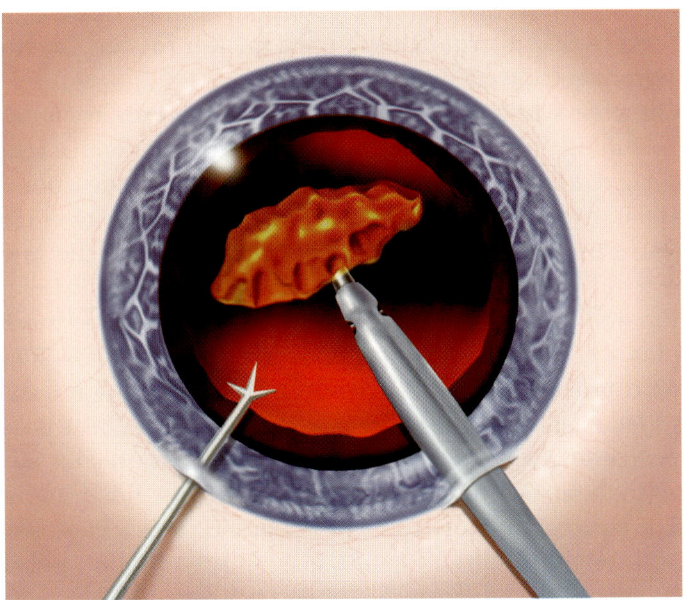

Fig. 10: Emulsification is completed in the iris plane

pole. Again, it is supported in the iris plane until the emulsification is completed. Alternatively the nucleus can be rotated and emulsified from the outside edge in, in a carousel or cartwheel type of technique. Finally, in some cases, the nucleus can be continuously emulsified in the iris plane if there is good followability until the entire nucleus is gone.

This a very fast and very safe technique, and as mentioned before, it is a modification of the iris plane technique taught by Richard Kratz, MD in the late 1970's and 1980's. It is basically "back to Kratz" with help from Brown and Maloney in the modern phacoemulsification, capsulorhexis, hydrodissection and viscoelastic era. Surgery times now range between four and seven minutes with this approach rather than ten to fifteen minutes for endocapsular phacoemulsification. In addition, our capsular tear rate has now gone under 1%. Therefore, we find this technique which to be easier, faster and safer. It is true that in this technique the phacoemulsification tip is closer to the iris margin and also somewhat closer to the corneal endothelium. There is, however, a significantly greater margin of error in regards to the posterior capsule. Care needs to be taken to position the nucleus away from the corneal endothelium and away from the iris margin when utilizing this approach.

If the nucleus does not tilt with simple hydrodissection, it can be tilted with viscoelastic or a second instrument such as a nuclear rotator, Graether collar button or hydrodissection cannula.

The dual function Bausch and Lomb Millennium ™ is excellent for all cataract techniques including "tilt and tumble." The vacuum is set with a range of 325 to 400 mm of Hg and the ultrasound power set in a pulse mode from 10 to 30%. The foot pedal is arranged such that there is surgeon control over ultrasound on the vertical or pitch motion of the foot pedal, and then on the yaw or right motion foot pedal, there will be vacuum control. This allows very efficient emulsification, and the Millennium ™ is currently our preferred machine. The microflow plus needle with a 30° angle tip works well with the Millennium.

Following completion of nuclear removal, the cortex is removed with the irrigation aspiration hand piece. We prefer a 0.3 mm tip and utilize the universal hand piece with interchangeable tips. A curvilinear tip is used for most cortex removal. Sub-incisional cortex can be aspirated with a Lindstrom right angle sand blasted tip currently manufactured by Rhein and Storz. If there is significant debris or plaque on the posterior capsule, one can attempt some polishing and vacuum cleaning but not so aggressively as to risk capsular tears.

The anterior chamber is reconstituted with viscoelastic and the intraocular lens is inserted utilizing an injector system.

Excess viscoelastic is removed with irrigation aspiration. Pushing back on the intraocular lens and slowly turn the irrigation aspiration to the right and left two or three times allows a fairly complete removal of viscoelastic under the intraocular lens.

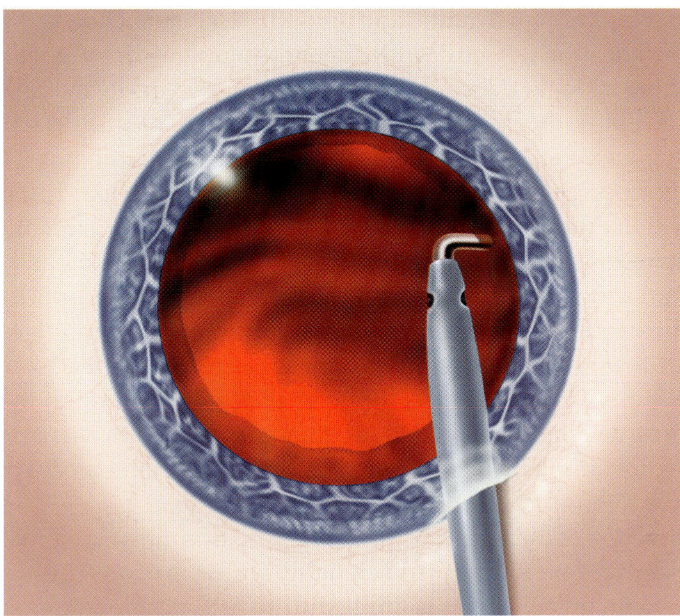

Fig. 11: Subincisional cortex is removed with a right-angled tip

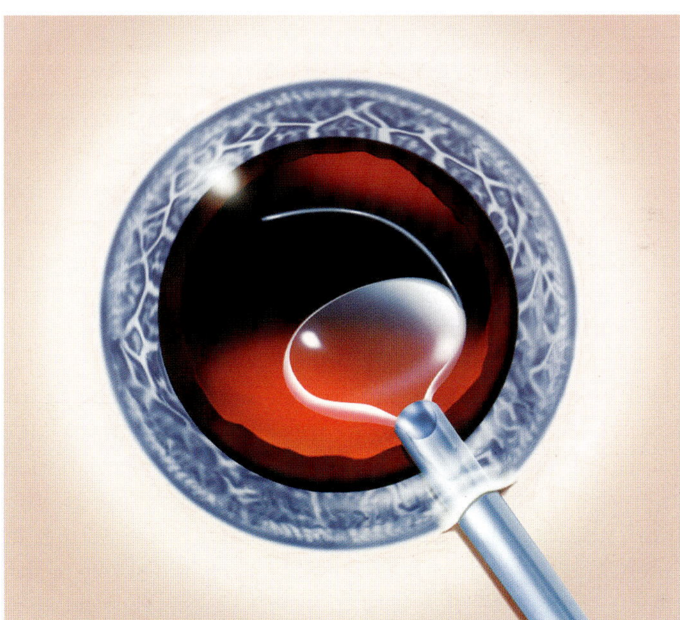

Fig. 12: The intraocular lens is inserted with an injector system

We favor injection of a miotic and tend to prefer carbachol over miochol at this time, as it is more effective in reducing postoperative intraocular tension spikes and has a longer duration of action. It is best to dilute the carbachol 5 to 1, or one can obtain an excessively small pupil which results in dark vision for the patient at night for one to two days. The anterior chamber is then refilled through the counter-puncture and the incision is inspected. If the chamber remains well constituted and there is no spontaneous leak from the incision, wound hydration is not necessary. If there is some shallowing in the anterior chamber and a spontaneous leak, wound hydration is performed by injecting BSS peripherally into the incision and hydrating it to push the edges together. We suspect that within a few minutes these clear corneal or posterior limbal incisions seal, much as a LASIK flap will stick down, through the negative swelling pressure of the cornea and capillary action. It is important to leave the eye slightly firm at 20 mm of Hg or so to reduce the side effects of hypotony and also help the internal valve incision appropriately seal.

At completion of the procedure another drop of antibiotic, steroid and non-steroidal, is placed on the eye. Additionally, one drop of an anti-hypertensive such as Betagan or Alphagan is applied to reduce postoperative intraocular tension spikes.

Postoperative Care

No patch is routinely utilized for the topical and intracameral approach. If a mini-block of the lids has been performed, this will wear off in thirty to forty-five minutes, and there is usually adequate lid function for a normal blink at the completion of the procedure. Patients are advised that they will have some erythropsia, meaning they will see a pink after image for the rest of the day, but usually this will resolve by the next morning. They are also told that their vision may be a little dark at night from the miotic, and not to be concerned if they wake up at night and their vision seems dimmer.

The patient is seen on the first day postoperative and then at approximately two to three weeks postoperative. At this time a refraction, slit lamp, and funduscopic examination is performed. If there is no inflammation, patients are seen again one year postoperative. If at three weeks there is still persistent inflammation, additional postoperative anti-inflammatory medications are recommended, and the patient is asked to return again at two to three months postoperative.

Topical antibiotic, steroid and non-steroidal, are utilized twice a day, usually requiring a 5 cc bottle and three to four weeks of therapy. Occasionally a second bottle of steroid and non-steroidal is necessary if flare and cell persist at the three week examination. There are minimal restrictions, including a request that there be no swimming and no very heavy lifting for two weeks. We consider

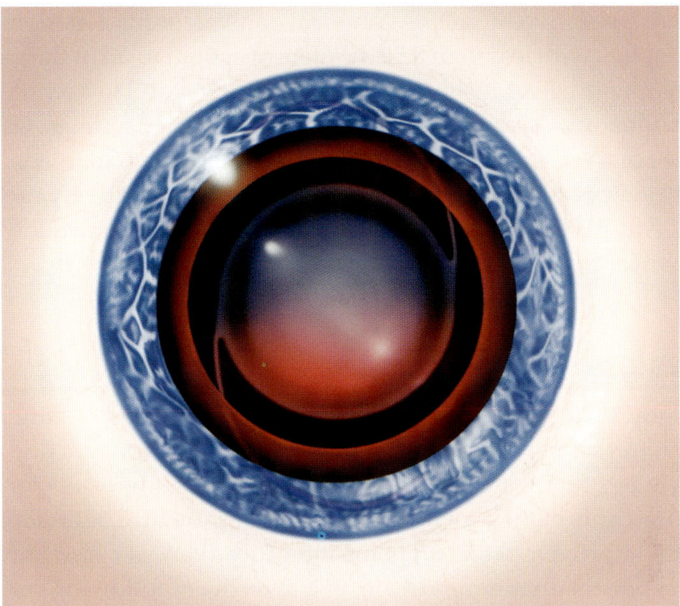

Fig. 13: The lens is centered in the capsular bag

the ideal postoperative refractive spherical equivalent for a monofocal lens to be –0.62 diopters with less than 0.50 diopters of astigmatism in the same axis as existed preoperatively. Most patients can see 20/30+ and J3+ with this type of correction. Monovision can be utilized in the appropriate settings. Good results can also be obtained accommodating or multifocal intraocular lens.

The second eye is done at 2 weeks or greater postoperatively except in rare situations. Any YAG lasers are deferred for 90 days in order to allow the blood aqueous barrier to become intact and capsular fixation to be firm.

Conclusion

We hope other surgeons will find this approach to cataract surgery useful. These techniques must be personalized, and every surgeon will find that slight variations in technique are required to achieve optimum results for their own individual patients in their own individual environment. Continuous efforts at incremental improvement result in meaningful advances in our ability to help the cataract patient obtain rapid, safe, visual recovery following surgery.

19

Small Pupil Phaco: An Innovative Technique

Boris Malyugin (Russia)

Introduction

In spite of several recent innovations in cataract surgery patients with small pupils are always challenging.

Poor pupil dilation we can be observed in cases complicated by pseudo-exfoliation syndrome, uveitis, posterior synechiae, trauma or previous intraocular surgery.

Significant amount of patients who present for phacoemulsification cataract surgery have pupils that do not respond adequately despite several pharmacological attempts with different mydriatic agents. Inadequate pupil dilation can decrease visualization during all stages of the phacoemulsification including capsulorhexis, hydrodissection, lens nucleus disassembly and IOL insertion. This compromises the surgery and increases the risk for complications.

Pharmacological therapy with the use of nonsteroidal eyedrops or strong mydriatics such as phenylephrine 10% sometimes lead to unwanted ocular and systemic side effects. Intracameral mydriatics is an effective, and safe addition to topical mydriatics in phacoemulsification. In some cases their use can simplify preoperative patients preparation and in certain high-risk groups, may reduce the risk for cardiovascular side effects.

Unfortunately present pharmacological approaches of managing a small pupil during cataract surgery have limitations. Most surgeons decide to dilate the pupil mechanically at the time of the surgery if pharmacological agents fail.

There is no general recommendation or solution to the small pupil problem because the strategies for pupil enlargement greatly depend on surgeon skill and preferences, as well as on intraoperative situation. There are four main dilation methods: the first is the synechiolysis, the second is mechanical stretching, the third is the cutting method and the fourth is the iris retraction.

In the first method the surgeon separates the adhesions between the iris, the lens capsule and/or the cornea. The technique of pupillary membranectomy with the forceps presented by R.Osher is also effective in some cases.

The second method—mechanical stretching of the pupil was introduced by Miller and Keener. It is usually effective for small pupils with the rigid iris tissue which is usually caused by prior miotic use, pseudoexfoliation, or posterior synechiae. Stretching can be achieved with the spatula, Sinskey hook or special instrument—Beehler pupil dilator. Usually a pair of hooks is introduced through 2 stab incisions in the cornea engage the iris sphincter. After that the hooks are pulled in opposite directions. This maneuver creates microscopic sphincter tears which enlarge the pupil aperture. The main advantage of this procedure is that it is relatively simple and requires no special instruments. Mechanical stretching of the pupil usually provides sufficient access to the lens and maintains the pupil diameter intraoperatively.

Sometimes iris stretching technique leads to instability of its papillary margin, which can compromise cataract surgery. In some eyes and stretching

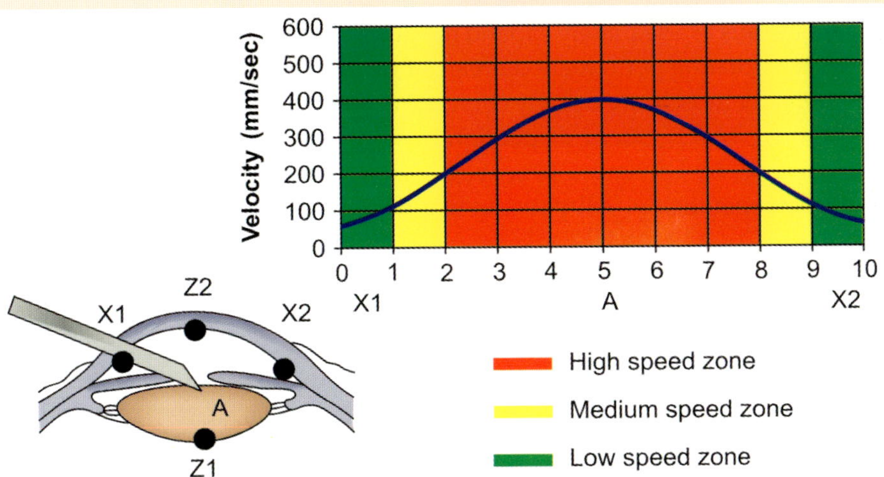

Fig. 1: Fluid velocity distribution along the line connecting the opposite points of the anterior chamber angle (X1 – X2) in case of US handpiece location in the middle of the anterior chamber at the iris plane

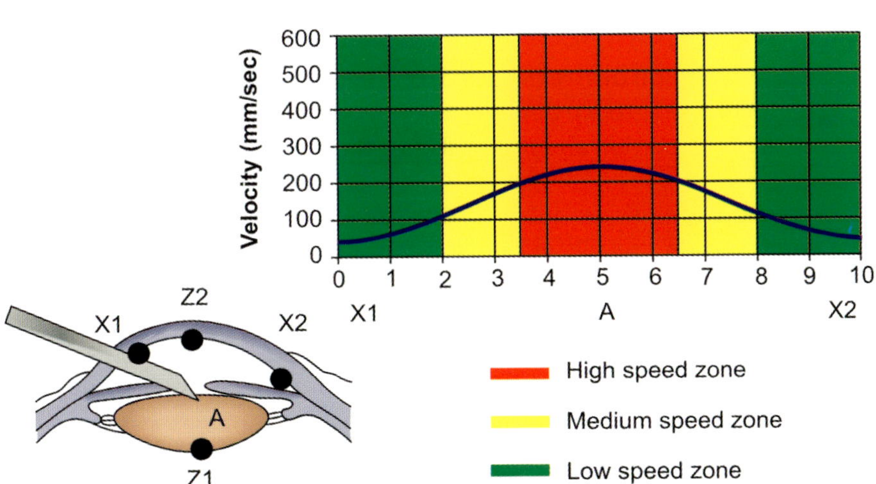

Fig. 2: Fluid velocity distribution along the line connecting the opposite points of the anterior chamber angle (X1 – X2) in case of US handpiece location in the middle of the lens nucleus

technique fails to adequately expand the pupil. The drawback of this technique is that it is creating permanent damage of the iris sphincter. The micro tears of the sphincter muscle are usually clinically asymptomatic but sometimes result in bleeding and pigment dispersion postoperatively. In a study of stretch pupilloplasty by Dinsmore 10% of 50 patients developed an enlarged atonic pupil postoperatively. All patients had a history of injury or inflammatory disease.

Partial-thickness iris sphincter cuts made with micro scissors is a common pupil enlargement technique. The cutting method is more controlled but requires multiple maneuvers of the scissors inside the anterior chamber which can result in corneal endothelial damage. The disadvantages are the same as those with the stretching method.

Suboptimal pupil dilation in response to the preoperative mydriatic protocols and minimal efficacy of pupil stretching techniques is a usual indication to the intraoperative use of iris hooks or other mechanical pupil dilation devices. For the iris retraction several devices have been introduced in the clinical practice. The main disadvantages of these devices include the bulkiness and rigidity. They are difficult to insert, remove, and manipulate through a small incision.

Graether developed a pupil expander that according to his data is superior to other methods of pupil enlargement, causing less sphincter trauma and fewer cases of permanent pupil size alteration. Pupil dilation technique with the hydrogel ring reported by Siepser has a potential benefits but very limited clinical use. The Perfect Pupil device (Milvella) is a disposable polyurethane ring with the 0.24 mm flanged groove throughout the length of the ring and an integrated arm that allows insertion and removal from the anterior chamber at the end of surgery.

Retracting the iris tissue rather than cutting it as in a classic sector iridectomy is much simpler and results in a much better postoperative pupil appearance. Mackool was the first one who described a 4-point iris retractor configuration for phacoemulsification. He developed metal iris retractors connected to small blocks of titanium. The latter allows for stabilization of the hooks during the retraction of the iris. This method was enhanced with the introduction of the flexible iris retractor by de Juan and Hickingbotham.

Traditionally, 4 evenly spaced retractors are placed through limbal paracentheses 90 degrees apart from one another. The corneal incision is centered on 1 of the 4 sides of the square. Some surgeons use iris retractors in a triangular pattern decreasing the number of additional corneal incisions. The use of the iris hooks may lead to the damage of the pupillary margin intraoperatively producing a semimydriatic nonreacting pupil postoperatively.

Modification of the original square retractor configuration is Oetting and Omphroy. The rotation of the square improves lens access in clear corneal phacoemulsification by orienting the phacoemulsification needle along the

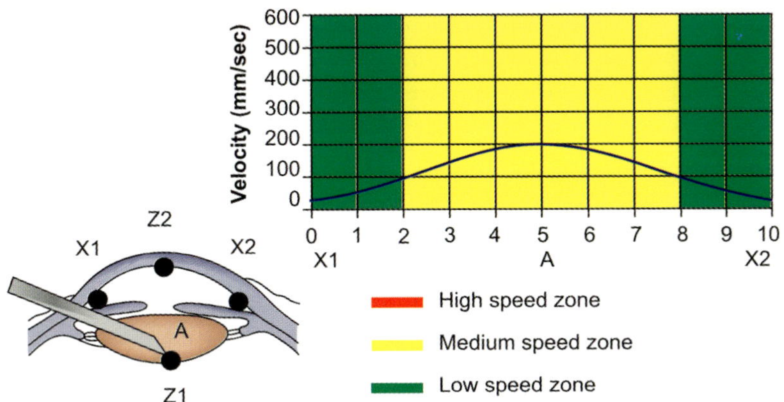

Fig. 3: Fluid velocity distribution along the line connecting the opposite points of the anterior chamber angle (X1 – X2) in case of US headpiece location close to the center of the posterior capsule

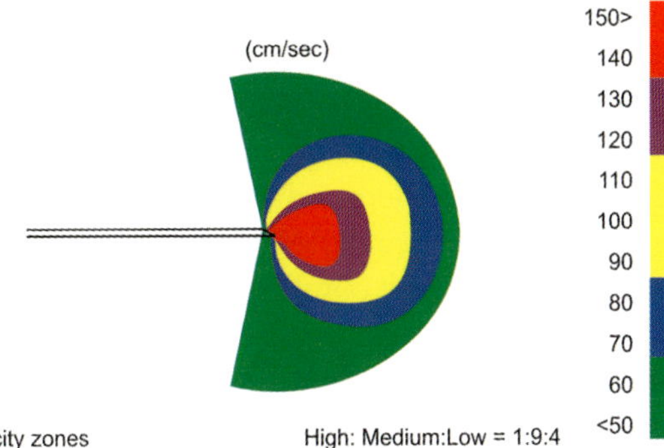

Fig. 4: Fluid velocity distribution around the tip of the US handpiece

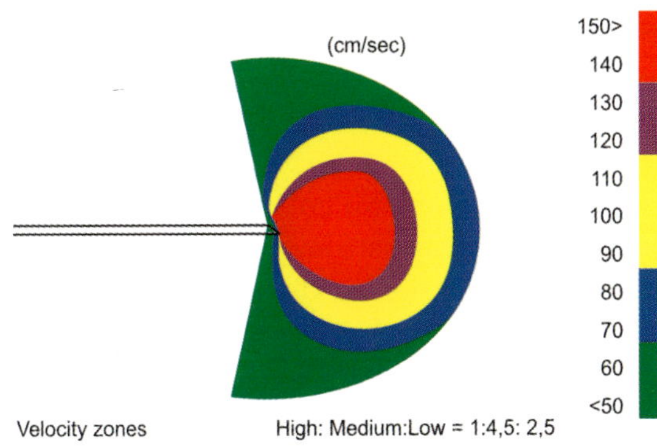

Fig. 5: Fluid velocity distribution around the tip of irrigating-aspirating handpiece

diagonal. This was called by Dupps and Oetting "diamond configuration" of retractors. Advantages of this technique include ease of conversion from phacoemulsification, optimal orientation of the maximum pupil diameter nucleus expression or intracapsular lens removal, and conservation of iris tissue.

Birhall assessed the effect on pupil shape and circumference of various flexible iris hook positions. He confirmed that malpositioned iris hooks may increase pupil stretching with possible deleterious effects on postoperative pupil function. He recommends using additional fifth hook to create a pentagonal pupil that reduces pupil stretching by 17%.

Masket and Yuguchi and coauthors recommends the pupil not be stretched by the hooks to larger than a 5.0 mm square because overstretching produces irregular atonic pupils postoperatively. Novak suggests the use of hooks with rigid pupils smaller than 3.0 mm (4.0 mm with a hard nucleus) and smaller than 4.0 to 5.0 mm for an inexperienced surgeon. In extremely small and rigid pupils he prefers combining the use of hooks with a radial sphincterotomy.

During engagement of the pupillary edge with the iris hook, it may catch and damage the capsule, leading to an anterior capsule tear that may extend to the periphery. To avoid this problem, a drop of viscoelastic material should be injected between the iris and the capsule before the hook is inserted. The other useful technique is to keep the hook parallel to the iris plane during the insertion and to tilt it slightly posterior right near the pupillary edge to engage the iris only. The iris hooks may become loosened during surgery. Their tips may become dislocated, no longer holding the pupillary edge. This can cause some problems including iris aspiration and chafing from contact with the phacoemulsification needle.

Small degrees of pupil dysfunction are common place after cataract surgery with and without iris manipulation but usually this causes no subjective symptoms. Halpern and coauthors found an incidence of postoperative atonic pupil of 1.1% after phacoemulsification, with pupil diameters ranging from 6.0 to 8.0 mm.

Most of the surgical maneuvers for enlarging the pupil and preventing its intraoperative constriction are not safe enough. They can lead to an increased risk of iris sphincter tear, bleeding, iris damage, posterior capsule tears, and loss of the vitreous body. The postoperative complications can include an atonic pupil of irregular shape with poor cosmetic result, and photophobia.

The rate of occurrence of iris prolapse has been reported between 0.3% and 1% in complicated cataract cases. Allan described one of the critical factors of iris prolapse during phaco which relates to fluid velocity. Allan's model considers the Bernoulli principle as the most important because when the velocity of fluid passing through the anterior chamber increases, the force exerted on the iris increases by the square of the velocity.

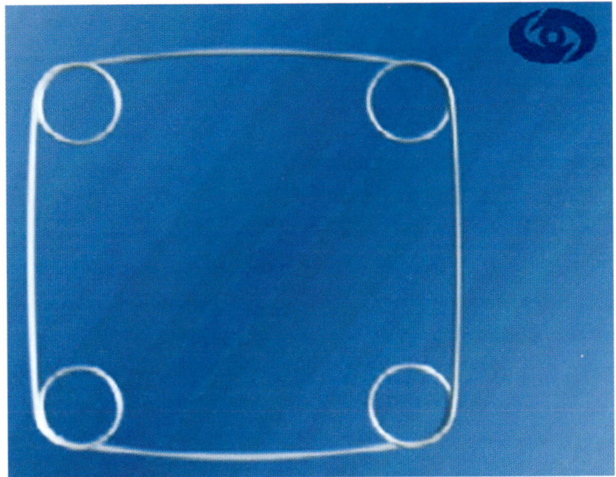

Fig. 6: The general view of IQ-ring

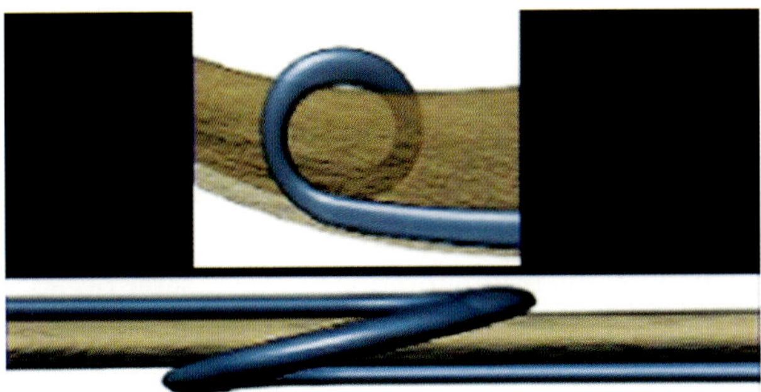

Fig. 7: The principle of iris pupillary margin fixation with the curl of IQ-ring

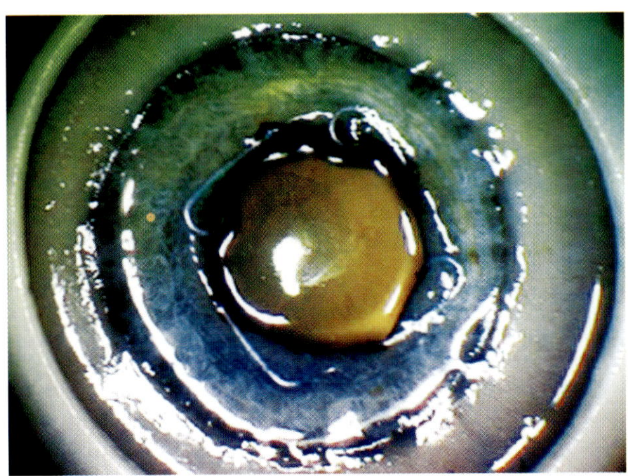

Fig. 8: IQ-ring implantation in the cadaver eye

We calculated the speed of the emulsion in the anterior chamber during the phaco procedure with the Millenium CCS (Bausch and Lomb) for US handpiece settings: 1.0 mm Microflow US needle, vacuum 300 mm Hg, bottle height 85 cm, and I/A handpiece settings: coaxial handpiece, 0.3 mm opening, vacuum 550 mm Hg, bottle height 90 cm. For the calculation we utilized the equation of Navie-Stocks. The calculations were performed for the two positions of the handpiece: in the center of the anterior chamber at the iris plane in the middle of the capsular bag and close to the center of the posterior capsule.

Figures represent the color coded map of fluid velocity distribution around the US and irrigating-aspirating handpiece. The areas of the highest currents are located in the angle of 40 to 60 degrees with the apex at the end of the aspiration orifice. Three zones of high (more than 120 cm/sec) medium (80-120 cm/sec) and low (80-cm/sec) fluid velocities are represented.

The pupil often dilates poorly in atrophic irises, with significantly decreased iris tone unable to withstand the fluidic currents in the anterior chamber and maintain the correct position of the iris. These calculations give us some conclusions. In small pupil iris tissue is located closer to the zone of the high fluidic currents that is why it is more likely to be aspirated into the US or IA handpiece. Decreasing of flow parameters is an important factor of preventing iris damage during phacoemulsification. Not only reducing the flow can make an appreciable difference in these cases, but also central positioning and minimal movements of the handpiece are also important to prevent iris damage. Endocapsular lens nucleus fragmentation is much safer because the areas of the highest fluidics currents are located inside the capsular bag away from the corneal endothelium and iris.

Chang and Campbell recently described the intraoperative floppy-iris syndrome (IFIS) associated with systemic administration of the α-1A antagonist tamsulosin (Flomax). The intraoperative diagnostic triad of this symptom is fluttering and billowing of the iris stroma, a tendency to iris prolapse through the main and/or side-port incisions, and progressive constriction of the pupil during surgery. Stretching of the pupil is ineffective in IFIS because the iris pupil margin remains elastic and the pupil immediately snaps back to its original size following attempts at stretching it.

Viscomydriasis with high viscosity OVDs such as Healon5 are very useful in small pupil phaco cases. S.Arshinoff described a technique using ophthalmic viscosurgical devices to perform cataract surgery in patients taking tamsulosin. This method uses a combination of the two OVDs. The lower-viscosity dispersive OVD which is highly retentive despite the presence of moderate fluid turbulence is injected in the periphery of the anterior chamber and covers the endothelial layer and the iris. The viscoadaptive central layer of Healon5, according to S.Arshinoff adds a relatively rigid OVD roof above the surgical space and adds rigidity to the OVD structure to keep the iris from moving and the Viscoat in

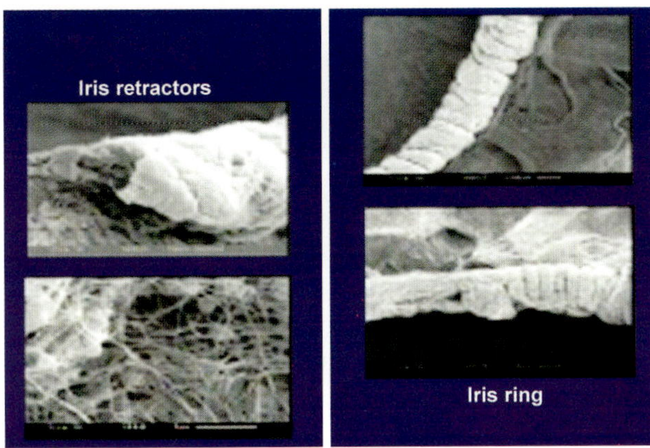

Fig. 9: Scanning electronic microscopy of the pupillary margin of the cadaver eye after implantation of the IQ-ring and conventional iris hooks

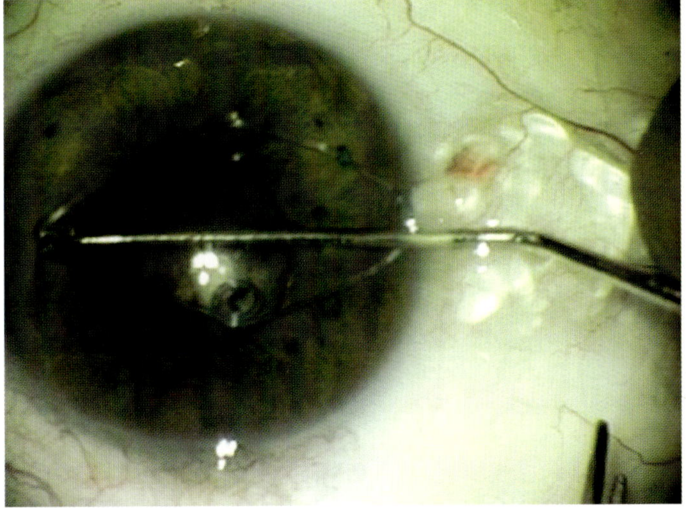

Fig. 10: IQ-ring is inserted through the main clear corneal incision

place. The BSS layer just over the pupillary space and below viscoadaptive central layer provides working space for the phaco tip. The surgeon is working in the endocapsular space and Healon5 is not attracted into the phaco tip and the OVD shell structure remains intact throughout the case. This technique gives satisfactory iris stability and permits uneventful surgery.

Cataract surgery in cases of iridoschisis may result in aspiration of iris fibers flowing in the anterior chamber. In these cases stretching the iris with various instruments or dilating the pupil with iris retractors may not prevent the danger contact of US needle with the iris tissue and aspiration of fibers.

Intraoperative iris manipulations may lead to severe postoperative fibrinoid reaction especially in eyes with pseudoexfoliation syndrome, chronic uveitis, glaucoma or diabetes. That is why cataract surgery in the presence of a small pupil remains one of the most difficult and challenging cases.

IQ-ring

"To enhance phaco surgery in complicated small-pupil cases we designed the new device which was called IQ-ring. It is used in cases of pupil miosis refractory to dilation protocols. The device is a square, O-shaped, temporary implant with four circular curls that holds the iris at equidistant points. One-piece design with the curls at each angle of the ring provides balanced stretching and gentle holding of the iris tissue. The main principle of iris pupillary margin fixation with the curl is represented on Figure."

The insertion of IQ-ring is carried out through the main incision. The pupil expander is positioned centrally and gently pushed at each angle with the help of a Sinskey hook to trap the iris in the four curls. Once in place, the ring expands the pupillary opening to 6.0 mm. The IQ-ring provides stable mydriasis with no trauma to the iris tissue and no need for additional paracentesis. It retracts the iris away from the flow currents and thus helps to prevent its incarceration into the US and I/A handpieces. As the result of the IQ-ring implantation we obtain a square, 6 mm pupil dilation that allows for safe and comfortable maneuvers during phacoemulsification.

The ring is usually inserted at the beginning of the phaco procedure through an unenlarged 2.8 mm clear corneal incision into the pupillary aperture. The surgeon can control the iris without significant changes of his accustomed technique.The capsulorhexis, hydrodissection, phacoemulsification, and injection of the intraocular lens are performed through the expanded pupil with the device in place. In case of necessity the ring can be inserted at any stage of the operation.

Cadaver eye study using scanning electronic microscopy showed that much less damage to the pigmented iris tissue was caused by the new instrument than by conventional iris retractors.

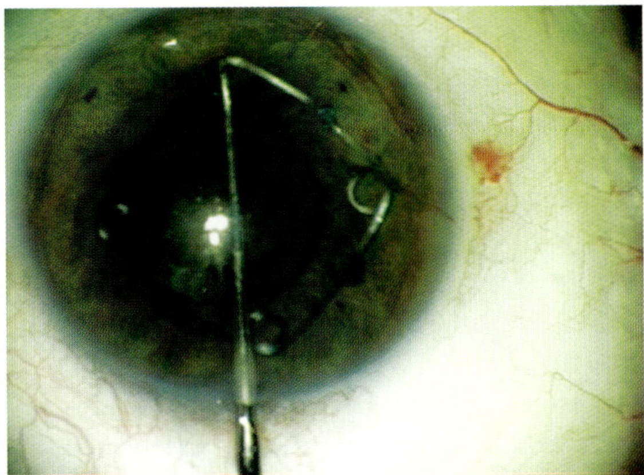

Fig. 11: The iris is fixated in the loops of the device

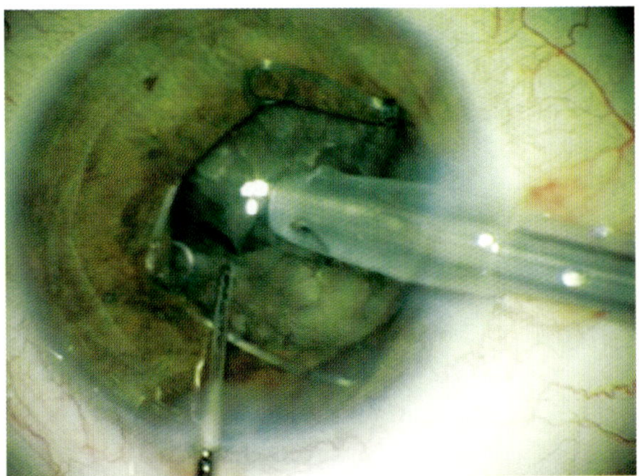

Fig. 12: Phacoemulsification of the nucleus with the IQ ring in place

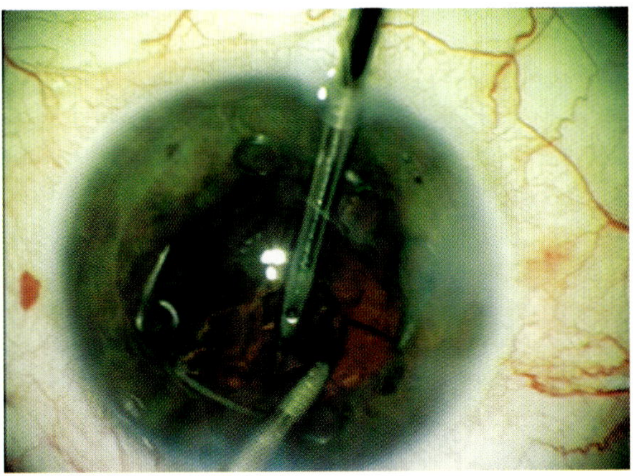

Fig. 13: Irrigation-aspiration after IOL implantation and removal of the device

Surgical Technique

Topical anesthesia is applied using 2% lidocain, and the paracentesis is done at 12 o'clock. A 2.8 mm temporal clear corneal incision is performed using the disposable metal blade. A dispersive ophthalmic viscosurgical device (OVD) is injected in the anterior chamber to stabilize it and protect the corneal endothelium. The IQ-ring is introduced into the AC through the clear corneal phacoincision using forceps and Sinskey hook. The device is placed in the AC and laid flat on the iris. It is then attached to the pupillary margin in a circular manner, resulting in a pupillary opening approximately 6.0 mm wide. Capsulorhexis is performed using forceps or a bent needle.

Hydrodissection and hydrodelineation are performed with BSS until the nucleus could be rotated freely inside the capsular bag. Phacoemulsification is done with the Millennium CCS phacoemulsifier (Bausch and Lomb) using a modified quick-chop technique (Microflow or Kelman US needle; 36% of linear US power; pulse 10 pps, duty cycle 80%; vacuum settings at 350 mm Hg; bottle height 85 cm). A deep but short central trench is made in cases of the hard nucleus cases. The step-by-step chop in situ and lateral separation technique allows nucleus division with minimal stress on the capsular bag.

Coaxial or bimanual irrigation/aspiration is used to clean residual cortical fibers from the capsular bag. The capsular bag is then filled with the cohesive OVD and foldable intraocular lens (IOL) is inserted using injector through unenlarged incision. "Forceps flexible IOL insertion usually requires incision enlargement from 3.5 to 3.75 mm."

Then the device is loosened from the pupillary margin using a Sinskey hook and laid on the iris. The ring is cut with the Vannas scissors and retracted from the anterior chamber through the clear corneal incision with the forceps. Aspiration is performed to remove the residual OVD. After viscoelastic removal, the clear corneal incision is hydrated with balanced salt solution (BSS).

On the first postoperative day, the eyes presented with minor cell and flare in the anterior chamber. The pupillary margin was minimally disturbed or undamaged and the IOL well centered. We usually treat patients with small pupils after the surgery more aggressively than uncomplicated patients with topical steroids, cycloplegics, and sometimes systemic steroids patients receive local antibiotic and steroid treatment for 4-6 weeks.

Conclusion

Adequate transpupillary access to the lens is essential to the success of phaco procedures especially in cases with zonular weakness and capsular inadequacy. We believe that our iris retraction technique with IQ-ring has several advantages.

First, the IQ-ring does not require additional incisions. This instrument is inserted through main incision, thus reducing surgical trauma and minimizing the risk of contamination and postoperative inflammatory reaction.

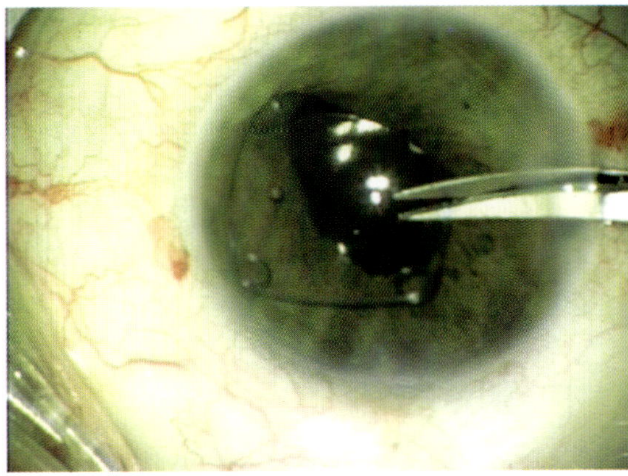

Fig. 14: The ring is cut with the Vannas scissors

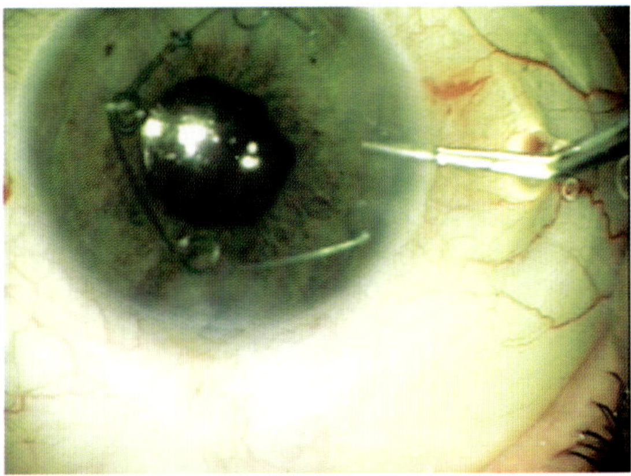

Fig. 15: The ring is removed from the anterior chamber through the clear corneal incision with the forceps

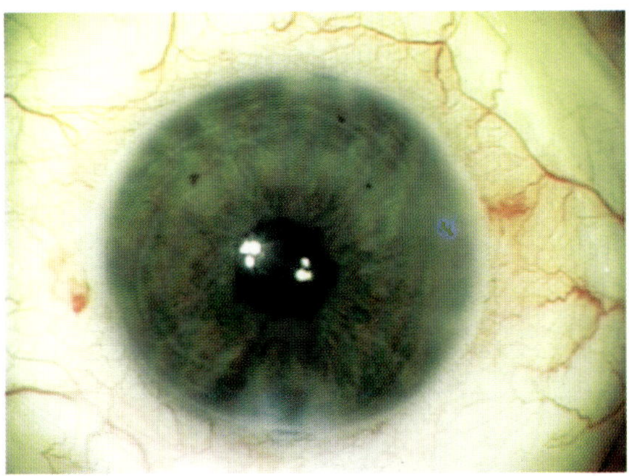

Fig. 16: Final situation after surgery

Second, the device is applying pressure to the sphincter muscle over an area which is wider than in cases of iris hooks. It is particularly useful in patients in which cutting or tearing of the iris tissue should be avoided. Especially in the presence of rubeosis, chronic anterior uveitis, or systemic coagulopathy. Iris rim is safely fixed in the loops of the ring and there is no risk of iris aspiration during phacoemulsification.

Third, compared to other long-in-use iris retractors IQ-ring has the advantage of being friendlier with the eye, due to the well-distributed stretching and gentle holding of the delicate iris tissue, and to the easier and less traumatic implantation. It has no sharp or pointed endings that can damage the eye.

Fourth, equidistant position of the loops that holds the iris tissue ensure correct position of the iris and prevents the effect of overstretching of the pupil observed in incorrect iris hooks position.

Fifth, IQ-ring provides sufficient room for nucleus fragmentation and removal. The device configuration and plate design allows surgeon to work in the deep lens layers below the iris plane and the square-shaped pupil formed by the ring. This provides enough space for grooving and cutting the nucleus and increased peripheral visualization during the chopping phase of the procedure.

In summary, different techniques of nucleus disassembly in small-incision cataract surgery requires wide and unobstructed view of the anterior portion of the lens as well as the instruments inserted in the anterior chamber. The other important factor is sufficient manipulability of the instruments which is critical for the successful completion the surgery. A pupil that fails to dilate makes cataract removal more difficult with added risk. The IQ-ring adequately dilates the pupil, prevents iris sphincter damage. It is easy to insert and remove. The ring expands the pupil to 6.0 mm, protects the iris sphincter during surgery, and allows the pupil to return to its normal shape, size, and function after the operation.

IQ ring is an important tool in phacoemulsification surgery. Careful intraoperative manipulation and insertion of the IQ-ring with liberal use of OVD can help prevent complications. After the surgery most of our patients had pupils almost indistinguishable from the appearance before surgery with the preserved functional activity. We consider IQ-ring among the most effective methods to increase the size of even very rigid small pupils during phacoemulsification surgery. We use it in cases with IFIS syndrome with a great success. The use of this method is highly recommended as it is likely to reduce postoperative abnormalities in pupil size and function.

20

Bimanual Microphaco versus Coaxial Miniphaco

Gian Maria Cavallini, Luca Campi,
Cristina Masini, Simone Pelloni (Italy)

Introduction

Cataract surgery nowadays, is considered both a therapeutic procedure to remove cataract and a refractive surgery, as patients often claim to obtain a post-surgical excellent visual rehabilitation. From 1967, year in which Kelman introduced the phacoemulsification technique, begun a new era for cataract surgery: more invasive procedures were abandoned, and we assisted in a decrease in incision size from the 10.0 mm required for the intracapsular cataract extraction to 7.0 for extracapsular cataract extraction and ultimately to the small incisions (3.2 to 2.8 mm) used for phacoemulsification. The use of smaller surgical instruments, flexible intraocular lenses (IOLs), and more advanced management software for the phaco units, further allowed to reduce incision size and tissue trauma and to promote faster functional recovery. Clinical trials have found that the length of the incision is directly proportional to the amount of induced astigmatism and inversely proportional to its stability over time.

In this chapter we will describe two different mini-invasive cataract surgery techniques: bimanual microphacoemulsification and coaxial miniphacoemulsification. The ***bimanual microincision phacoemulsification technique*** is a less invasive variation of traditional coaxial phacoemulsification and allows cataract extraction through incisions of 1.5 mm or smaller. Notwithstanding the increasing success of bimanual microincision phacoemulsification and its increasing acceptance by the international surgical community, skepticism remains. Perhaps this is more related to the difficult of giving up a technique such as coaxial phacoemulsification rather than to actual limitations or disadvantages of the new procedure. The ***coaxial miniphacoemulsification technique*** is a minimally invasive coaxial phacoemulsification technique using incisions smaller than those in traditional coaxial phacoemulsification (2.2 mm versus 2.8 mm) allowing surgeons to use the same surgical approach.

We describe below the two different surgical techniques, and present the results of our clinical trial that compared bimanual microphacoemulsification and coaxial miniphacoemulsification, in order to determine whether one technique has advantages over the other.

Bimanual Microphacoemulsification

ANESTHESIA

Although all types of anesthesia are compatible with bimanual phaco, local anesthesia remains the most reasonable alternative as compared to locoregional or general anesthesia in microincision cataract surgery.

The commonly used eyedrops for topical anesthesia are Ropivacaine 10 mg/ml and 2% Lidocaine, instilled 3-4 times every 5 minutes before surgery.

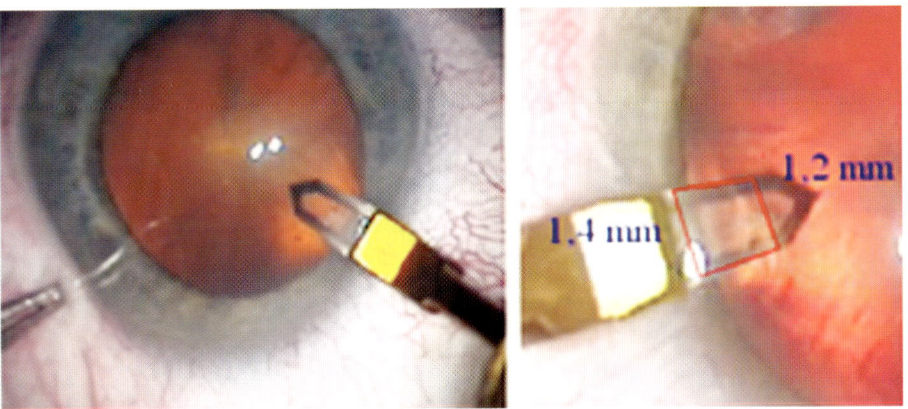

Fig. 1: Microincision with precalibrated diamond knife in the clear cornea at 10 O'clock and particular of trapezoidal incision

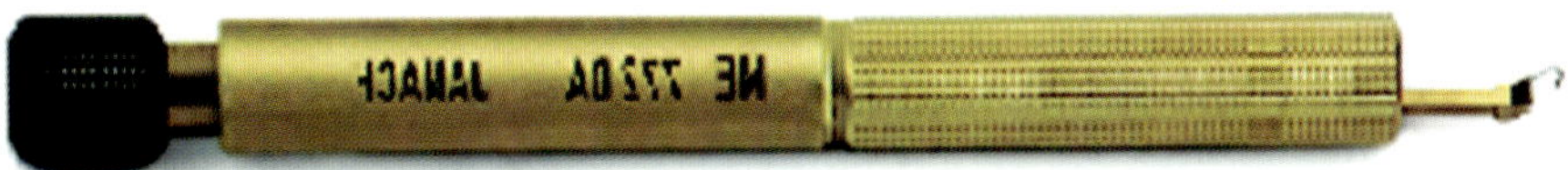

Fig. 2: Diamond knife with trapezoidal shape (e.Janach, Como, Italy)

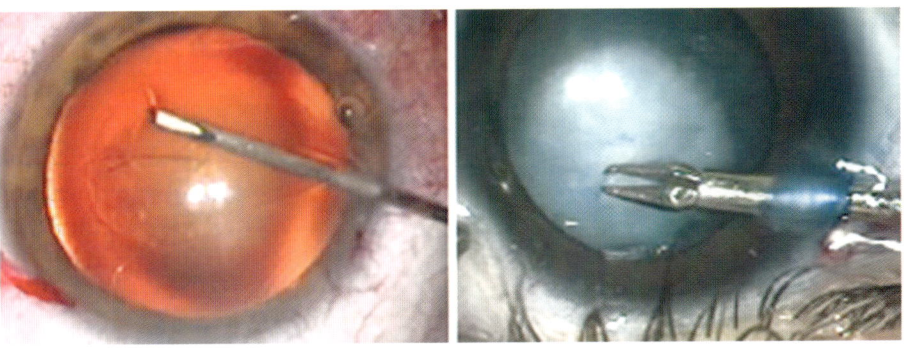

Fig. 3: Capsulorhexis with cystotome 26 G needle, and with specific bimanual capsulorhexis forceps (Duet)

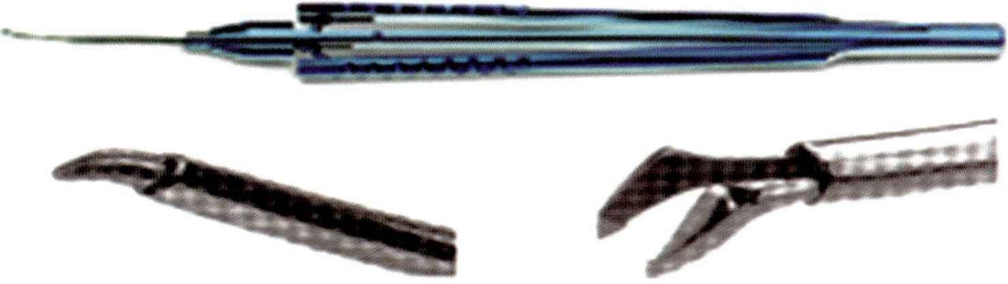

Fig. 4: Specific bimanual capsulorhexis forceps with the particular of squeeze-handle mechanism (Duet)

INCISIONS

It's a crucial point of the microphaco surgical technique, as microincisions must be created in order to prevent leakage and enable easy insertion of the instruments to be used. The width of the incision must be perfectly adapted to the instruments used by the surgeon to prevent tension and deformation of the incision, while preventing leakage. Ideally, the incision should have a trapezoidal shape with an inner corneal incision of 1.2 mm and an external limbic base of 1.4 mm. I usually perform two 1.4 mm trapezoidal incisions in the clear cornea at 10 O'clock and 2 O'clock with a precalibrated diamond knife (e. Janach, Como, Italy).

CAPSULORHEXIS

Since its introduction in 1985 by H Gimble and T Neuhann, capsulorhexis is a key phase of any safe phacoemulsification procedure. It can be performed, as I usually do, with cystotome 26 G needle, but it's may be easier by using capsulorhexis forceps, that enables perfect control of the circular cutting of the anterior capsule, or by distal control forceps, such as a vitreoretinal surgery forceps with a smooth tip. Besides, there are specific bimanual capsulorhexis forceps (Duet) which can be introduced through an incision of less than 1 mm, with a short beak and a smooth introduction tip, facilitating manipulation inside a microincision. A viscoelastic device combining both dispersion and cohesion agents, is particularly appropriate for bimanual microphacoemulsification. The correct capsulorhexis diameter in order to avoid surgical difficulties and complications, is between 5 mm and 6 mm.

HYDRODISSECTION

This surgical step does not require specific instruments for bimanual microphaco, as it can be used a normal 26 G cannula properly introduced through microincision, placed under the capsulorhexis and slightly lifted to create a small tent under the anterior casule to facilitate the progression of BSS. This surgical step is essential to create a cleavage between the lens capsule and the cortex, and to verify if the nucleus rotates properly within the bag. If the nucleus does not turn, the surgeon must repeat the procedure in the opposite quadrant.

PHACOEMULSIFICATION

This surgical step needs dedicated instruments for microphaco: an irrigating chopper, a sleeveless 21 G phaco-tip, and phaco machines with ultrasound power modulation technologies, which enable discontinuous US emission and avoid thermal burns in the corneal tunnel. One of the most diffuse phaco machine, that I use, is the AMO-Sovereign phacoemulsificator with White-Star

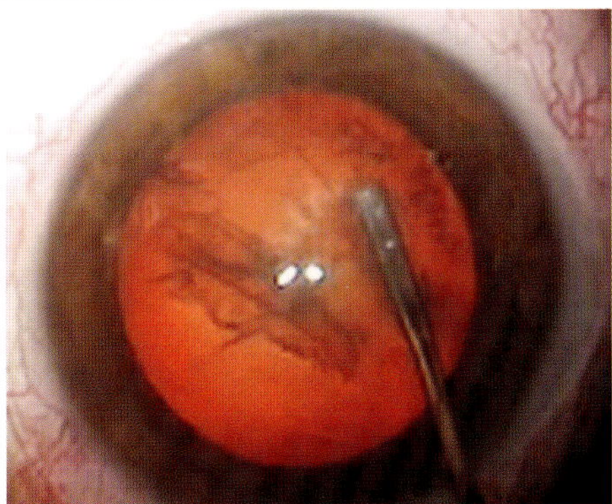

Fig. 5: Hydrodissection with 26 G cannula

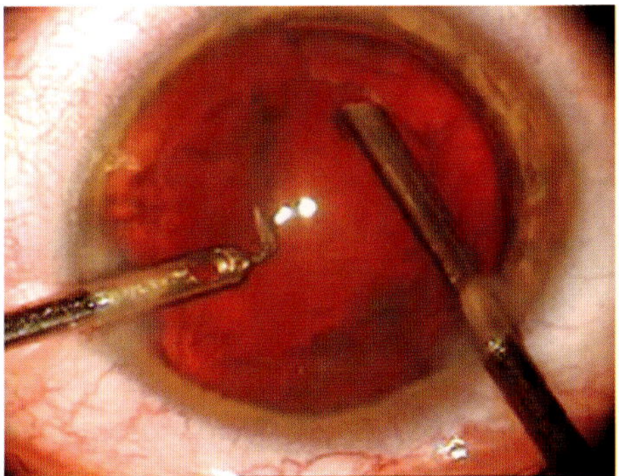

Fig. 6: Irrigating chopper

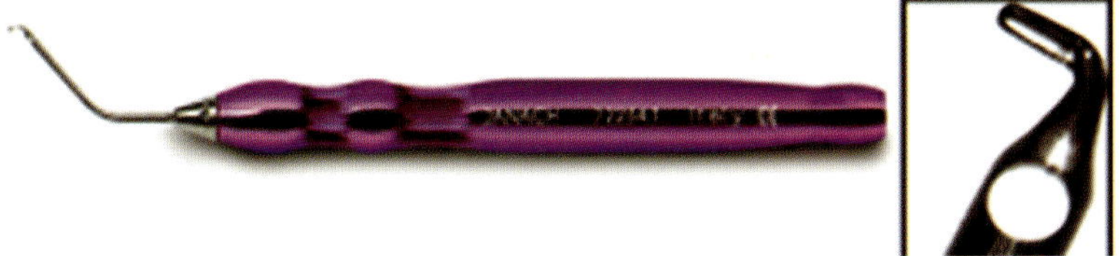

Fig. 7: Irrigating Chopper 21 G with the particular of the irrigant point (e. Janach, Como, Italy)

technology for micropulsed US emission, but there are also other machines (Oertli OS-3, Alcon Legacy 2000, Alcon Infiniti, the new Bausch & Lomb Stellaris, Nidek CV24000, Optikon Pulser) that allow the optimization of ultrasound power with different technologies.

For phacofracture we can adopt the usual techniques, but I suggest to use the "divide and conquer" or "stop and chop" technique for normal nuclei, and "vertical phaco-chop" for harder ones.

Whatever is the phacofracture procedure, the great advantages of the bimanual technique are:

- The use of an irrigating chopper, that allows to direct the nucleus fragments towards the phaco-tip, with better followability and less turbulence in anterior chamber (AC);
- The optimization of fluidics, that allows a great AC stability;
- A greater visibility of the surgical field for the minimal size of the surgical instruments, that make this technique ideal for microphthalmos and infantile cataracts.

IRRIGATION/ASPIRATION

Aspiration of cortical material is greatly facilitated by the bimanual technique. The separated aspiration and irrigation probes are introduced through microincisions into the AC, with the aspiration probe in the dominant hand, that is positioned under the anterior capsulorhexis to aspirate the cortical remnants. The infusion probe in the other hand works in a continuous infusion mode, in order to avoid AC collapse, and helps to direct the cortical material towards the aspiration probe minimizing turbulence. After having performed aspiration of material on the opposite half of the entry point of the aspiration probe, the surgeon changes hands and keeps the aspiration probe with the other hand in order to perform aspiration of material in the other half. I usually use 20 G probes with oval section (AMO), that perfectly fit with the trapezoidal microincisions.

IOL IMPLANTATION

Currently, I insert the IOL through a third incision at 12 O'clock performed between the two microincisions, but it is also possible to enlarge one of the two incisions for the implant. There are now available many IOLs for microincisions (Acriflex MICS 46 CSE; Acri.Smart 48S; Acri.Twin 447 D/443D; SmartLens-Medennium; and the new Akreos MI 60), that can easily be introduced in posterior chamber with a dedicated injector through the microincisions.

At the end of the implant I usually perform a simple suture hydration, but it's also possible to suture the major incision with Nylon 10-0.

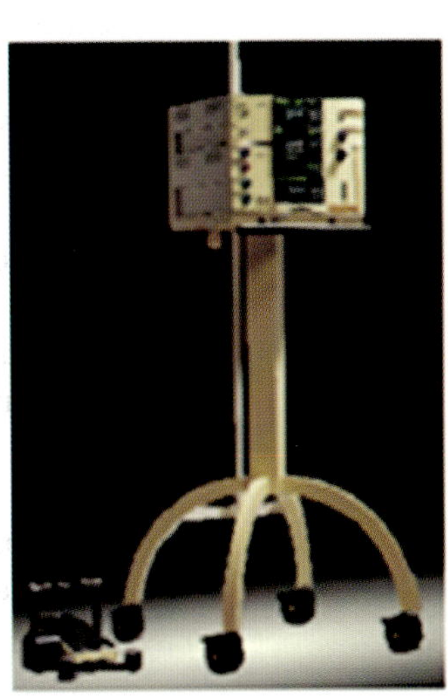

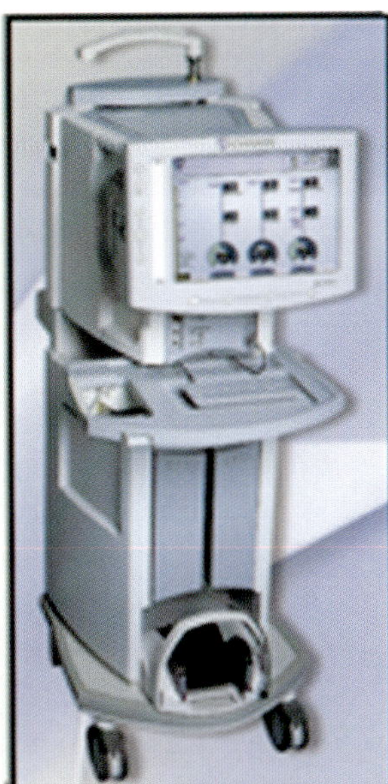

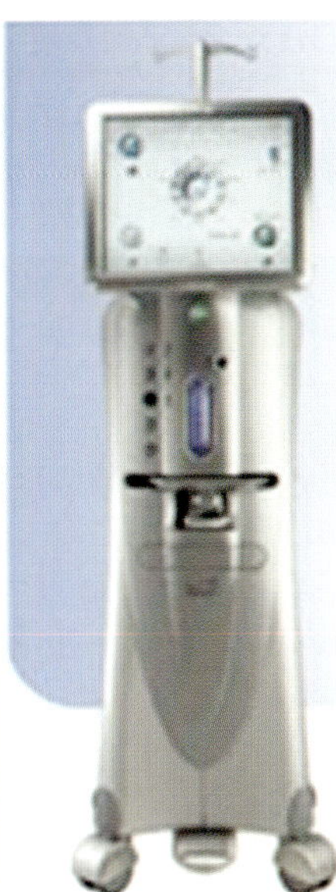

Fig. 8: Oertli OS-3, AMO-Sovereign with White-Star technology and the new Bausch & Lomb Stellaris phacoemulsificators

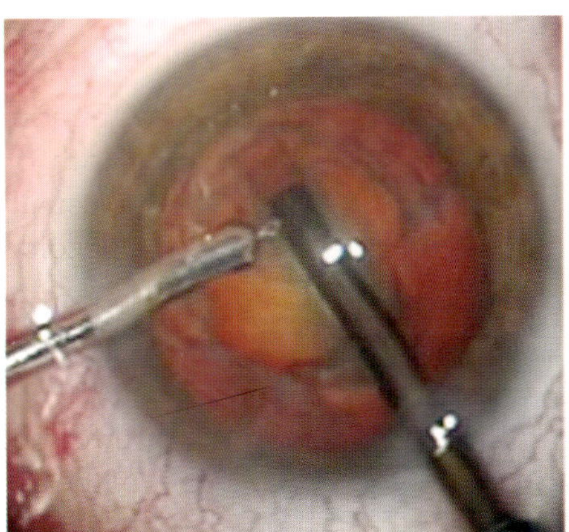

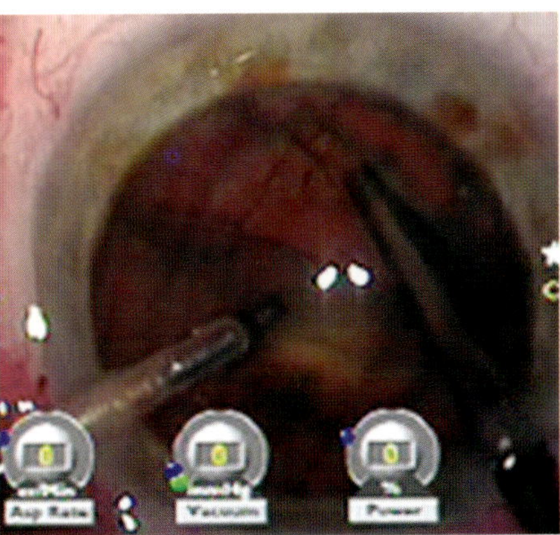

Fig. 9: Culture and cracking of cataract with techniques of "divide and conquer"

Coaxial Miniphacoemulsification

It is a minimally invasive coaxial phacoemulsification technique using incisions smaller than those in traditional coaxial phacoemulsification (2.2 mm versus 2.8 mm). So, the only difference from the traditional coaxial phaco is the use of a phaco-tip with a 21-G Ultrasleeve, that allows the insertion of the instrument through a 2.2 mm incision.

My personal technique for minicoaxial phaco is the following: after local ***anesthesia***, I perform two 1.4 mm ***incisions*** in clear cornea at 10 O'clock and 2 O'clock with a precalibrated diamond knife; then, I create a ***capsulorhexis*** with a cystotome. After ***hydrodissection***, I enlarge one of the incisions to 2.2 mm with a precalibrated steel knife and perform ***phacoemulsification*** with a 20-gauge, 30-degree-angled probe with Ultrasleeve (Alcon Surgical). I use the same 20-gauge chopper as in the bimanual technique, although it is closed and not linked to the irrigating source. Finally, I perform ***bimanual I/A*** of the residual fragments with a 20-gauge probe with an oval section, and ***implant the IOL*** through the 2.2 mm incision used for phacoemulsification. Then I finish with suture hydration.

Bimanual Microphaco versus Coaxial Miniphaco: A Clinical Study

In a controlled, prospective clinical trial 100 eyes of 50 patients with nuclear or corticonuclear cataract of grade 2 to 4 on the Lens Opacities Classification System III had phacoemulsification between January 2006 and July 2006 at the Institute of Ophthalmology, University of Modena. Fifty eyes were randomized to have surgery by the bimanual technique and 50, by the coaxial technique. All surgeries were performed by the same surgeon (GMC) using the same machine (Sovereign WhiteStar, American Medical Optics). All patients provided informed consent before surgery.

INCLUSION CRITERIA

1. Transparent central cornea
2. Good preoperative pupil dilation
3. No pseudoexfoliation
4. No history of previous eye surgery or glaucoma
5. No history of retinal disease
6. Endothelial cell count of 1600 cell/mm^2 or greater
7. Astigmatism lower than 3.0 diopters (D).

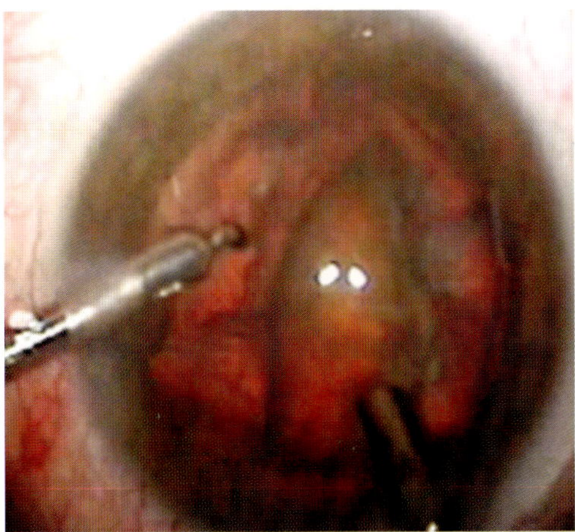

Fig. 10: Techniques of “stop and chop” on an eminucleous

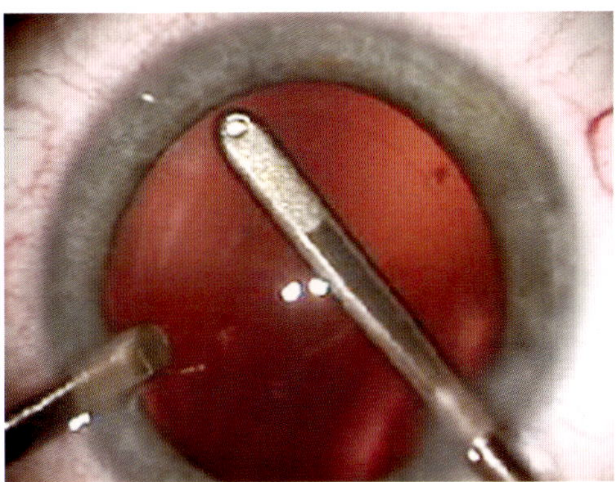

Fig. 11: Separated aspiration and irrigation 20 G probes with oval section (AMO)

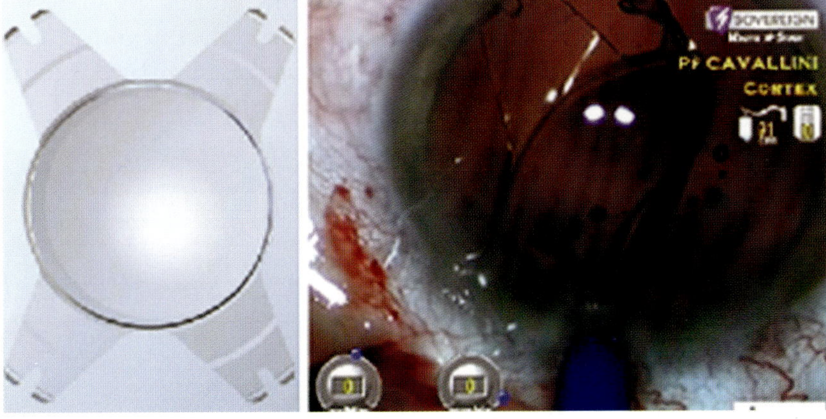

Fig. 12: New Akreos MI60 IOL for microincision implanted trough a third 1.8 mm incision at 12 O’clock

PRE- AND POSTOPERATIVE EXAMINATIONS

Preoperative

The same surgeon (GMC) performed all preoperative examinations. Examinations included:

1. Snellen visual acuity
2. Biomicroscopy of the anterior and posterior segments
3. Echobiometry for IOL power calculation
4. Endothelial cell count by specular microscopy (Noncon Robo-CA, Konan)
5. Corneal thickness by ultrasound pachymetry (IOPac, Heidelberg Engineering)
6. Astigmatism by corneal topography (CT1000, Shin-Nippon).

Postoperative

Postoperative control visits were at 1 day, 1 week, and 1 and 3 months by the same surgeon who performed the preoperative evaluations. Examinations included:

1. Best corrected visual acuity
2. Intraocular pressure measurement
3. Fundus evaluation
4. Complete biomicroscopy of the anterior segment.

SURGICAL TECHNIQUE

Patients had surgery by the bimanual technique in 1 eye and the coaxial technique in the fellow eye; thus, there were 50 eyes in each group. Eyes were randomly assigned to surgical technique.

All surgery was performed by the same surgeon using the same phaco machine (Sovereign White-Star, AMO); shows the settings. In all eyes, the incision was made in clear cornea in the superior sector and a flexible hydrophobic acrylic IOL (Acri.Smart 48 S, Acri.Tec) was implanted using a 2.0 mm injector (Acri.Tec).

TABLE 1: Surgical parameters for the Sovereign WhiteStar set-up by group

Parameter	Bimanual group	Coaxial group
Power (%)	20-25	20-25
Aspiration flow (cm³/min)	24-28	24-28
Vacuum (mm Hg)	60-250 (unocclusion) 80-300 (occlusion)	60-250 (unocclusion) 80-300 (occlusion)
Cortical remnant I/A (mm Hg)	450	450

I/A = Irrigation / aspiration

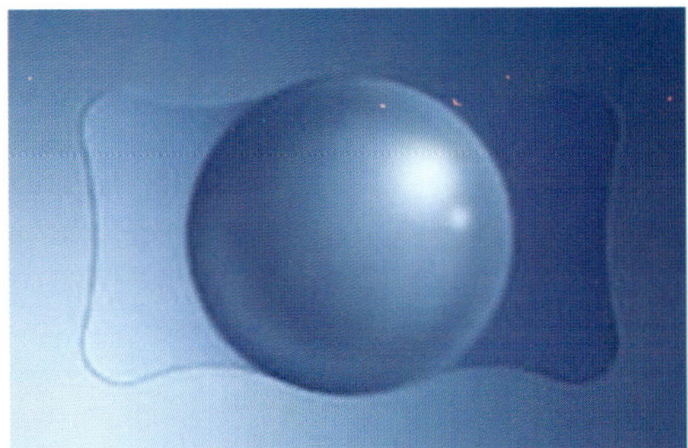

Fig. 13: Acri.Smart 48 S

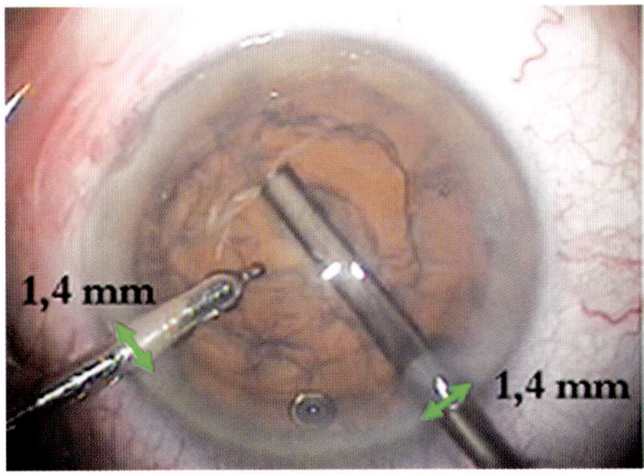

Fig. 14: Bimanual microphaco technique

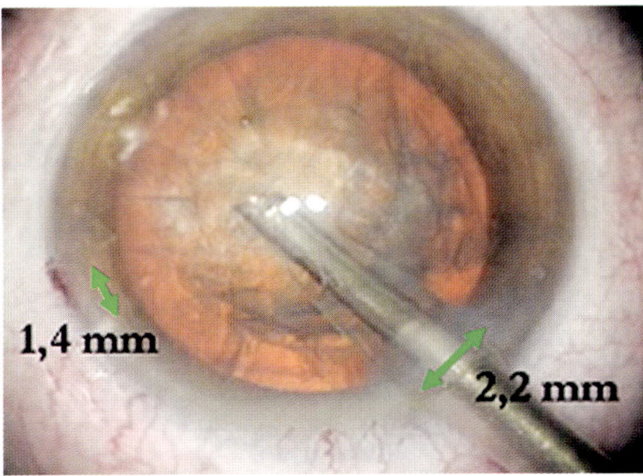

Fig. 15: Coaxial miniphaco technique

Bimanual Group

Two 1.4 mm trapezoidal incisions were made in the clear cornea at 10 O'clock and 2 O'clock with a precalibrated diamond knife (E Janach). A continuous curvilinear capsulorhexis (CCC) with a diameter between 5.0 mm and 6.0 mm was made with a cystotome. Hydrodissection was performed with a 26-gauge cannula and phacoemulsification, with a 20-gauge, 30-degree-angled sleeveless probe and an irrigating chopper (E Janach). Phaco fracture was by the stop-and-chop technique. Irrigation/aspiration (I/A) was performed with a 20-gauge probe with an oval section (American Medical Optics) introduced through the microincisions. Gradual suction of the cortical remnants and epinucleus was done with the aspiration probe in the dominant hand and the irrigation probe in the other, using the continuous infusion mode to avoid sudden collapse of the anterior chamber. With the irrigation probe, the lens fragments were directed toward the aspiration probe to simplify the procedure and lower turbulence in the anterior chamber. After the half of the capsular bag opposite the entry site was polished with the aspiration probe, the instruments were passed from one hand to the other, retracting the aspiration probe first. The remaining capsular bag was cleaned in the same way. Then, the IOL was inserted through a third incision created at 12 O'clock.

Coaxial Group

Two 1.4 mm incisions were made in clear cornea at 10 O'clock and 2 O'clock with a precalibrated diamond knife. A CCC was created with a cystotome. After hydrodissection, the incision was enlarged to 2.2 mm with a precalibrated steel knife and phacoemulsification was performed with a 20-gauge, 30-degree-angled probe with Ultrasleeve (Alcon Surgical). The same 20-gauge chopper as in the bimanual technique was used, although it was closed and not linked to the irrigating source. Finally, bimanual I/A of the residual fragments was done with a 20-gauge probe with an oval section, and the IOL was implanted through the 2.2 mm incision used for phacoemulsification.

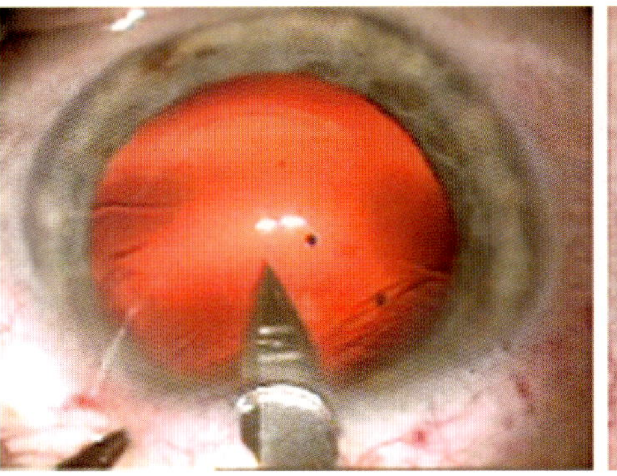

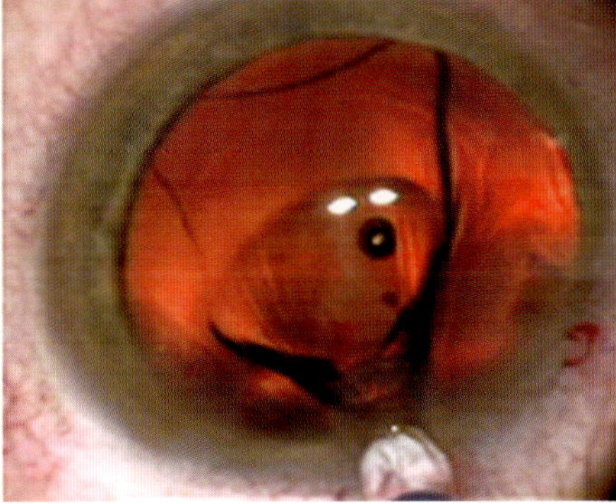

Fig. 16: A third clear corneal incision of 2,2 mm is created at 12 O'clock with a precalibrate steel knife. The IOL is implanted trough the third incision

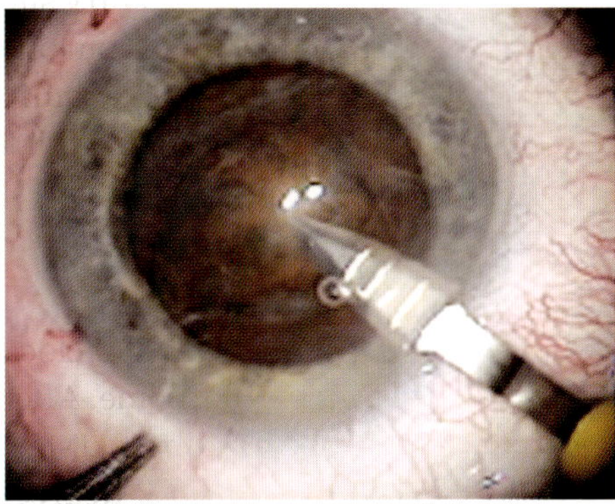

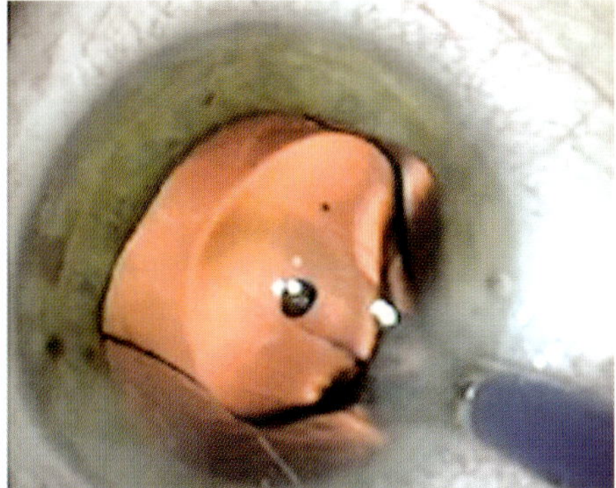

Fig. 17: The phaco tip with Ultrasleeve and the IOL injector are inserted trough a 2,2 mm clear corneal trapezoidal incision. The IOL is implanted trough the incision at 10 O'clock

Both Groups

In both groups, surgery ended with hydration of the incisions. Postoperative therapy included a topical combination of neomycin and dexamethasone 3 times a day for 2 weeks, which was gradually tapered to 2 times a day for 10 days.

INTRAOPERATIVE AND POSTOPERATIVE PARAMETERS

1. Mean phacoemulsification time
2. Total phacoemulsification percentage
3. Effective phacoemulsification time (EPT)
4. Total volume of the balanced salt solution (BSS) used
5. Total surgical time (from the first corneal incision to hydration of the wound)
6. Final size of the corneal incision.

For each parameter, statistical analysis between the bimanual group and coaxial group was done using the Student t test. A P value of 0.05 or less was considered statistically significant.

Results

Of the 50 patients, 15 were men and 35 were women. The mean age of the patients was 77.25 years ± 5.36 (SD) (range 69 to 86 years). No early intraoperative or postoperative complications occurred that required a change in the therapy, and no complications were reported during the postoperative follow-up. No eye showed the signs of corneal thermal burn, zonular dehiscence, capsule rupture, or iris damages; there were no cases of endophthalmitis.

In 2 cases (1 in each group), the IOL partially ruptured but did not require removal. In 2 cases (1 in each group), the IOL ruptured completely and required removal and replacement with another IOL. Table 2 shows the results of the statistical analysis of the parameters in both groups. The only statistically significant difference between the 2 groups was the total volume of the BSS used (P = 0.004) and total surgical time (P = 0.045).

Discussion and Conclusions

The current clinical trial compared bimanual microphacoemulsification and coaxial miniphacoemulsification. Using a 20-gauge phaco tip with an Ultrasleeve, coaxial phacoemulsification was performed through incisions of approximately 2.2 mm, smaller than the 2.8 mm incisions used in conventional phacoemulsification. This allows the surgeon to use the same methods as the conventional technique but with smaller incisions, decreasing surgical induced astigmatism (SIA). We did not find any statistically significant difference

TABLE 2: Results of the statistical analysis on the intraoperative and postoperative parameters

	Bimanual group	*Coaxial group*	*P value* *
Cataract grade (LOCS III)	2.8 ± 0.82	2.6 ± 0.71	0.982
Final incision size (mm)	2.24 ± 0.04	2.29 ± 0.08	0.053
Endothelial cells loss (cells/mm^2) after 3 months	11.9 ± 15.2	10.07 ± 11.71	0.692
Total surgical time (sec)	637.32 ± 142.33	736.43 ± 173.52	0.045
EPT (sec)	3.86 ± 2.91	4.94 ± 2.99	0.232
Total phaco %	77.51 ± 38.72	90.82 ± 28.23	0.201
Mean phaco time (sec)	4.16 ± 1.81	5.24 ± 1.95	0.066
Total BSS volume (mL)	114.51 ± 32.23	147.42 ± 39.53	0.004
Corneal pachimetry (μm)			
Preoperative	566.94 ± 31.93	564.72 ± 28.13	0.812
3 mo postop	563.72 ± 28.42	555.33 ± 24.14	0.341
BCVA[1]			
1 d	0,88 ± 0,11	0,87 ± 0,16	0.912
7 d	0,91 ± 0,15	0,93 ± 0,09	0.644
1 m	0,98 ± 0,04	0,98 ± 0,03	0.813
3 m	0,99 ± 0,04	0,99 ± 0,03	0.964
Flare/cells in AC[2]			
1 day	0,69 ± 0,63	0,60 ± 0,65	0.702
7 days	0,34 ± 0,48	0,35 ± 0,47	0.833
1 month	0,17 ± 0,38	0,26 ± 0,44	0.302
3 months	0,08 ± 0,28	0,13 ± 0,34	0.681

AC = Anterior chamber; BVCA = Best corrected visual acuity; BSS = Balanced salt solution; EPT = Effective phacoemulsification time; LOCS III = Lens Opacitioes Classification System III

* Student *t* test

[1] BCVA expressed in decimals on a 10/10 = 1 scale basis (1/109 = 0.1,2/10 = 0.2, etc.)

[2] Flare and cells were measured according to 0 to 4 + grading scale standardized by Hogan et al.

between the 2 techniques in SIA or postoperative visual acuity. Therefore, we conclude that the 2 phacoemulsification techniques are equally valid as postoperative visual rehabilitation was quick and satisfactory in both groups. Similarly, there were no significant differences between techniques in postoperative inflammation, endothelial cell loss, or corneal thickness. The only significant difference between techniques was the total volume of the BSS used and total surgical time. Both values were lower in bimanual microphacoemulsification group. The statistical difference between the 2 groups in total BSS volume may be related to the instruments and technique used for coaxial miniphacoemulsification. The 1.4 mm incisions are well suited to the 20-gauge bimanual I/A cannula, and using a 20- gauge cannula with a 2.2 mm incision in the coaxial technique results in greater wound leakage and therefore greater use of BSS.

The difference in BSS volumes between the 2 techniques, although statistically significant, was not clinically relevant and did not affect the endothelial cell count, pachymetry, or inflammation. The continuous improvement in bimanual microphacoemulsification technique in terms of control of fluidics and intraoperative leakage could result in further reduction of intraoperative corneal damage compared with the coaxial technique. Although not statistically different, the EPT values were lower in the bimanual microphacoemulsification group (mean 3.86 ± 2.91 seconds versus 4.94 ± 2.99 seconds).

In conclusion, we can assert that bimanual microphacoemulsification and coaxial miniphacoemulsification were both effective and safe techniques for cataract surgery. However, bimanual microphacoemulsification seems to be superior as gives the surgeon greater control of the fluidics and reduces surgical times. Further clinical trials are necessary to confirm these data; anyway, I think that bimanual microphacoemulsification is really the technique of the future as it opens the door to the possibility of performing cataract surgery through increasingly smaller incisions. The advancing technology and the development of new IOLs that can be introduced through smaller and smaller incisions will make this possible.

21

Implantation of a New HOYA-IOL, Y-60H, through a 1.7 mm Corneal Incision

Hiroshi Tsuneoka (Japan)

Introduction

Hoya Corporation (Japan) manufactured a new hydrophobic foldable IOL, Y-60H, which can be inserted through a 1.7mm corneal incision. Here, the author introduces surgical techniques for inserting a new IOL after removing a lens with a bimanual micro phacoemulsification.

After a 1.4 mm incision at 2 locations on the cornea is made, CCC and hydrodissection are performed.

A 20-gauge Tsuneoka irrigating chopper is inserted through the left incision, and a 20-gauge phaco tip is inserted through the right incision, and bimanual micro phaco is used to emulsify and aspirate the nucleus. First a "slice chop" is used to divide the nucleus into two sections.

After rotating the nucleus 90°, a "vertical chop" is used to cut the nucleus into 4 sections. At this point, the bottle height is 60 cm, flow rate is 25 ml/min, and maximum aspiration pressure is set at 200 mmHg.

To emulsify and aspirate the second half of the nucleus, this half nucleus is rotated 180° and a vertical chop is used to cut it into quarter. The openings of the irrigating chopper and the phaco tip are angled downwards while emulsifying and aspirating the nuclear fragments. This prevents the nuclear fragments from being dispersed in the anterior chamber and the nuclear fragments are phaco-emulsified only within the lens capsule (in-the-bag phaco).

When almost all of the nuclear fragments have been phacoemulsified and aspirated, the phaco tip is withdrawn and the aspiration cannula is positioned in the anterior chamber to aspirate any residual cortical fragments.

After a viscoelastic material is injected into the anterior chamber, and the lens capsule is expanded, a 1.7 mm wound-enlarging knife is used to enlarge the initial incision to 1.7 mm.

The tip of a specialized HOYA F-1 cartridge is inserted through the incision and into the anterior chamber. At this point, the aspiration cannula inserted through the side port is used to hold the eyeball in place and prevent any movement. By rotating the cartridge slightly to the left and right as the tip is inserted into the eye, then after the aspiration cannula is withdrawn the injector plunger is rotated to insert the HOYA-IOL Y-60H into the eye. After the optics of the IOL has entered the eye, the cartridge is withdrawn. A push and pull hook is used to position the trailing loop within the lens capsule.

After IOL insertion, the incision is measured using inner calipers. The 1.7 mm and 1.8 mm calipers will fit, but not the 1.9 mm caliper. This indicates that insertion of an IOL through a 1.7 mm corneal incision resulted in a final incision of 1.8 mm.

Up to this point, HOYA has marketed an acrylic hydrophobic IOL having an optic diameter of 6 mm. By using an E-1 cartridge, it was possible to insert that IOL through a 2.3 mm corneal incision. In order to enable slightly smaller incisions, they tried placing a slight depression at the base of the loop on

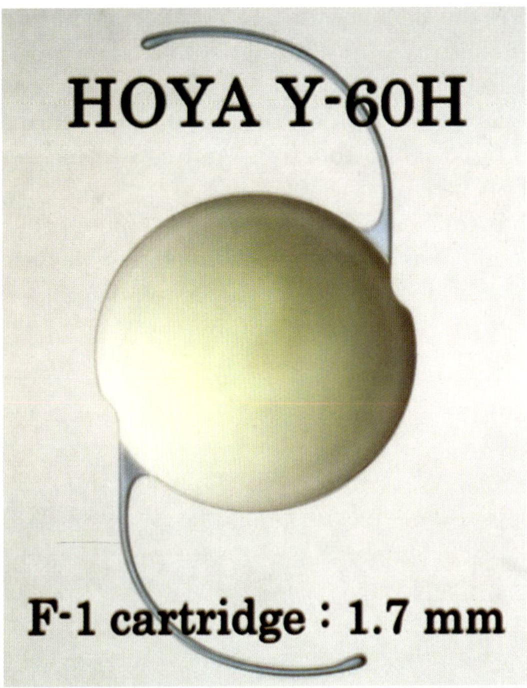

Fig. 1: The new HOYA-IOL, Y-60H

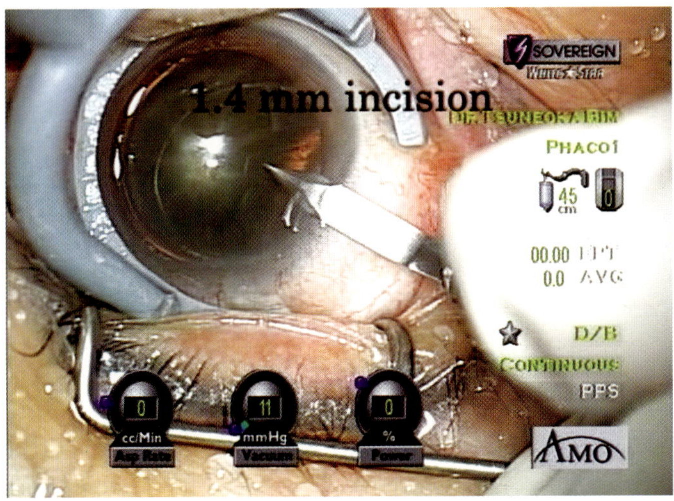

Fig. 2: 1.4 mm corneal incision

one side. Changing the shape of the lens and using a narrower F-1 cartridge made it possible to insert the lens through a 1.7 mm incision.

The acrylic hydrophobic IOL with a 6 mm optics is known worldwide for its extremely high reliability. The procedure I introduced here makes it possible to insert this IOL, HOYA Y-60H through a 1.7 mm corneal incision. After insertion, the incision has only increased to 1.8 mm.

Here is a slit lamp microscope view of the eye 1 month after surgery. Central positioning of the IOL was satisfactory, with no notable dislocation. With the 1.7 mm corneal incision, one month after surgery we detected only slight changes at the incision site in the corneal topography.

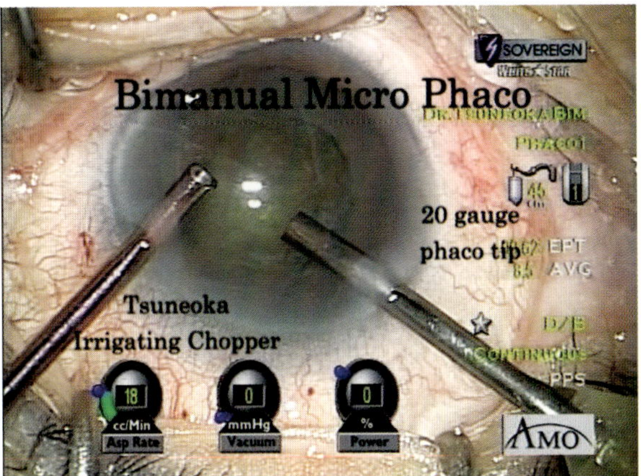

Fig. 3: The irrigating chopper and the sleeveless phaco are inserted through corneal incisions

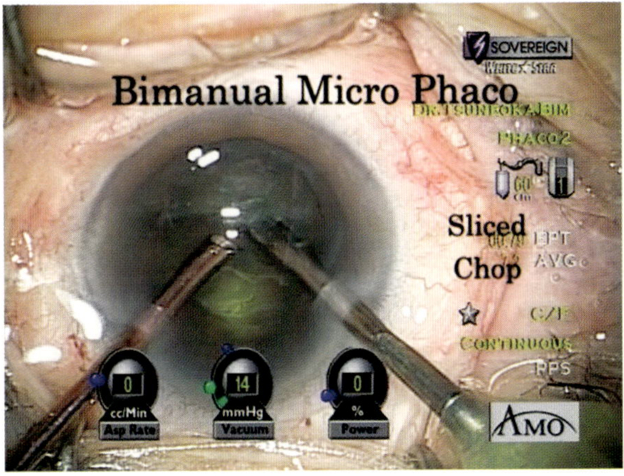

Fig. 4: Nucleus is divided in half using "slice chop" technique

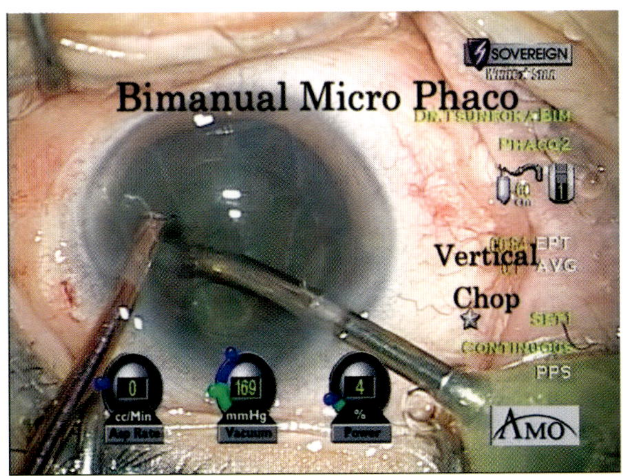

Fig. 5: Vertical chop is used to cut the nucleus into quarter

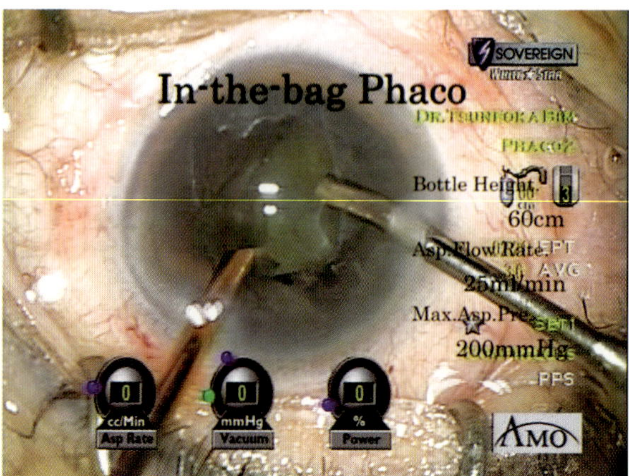

Fig. 6: In-the-bag phaco

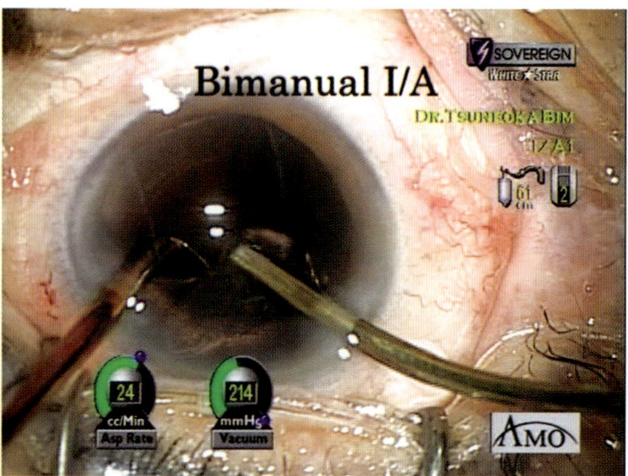

Fig. 7: Aspiration of the residual cortex

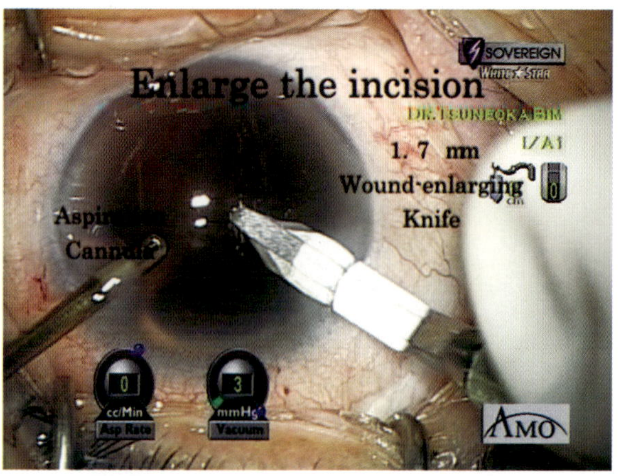

Fig. 8: Enlarging the initial incision to 1.7 mm

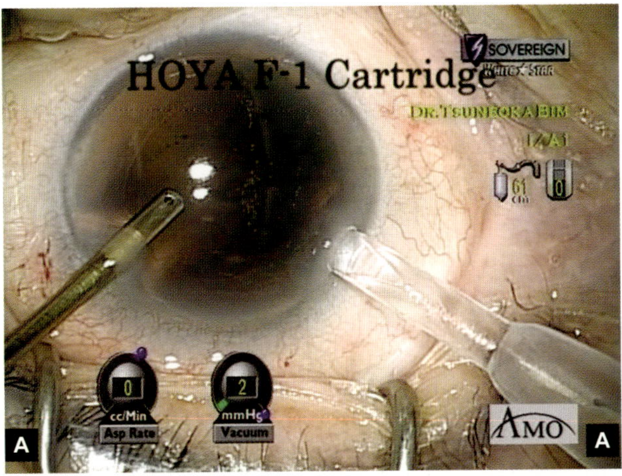

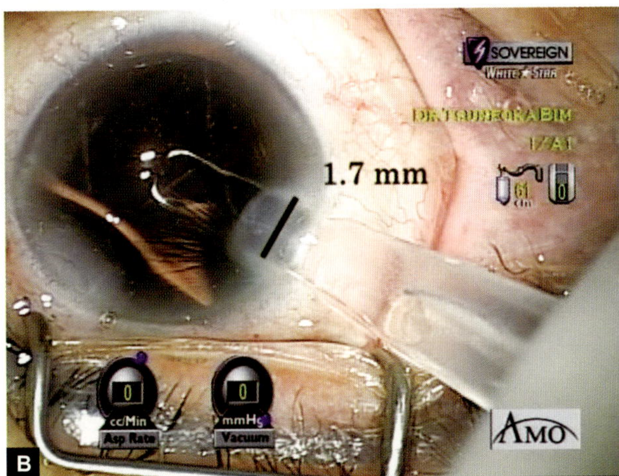

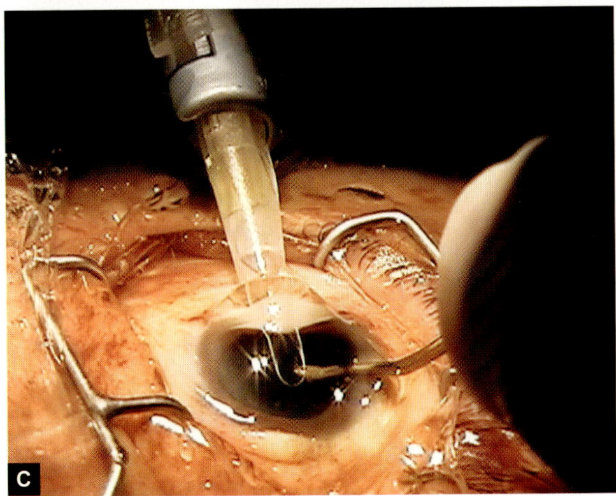

Figs 9A to C: Insertion of the F3 cartridge

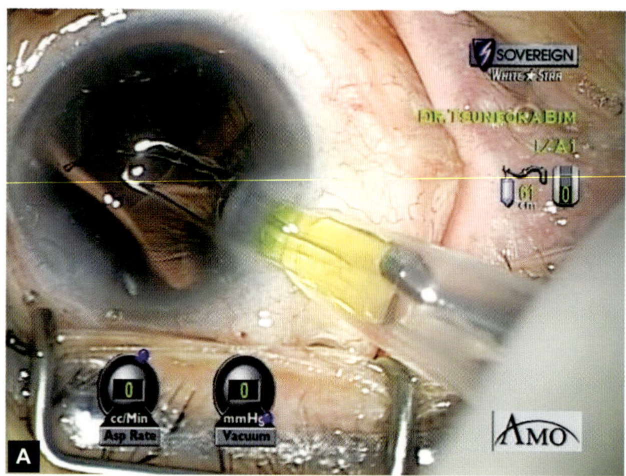

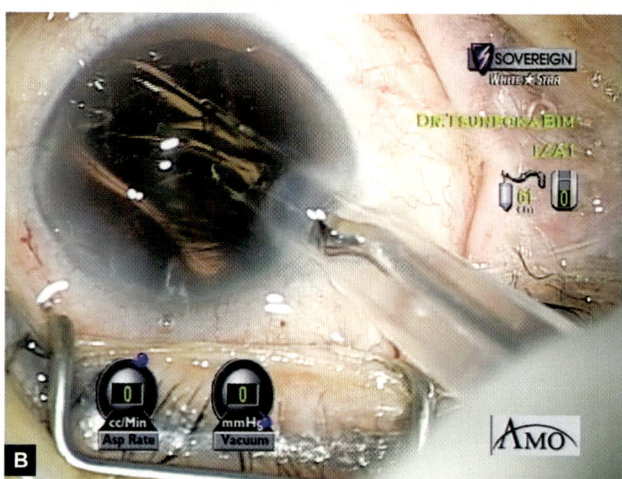

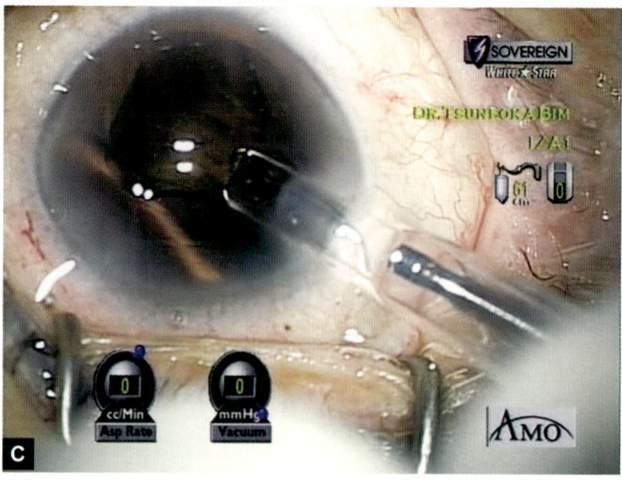

Figs 10A to C: Implantation of the Y-60H

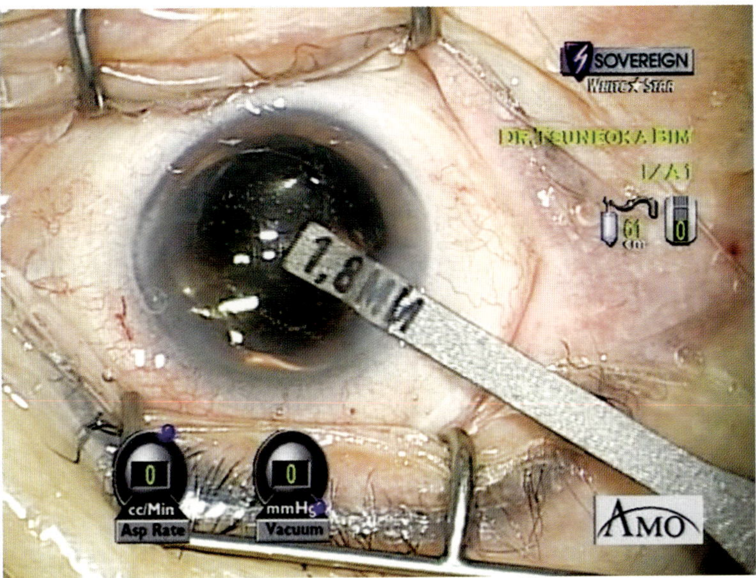

Fig. 11: Final incision size is enlarged into 1.8 mm

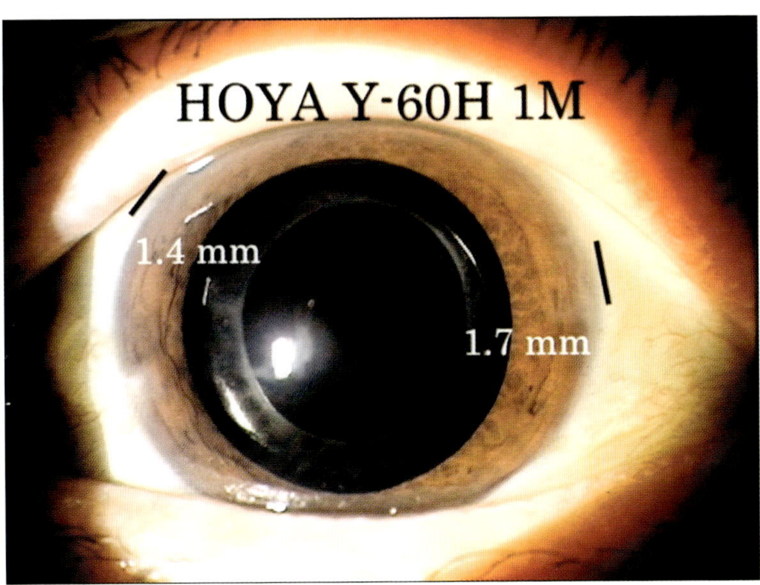

Fig. 12: Slit lamp photograph of Y-60H IOL 1 month after surgery

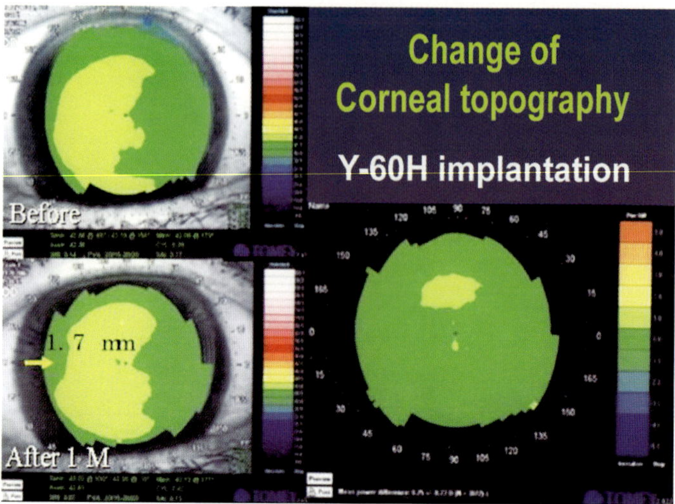

Fig. 13: The change of the corneal topography 1 month after surgery

22

Microphakonit for Refractive Lens Exchange (MIRLEX): A New Technique

Arturo Pérez-Arteaga (Mexico)

Summary

Microphakonit is a technique described by Amar Agarwal MD to perform a Bimanual Cataract Surgery through 20.7 mm ports with 700 microns cannulas and phacotips. It is until now, the smallest instrumentation to perform a cataract surgery.

What we are going to describe here is the use of these 700 microns instrumentation and technique to perform Refractive Lens Exchange (RLE). The advantages of this technique over the traditional coaxial RLE and over the traditional 1.0 mm Phakonit are first to be minimally invasive and second to have a complete control of the eye and over the anterior chamber stability during the entire procedure.

History

Refractive Lens Exchange (RLE) started as a high controversy technique because the potential consequences of aphaquia. In the early days of Intracapsular and Extracapsular techniques it appeared to be crazy to introduce a patient to all the nightmare of cataract surgery just for refractive purposes; the price at that time was very high. So other refractive procedures gain popularity like Incisional Surgery, Excimer Laser Ablations and Phaquiq Intraocular lenses.

I started my surgical practice in 1990; at that time I learned a bimanual technique to perform Clear Lens Extraction for Refractive purposes from Ignacio Barraquer MD from Colombia, trough Enrique Ariza MD and Guillermo Lieja MD from México. The technique was performed trough two side port 1.0 mm incisions, with irrigation/aspiration with two "hand made" 21 gauge cannulas.

At that time we used a very high bottle of intraocular solution and gravitatory force for irrigation and a peristaltic pump for aspiration. With the time we started to use the Irrigation/Aspiration (I/A) system of the Phacoemulsification equipments. The incisions were made only for I/A, so at the end a 3rd incision was done to introduce the intraocular lens (IOL). No ultrasonic power was needed, because no cataract was present; if some nucleus was very hard to aspirate by it self, a mechanical phacofragmentation between the two canulas was very easy to perform in order to obtain small pieces of nucleus easy to aspirate. We described our rate of complications with this technique.

This Bimanual I/A technique we used for many years even for cataract surgery; we did a traditional coaxial phacoemulsification, and after that the cortical material was aspirated with this technique. It was very safe, very stable and more efficient to obtain small pieces of cortical material in all positions of the eye, in comparison to traditional coaxial I/A, were the surgeon can experience troubles with the cortical material at 12 o'clock position.

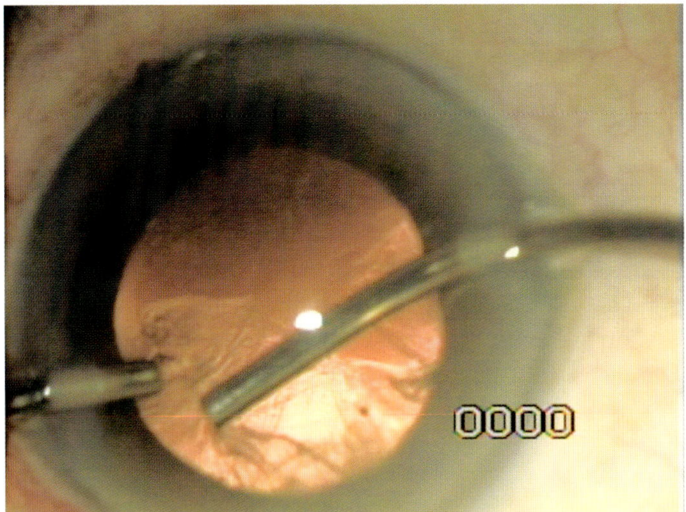

Fig. 1: Bimanual irrigation/aspiration through two 21 gauge cánnulas

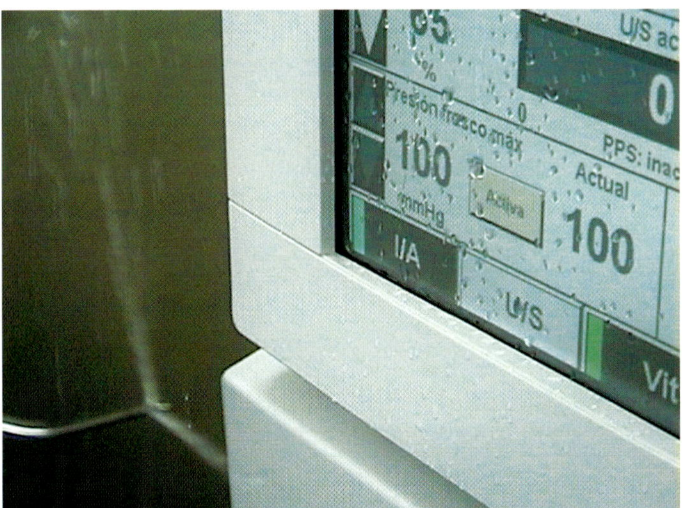

Fig. 2: Internal forced infusion obtained with the Millennium system

Then Prof. Amar Agarwal came with Phakonit. The entire concept for us changed, because it was not more needed to switch from a coaxial system for nucleus extraction, to a bimanual mode for cortical I/A.

These concepts were fast adopted to RLE patients. We started to use new instrumentation like the Duet system, new techniques like forced infusion and new parameters and ultrasonic power modulations. So, an exciting new era for RLE based in the Phakonit technique started.

We published by first time the concept MIRLEX (Microincisional Refractive Lens Exchange) to describe the extraction of the clear lens and the implantation of a microincision IOL with the ultrasmall incision techniques (Phakonit) only for refractive purposes. As the refractive surgeons worldwide found limitations of Laser procedures and phakic IOL´s implantations and at the same time a lot of new models of refractive IOL´s has arrived to the refractive field, RLE has regained popularity; many bimanual phaco surgeons have found safety in the Bimanual Lensectomy. In fact we do believe it is the time for a new born of this technique with a lot of improvements in the clear lens extraction and in the IOL technology.

At this time there is not an IOL that can go inside the eye safe trough a 1mm incision or less, even so this Bimanual Technique for RLE is gaining popularity because their advantages in stability even there is the need to open a third incision to implant any kind of IOL the surgeon wants.

Last year Amar Agarwal MD described Microphakonit, the Bimanual phacoemulsification technique performed with two 0.7 mm cannulas and phaco tip, breaking so the barrier of 1.0 mm incision for cataract surgery. So, we started also to perform MIRLEX trough 0.7 mm finding safety and efficacy in this minimally invasive procedure. This is the technique that the reader will find in this chapter.

Surgical Technique

INSTRUMENTATION

Very few instrumentation is needed to perform this technique:

1. Phacoemulsification machine with Internal or External forced infusion.
2. 0.7 mm infusion cannula: we believe that the double ended irrigating cannula provide the best irrigation and anterior chamber stability for this procedure. The one opened cannula can reject the nuclear and cortical pieces and this is why we do not use it. There is not need to have irrigating choppers because the nucleus is soft and there will be not need to chop. Even if the surgeon finds a hard nucleus there is not need to use irrigating choppers and a no-irrigating chopper technique can be used.

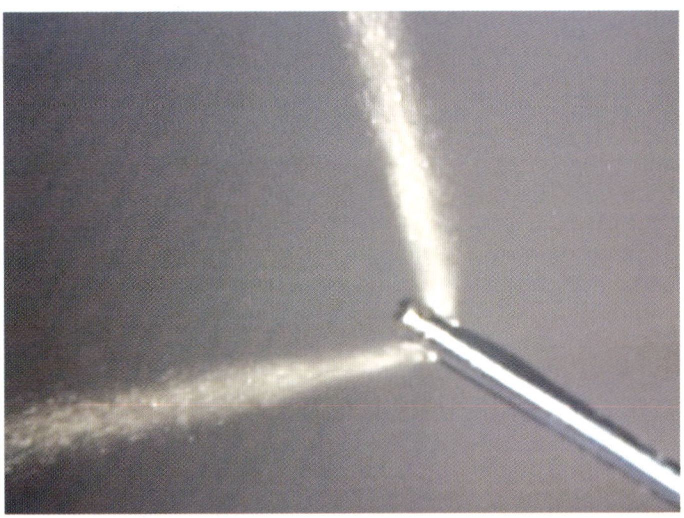

Fig. 3: Forced infusion through a double ended 0.7 mm irrigating cannula

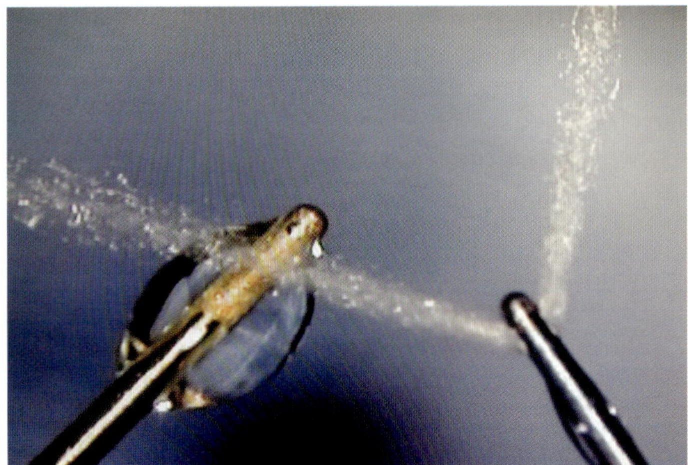

Fig. 4: Aspirating and irrigating 0.7 mm system of cannulas

3. 0.7 mm aspirating cannula: we believe a one-superior opened aspirating cannula is the best for this technique because the hole is in the opposite side of the posterior capsule and is always in the field of view of the surgeon.
4. Microphakonit tip (0.7 mm Phacotip) is not needed in most of the cases, because the nucleus is soft, so only the vacuum is needed to aspirate it and no ultrasonic force is used. This is only an irrigating-aspirating technique with an air pump at one side (forced infusion) and aspiration (vacuum or peristaltic pump) in the another side.
5. 0.7 mm diamond or saphire blades. It is important to be sure that the incision will be made with the exact size for this technique. It is almost a closed environment in the anterior chamber and will be possible only with the proper incisions. A large incision will lead to surge even if forced infusion is used, complicating so the procedure.
6. Microphakonit capsulorrhexis forceps. You can use any model you want, just be sure that your 0.7 mm incision is enough to permit the entrance of the instrument to the anterior chamber.
7. Forceps, viscoelastics, anesthetic eyedrops, IOL implantation devices, etc.

PATIENT PREPARATION

Before start the surgeon must be sure to have the following data:

1. *Refraction:* Because it is a refractive procedure the surgeon must be sure of the exact refractive state of the patient.
2. *Corneal topography:* We believe that the astigmatism can be reduced with the implantation incision placed at the steepest corneal meridian.
3. *IOL power calculation.* We believe for these refractive cases the best tool is the Interferometry Biometry (IOL Master Calculation)
4. Preoperative investigation of the health of the patient (diabetes, hypertension, renal diseases, etc.)
5. Signed informed consent about a RLE procedure and it´s potential complications. Complete knowledge about the procedure and about the IOL to be used (multifocal, monofocal, pseudo-accomodative, etc.). Also the signed possibility of a second procedure (posterior capsulotomy, astigmatic relaxing incisions, photorefractive procedures, IOL exchange).

Finally a preoperative preparation as the surgeon use to perform the cataract procedures with topical anesthesia in the operative room. We do believe that topical anesthesia must be the rule in RLE and of course in 0.7 mm MIRLEX, because the advantage for the patient that will be able to see just leaving the operating room, the early use of eyedrops to avoid inflammatory complications and the painless of a minimally invasive procedure.

SURGICAL STEPS

1. Place sterile drapes over the eye as usual.
2. Place some eyedrops of anesthetic and give the instruction to the patient to see the microscope light always with this eye. If you find a photophobic

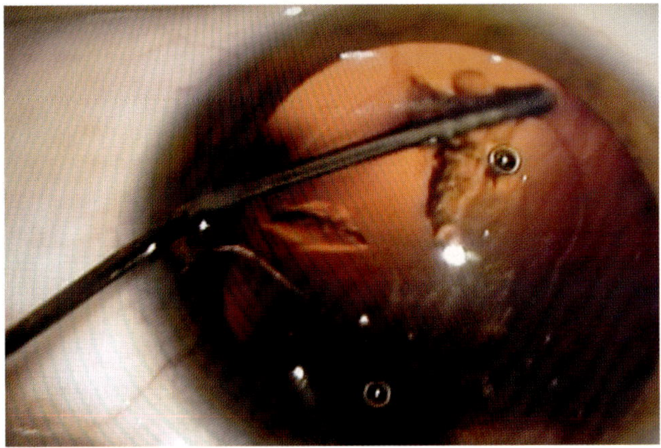

Fig. 5: Hydrodissection through a 0.7 mm sideport

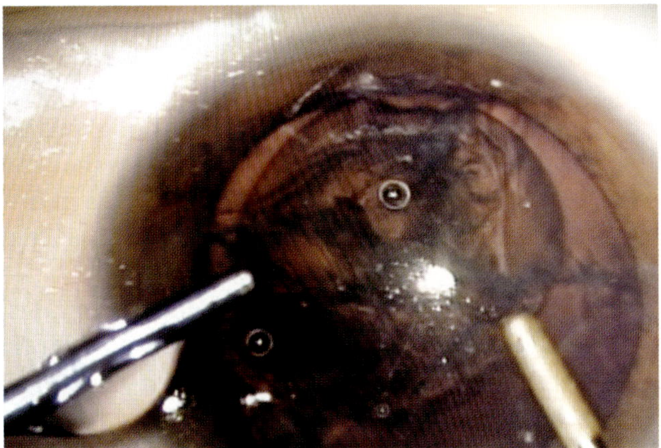

Fig. 6: 0.7 mm irrigation/aspiration system ready to go afted hydrodissection has been completed

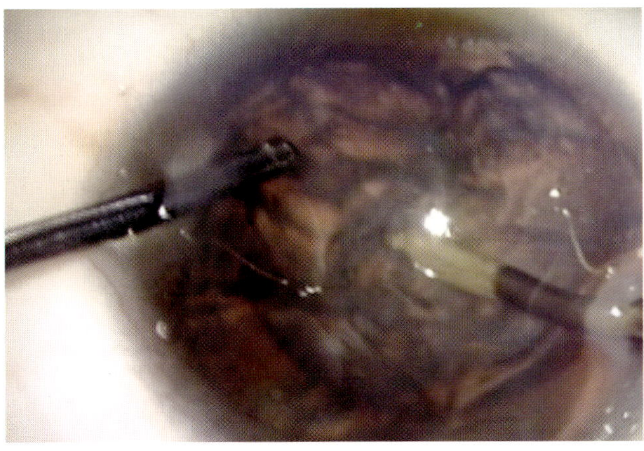

Fig. 7: Nuclear material 0.7 mm bimanual aspiration

patient, decrease the light of the microscope for your first incision, place intracameral lidocaine and then you can increase the intensity of your light safety because of the effect of the intracameral anesthesia.

3. Place your self at the meridian of the eye of your implantation incision. It means that if your patient has an astigmatism with the rule (at 180° or near) you must perform the implantation incision at 90°, so this is the place where the surgeon must seat. The irrigation-aspiration incisions will be at 3 and 9 o´clock position and will be astigmatically neutral.
4. Hold the eye very soft with a forceps with one hand and perform with the 0.7 mm blade the first incision at 3 o´clock position with the another hand. To be sure it will be a self sealed incision first go directly perpendicular to the cornea and before entry the anterior chamber change the direction parallel to the iris plane. Do it with a single movement, and be sure not to open more your incision when you retire your blade.
5. If you want you can place intracameral anesthetic and/or adrenergic drugs to obtain good mydriasis. After this, fill the anterior chamber with viscoelastic material. The main goal of this technique is to maintain the anterior chamber always open.
6. Use the viscoelastic cannula to hold the eye with your left hand trough this first incision. The advantage of a bimanual technique is that you can control always the eye movements with two hands during the entire procedure. Also it avoids the use of forceps over the conjuntiva to avoid surface damage or pain sensation.
7. Une the right hand to perform a second side port incision at 9 o´clock position at the same plane holding the eye with the vscoelastic cannula inside the first incision. Do it in the same plane that the first one. Both incision must be made aprox 1 mm inside the limbus, totally over the cornea. Some of these patients are soft contact lenses users and with a lot of limbal vascularization.
8. Keep holding the eye with the viscoelastic cannula at your left hand and introduce the cystitome trough the second incision to cut the anterior capsule. Perform capsulorrhexis with cystitome or forceps trough the second incision with your right hand while holding the eye with the viscoelastic cannula with the left. If you want during the rhexis you can switch hands to help your procedure; you can re-fill the chamber with viscoelastic any time you need.
9. Once the capsulorrhexis is done (the size will depend the IOL you will use), perform hydrodissection and hydrodelamination of the nucleus. Start just below the anterior capsule to separate first the cortex from the capsule, decreasing so the aspiration time, and then follow with epinucleus and nucleus.
10. Once you are sure all the lens material has been hydrodissected you prepare to insert the 0.7 mm irrigation/aspiration cannulas. Be sure of your forced infusion; we use 130 to 160 cm of H_2O for positive pressure with the 700

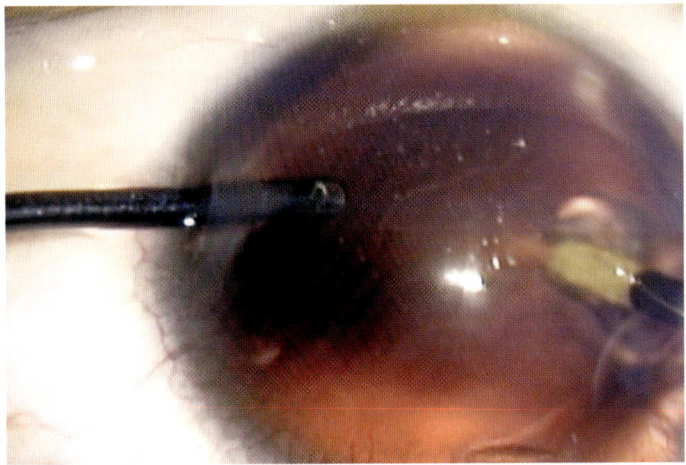

Fig. 8: Cortical material 0.7 mm bimanual aspiration

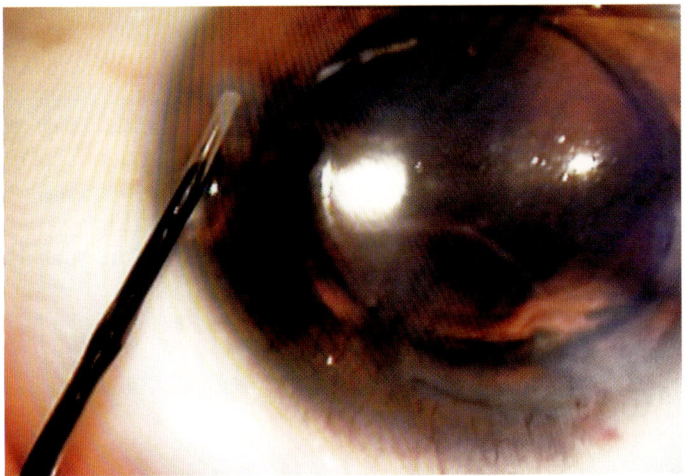

Fig. 9: Incisional edema and viscoelastic extraction

microns system. We suggest also, high vacuum levels (400 mmHg) with this system because the small diameter of the aspirating cannula. You must test these parameters before enter the anterior chamber, otherwise this system will not work properly.

11. Introduce the irrigating 0.7 mm cannula first with the irrigation on. You can introduce your irrigation directly to the nucleus to complete separate the layers of it. A small amount of viscoelastic material can fluid trough the incisions. Then introduce the 0.7 mm aspirating cannula trough the second sideport.
12. Control your aspirating force with the footpedal. Go first for the nucleus, then the epinucleus and finally the cortical material. There is not need to move so much your hands; if you have your correct parameters the hydrodinamic forced will do the surgery for you. Just be sure to aspirate near the iris plane to avoid the posterior capsule.
13. With the same 0.7 mm cannula you can pulish the posterior and anterior capsule after the cortical material has been removed.
14. Take out the aspirating cannula keeping the irrigating one inside the eye and with continuous irrigation to keep the anterior chamber wide open. Switch with your right hand from the aspirating cannula to the viscoelastic material and introduce it trough the aspirating incision. Slowly fill the anterior chamber with viscoelastic and stop the irrigation. Once your anterior chamber is totally fill with viscoelastic you are able to take out the irrigating cannula. This maneuver will help you to keep an anterior chamber formed all the time.
15. Now you can do your implantation incision at the meridian you need. Do it clear cornea,in two steps just like the side ports, with an exact size of your blade according your implant, and holding the eye with your left hand trough your irrigating sideport with the viscoelastic cannula in order to avoid forceps.
16. Do your IOL implantation and remember that you have two side ports to help you to manipulate the IOL.
17. Perform hydratation of the cornea with pressure enough to take out the viscoelastic material. Do not aspirate the viscoelastic, you can have an unestable anterior chamber after this; just with the pressure of a 10 cc syringe you can hydratate the peri-incisional strome and take out the viscoelastic material at the same time.
18. Place a soft bandage contact lens, some intracameral antibiotic and you are ready to go.

AVOIDING COMPLICATIONS

Most of the complications become when the technique is done improperly.

- Inappropriate wound construction will lead to leakage and surge. In this case the best solution is to close this wound with stromal hydratation and perform another.
- Bad programmation of parameters. For 700 microns technique Forced Infusion is mandatory; gravitatory force will be never enough to fill the

anterior chamber and avoid surge. It is also mandatory because high vacuum levels are also mandatory to be able to aspirate trough 700 microns aspirating cannula.

- Unexpected eye movements are easy to avoid using the viscoelastic cannula as a stabilization instrument with the left hand while performing maneuvers with the right hand. Be sure to perform "bimanually" almost all our maneuvers; it is one of the main advantages of the technique.
- Inappropriate instrumentation; be sure to have 700 microns system. At the time of writing this chapter only the Duet system from Microsurgical Technology (MST) is available.
- Inappropriate hydrodissection; be sure to perform it many times. The clear lens is soft so if you perform vigorous hydrodelamination, your aspirating time will be reduced and your movements inside the eye also will be less. Be sure to aspirate far away from the corneal endothelium, posterior capsule and iris in order to avoid damage to intraocular structures.
- Learn to use your both hands; it is a bimanual technique and also minimally invasive. You have the advantages that the eye is always in your control, so there is not need to perform "one hand maneuvers"; also you have the advantage to have an "always formed" anterior chamber. Learn to switch your instruments between both hands in order to take the maximum advantage from a "no-collapse technique".
- If posterior capsule is broken follow this steps:
  1. Keep with the irrigating cannula inside the eye with the irrigation on, but decrease the irrigation force to 100 cm H_2O.
  2. Take out the aspirating cannula with your right hand and switch it fast for your vitrectomy system. If it is not ready, fill the chamber with viscoelastic trough your aspirating sideport before take out the irrigating cannula.
  3. You might need to enlarge to 1 mm the aspirating incision because your vitrectomy system can be larger that 700 microns.
  4. Perform bimanual vitrectomy with 100 cm H_2O of irrigation force, 800 cuts per minute and 200 to 250 mmHg of vacuum, keeping the system closed. It is your main advantage, a bimanual vitrectomy in a closed chamber.
  5. Take out your vitrector while keeping the irrigation on and fill the anterior chamber with vicoelastic material trough your aspirating port. Do not stop and take out the irrigation cannula until you are sure your eye is filled with viscoelastic.
  6. Avoid the vitreous from the incisions and place your IOL in the sulcus. Use miotic intracameral medication to be sure there is not vitreous trough the incisions.

POSTOPERATIVE CARE

The postoperative care of your patient will be easy if the technique was done properly. It will include anti-inflammatory, antibiotic and anti-hipertensive eyedrops since the first day. The bandage contact lens can be retire the day after the surgery.

Monitoring the intraocular pressure is key; you have access to the anterior chamber trough the side port incisions at the slit lamp any time during the inmediate postoperative period to decrease intraocular pressure if needed; it is another advantage of a bimanual technique.

The refraction will be very stable during the first 4 to 6 weeks; remember that your implantation incision was made only for this purpose, implantation; no other maneuver has been done trough this incision (like exposure to ultrasonic power, enlargement in two planes), so it will be very stable soon. The side port incisions are astigmatically neutral so you will be ready to obtain a final refraction very soon and decide if you need an additional refractive procedure.

Your patient will feel like a LASIK patient; a 10 minute procedure done under topical anesthesia and in mediate visual recovery. So you have to be in communication and make see him or she that it was an intraocular procedure and must be taking care in the postoperative period.

FINAL COMMENTS

The main goal, and also the main advantage of this technique, is to keep an anterior chamber wide open all the time, in a closed environment. The no surge and no collapses technique has many advantages:

- No endothelial cell damage.
- Maneuvers far away from the posterior capsule.
- No vitreous movement: this is of particular importance in the miopic patient where a collapse can be the key to a retinal detachment.
- Always you have a positive pressure avoiding choroidal effusions
- Wide open pupil because there are not changes in intraocular pressure that can produce miosis.
- No flat chamber even in case of vitreous loss.

The forced infusion (positive pressure), also mandatory, has many advantages:

- Wide anterior chamber; this is of particular importance in the hyperopic patient where the anterior chamber is too shallow.
- Tense and "far away" posterior capsule.

The reader, and new bimanual surgeon, can think that the forced infusion can lead to a lot of irrigation inside the eye, but you will experience that the entire surgery is done with less that 100 cc of intraocular solution with this 700 microns system. In fact with the time, when you currently perform this technique for all your RLE patients, you will see that no more than 50 to 60 cc per case will be need.

We do believe that this is a very safe technique for your RLE patient; it also is a very safe technique for the surgeon, it is relatively easy and reproductible, so he or she can be sure that the patient is doing fine. The surgeon can sleep well.

23

Capsular Bag Refilling Using Capsulotomy: Capturing Intraocular Lens

Okihiro Nishi, Kayo Nishi,
Yutaro Nishi, Shiao Chang (Japan)

Introduction

Refilling the lens capsule with an injectable material, while preserving capsular integrity including zonules and ciliary muscles, offer a potential to restore ocular accommodation. The greatest technical challenge in this procedure was primarily preventing the leakage of injectable IOLs.

To prevent leakage, we developed a silicone plug to seal the capsular opening. We could confirm some accommodation in the young macaca monkies. Figure shows the Scheimpflug photographies of the eye of a monkey before and after surgery, showing evidence of some accommodation being obtained. After application of 4% pilocarpine, there is thickening of the lens with steepening of the anterior capsule and shallowing of the anterior chamber, both before and after surgery, although the findings were much less marked after surgery.

From these experiments, we have concluded that refilling the lens capsule is technically quite fasible. It is suggested that the procedure may restore ocular accommodation in humans. However, there are some essential problems to overcome: Refining and simplifying the technique; Prevention of anterior capsule opacification (ACO) and posterior capsule opacification (PCO); Reducing surgically-induced astigmatism because the unilateral CCC, though tiny, caused a great astigmatism (unpublished data).

Here, I will demonstrate a completely new concept and novel lens refilling procedure that may solve these problems. We had this concept already in 1989[9] and resumed the technique, because endocapsular balloon technique and the capsular plug technique will not be supposed to be applied clinically, and the technique will solve the problems mentioned above.

Refilling the Lens Capsule with Capsulotomy-Capturing Intraocular Lens

IOL

The IOL shape is similar to that of a conventional IOL, but the optic has small narrow grooves over its entire circumference. The CCC edge is put in this groove, which chokes the IOL, preventing leakage of the injected material. Figure 5 illustrates the procedure. Figure 6 shows the most recent foldable version of the IOL.

SURGICAL PROCEDURE

As in conventional cataract surgery, CCC, around 4 mm in diameter, is created in the middle of the anterior capsule. After phacoemulsification aspiration, viscoelastics are injected into the capsular bag in the usual manner. The folded IOL is introduced entirely into the capsular bag. A Sinskey hook is introduced

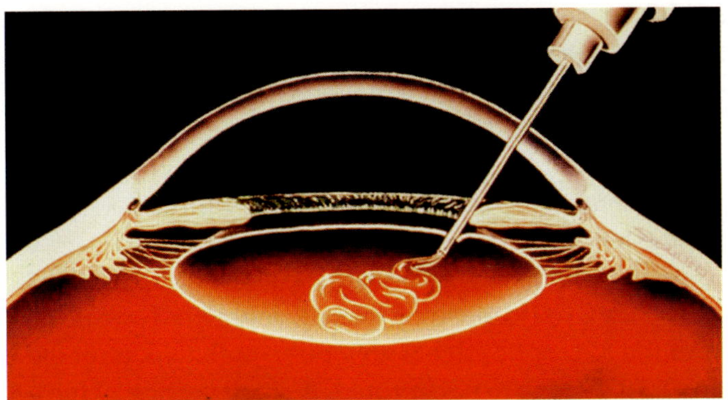

Fig. 1: Schematic illustration of the lens refilling procedure (*Courtesy: DJ Apple*)

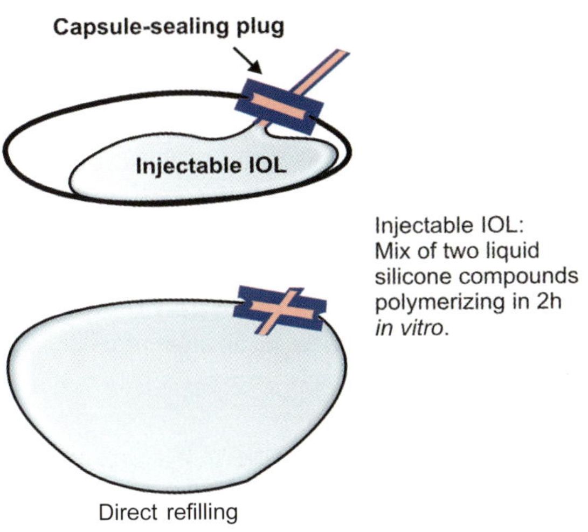

Fig. 2: Lens refilling technique using a silicone plug (*Reprinted by permission of Archives of Ophthalmology*)

underneath the IOL, and the IOL is lifted by the hook, so that the optic edge groove of the lower half of the IOL is captured by the lower half of the CCC. The lower half of the groove is captured almost automatically while lifting the lower half of the IOL, because the IOL is firmly fixed in the middle by both haptics remaining in the capsular bag. Then, the viscoelastics are completely removed by aspiration, during which an I/A cannula is introduced underneath the upper half of the IOL, which is now outside of the capsular bag. Viscoelastics are injected into the anterior chamber onto the IOL. The upper half of the IOL is then captured by the CCC by pushing the IOL downward and posteriorly at the middle part of the IOL optic edge with a push-pull hook until the upper IOL clears the upper CCC edge to be captured. A small portion of the CCC edge at the optic groove is now hooked with the Sinskey hook and pulled slightly to introduce the injection cannula. The injectable material, actually a mix of two liquid silicones is then injected into the capsular bag. It polymerizes in 2h *in vitro*.

Results and Discussions

We have refilled many pig cadaver eyes and rabbit eyes using this technique. After the IOL was correctly captured by the CCC, there was no leakage of the injected silicone. Thus, the apropriate size for the CCC, not too small to capture but not too large to capture firmly the IOL, is crucial for surgical success. If the CCC is appropriately sized, the procedure is highly reproducible. We marked a 5 mm circle on the cornea using a Hoffer optic zone marker for 5 mm, according to the technique described by Wallace, and used this mark as a guide for an appropriate CCC diameter around 4 mm.

EXPECTED MECHANISM OF ACCOMMODATION

The expected mechanism of accommodation involves forward-movement of the IOL and thickening of the lens.

These expected mechanisms are based on two recent studies. Nawa and his co-workers demonstrated the accommodation-amplitude obtained per 1 mm forward movement of the IOL. For this purpose, a ray-focusing equation for pseudophakic eyes was established using the ray-tracing method with dedicated computer software. It was found that the amplitude depends on axial length and corneal power. In eyes with an axial length of 21 mm and an IOL with 30 diopters, 1 mm forward movement yields 2.3 D of accommodation. Accordingly, in an eye with a length of 23 mm and 24 diopters, 1.6 D of accommodation will be obtained, while only 0.8 D will be obtained with values of 27 mm and 11 diopters. These findings indicate that improvements may be obtained with the recently developed accommodating IOL such as the Crysta lens or 1CU, specifically in hyperopic eyes with a short axial length.

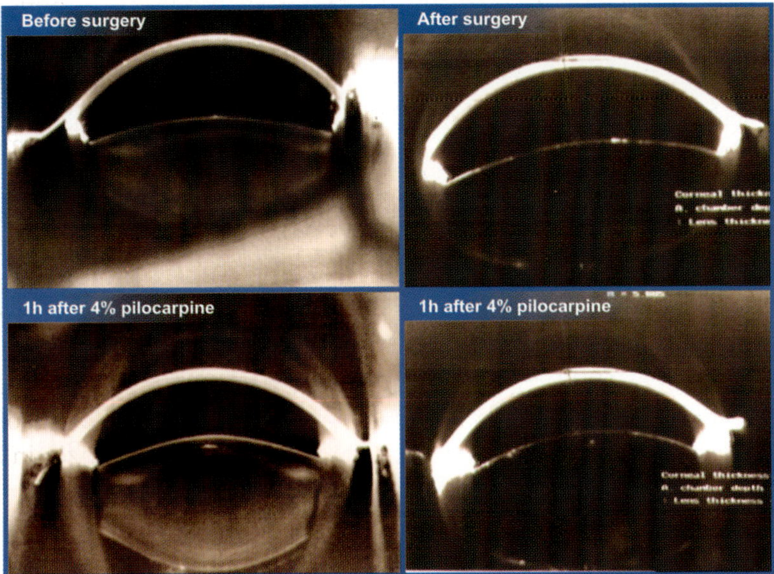

Fig. 3: Scheimpflug photographs of a monkey eye before and after refilling the lens capsule. Note that there was thickening of the lens with steepening of the anterior capsule and shallowing of the anterior chamber. After surgery (right), there were similar findings, though less remarkable. Note also that there were discontinuous zones in the lens before surgery, while the refilled lens was optically empty due to the silicone compound

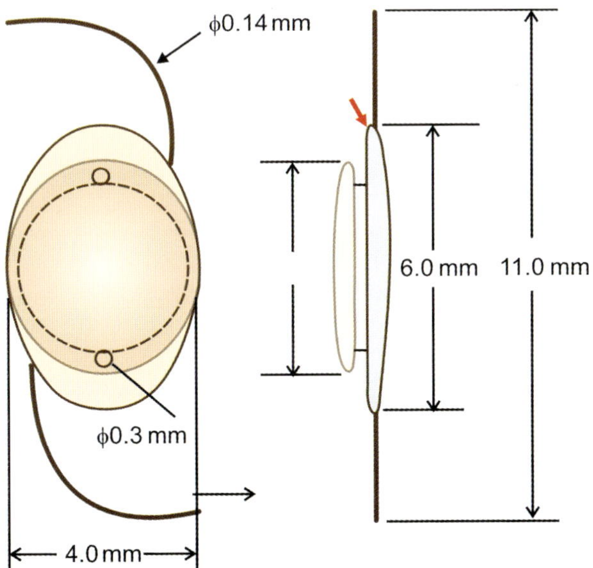

Fig. 4: Anterior capsule-supported IOL for sealing CCC. The arrows show the small narrow, grooves at the optic (*Reprinted by permission* of *Nishi O, Nishi K,* Graefe's Archives of Clinical and Experimental Ophthalmology)

Van der Heijde and co-workers measured microfluctuations of steady-state accommodation using ultrasonography, and demonstrated that fluctuations in accommodation are mainly caused by fluctuations of lens thickness. They found that on average, the lens increases by about 56 µm in thickness per diopter during fluctuation. That means that 3 diopters could be obtained by about 0.17 mm change in thickness.

ENHANCEMENT OF ACCOMMODATION-AMPLITUDE AND PCO-PREVENTION BY DUAL-OPTIC

To prevent PCO and possibly to augument accommodation-amplitude being attained, we have drafted a dual-optic concept, as Figure shows. First, a conventional foldable IOL with sharp edges and the enhanced haptic angulation is implanted into the capsular bag. It has a concave optic with a minus dioptric power, which may imperatively give a greater power to the anterior optic, achieving emmetropia. During accommodation, the anterior capsule moves forward, while the posterior capsule stays relatively unmoved, so that an anterior optic with a greater power may enhance the accommodation-amplitude attained. A large angulation of the haptic will press the sharp optic edge against the posterior capsule to create a strong compression on it for the prevention of PCO. The injected silicone mix will additionally press the IOL onto the posterior capsule. As an alternative technique, the same CCC-capturing IOL can be implanted after a posterior CCC is performed. Then, a CCC-capturing IOL is introduced into the capsular bag which contains the IOL being implanted previously and captured by the anterior CCC, as already described. To refill the bag, silicone mix is injected between two IOLs that are captured by the anterior and posterior CCCs.

Summary

To summarize, the novel anterior capsule-supported IOL is technically quite feasible. Some accommodation might be obtained by forward-movement and

TABLE 1: The relationship between AL and dioptric power of an MA30BA IOL and amount of accommodation per 1.0 mm forward movement

	Axial length (mm)						
Parameter	21.0	22.0	23.0	24.0	25.0	26.0	27.0
IOL power (IOL)	30.0	27.0	24.0	20.0	17.0	14.0	11.0
Accommodation per 1.0 mm forward IOL movement (D)	2.3	1.9	1.6	1.3	1.1	0.9	0.8

(*Reprinted by permission* of J Cataract Refract Surg.)

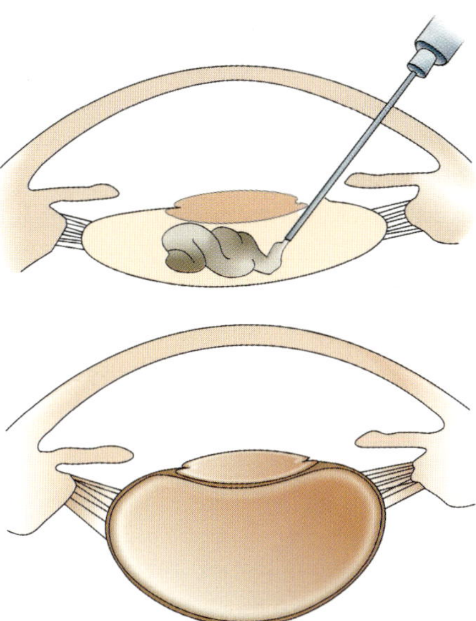

Fig. 5: Surgical lens refilling procedure using anterior capsule-supported IOL (*Reprinted by permission* of Graefe's Archives of Clinical and Experimental Ophthalmology)

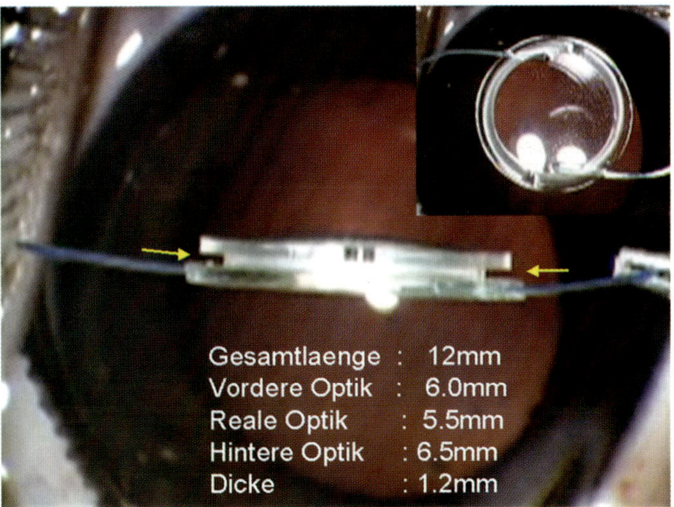

Fig. 6: Anterior capsule-supported foldable IOL and its dimensions

thickening of the lens. We will test this procedure in primate eyes. Anterior and posterior capsule opacification at least in the optical axis can be avoided. Postoperative emmetropia is supposed to be achieved more easily due to the predetermined optic. One of the advantages is that postoperative *in vivo* power change may be possible using an adjustable IOL.

In conclusion, restoration of accommodation by refilling the lens capsule is a goal of refractive cataract surgery. Technical feasibility has been repeatedly demonstrated by obtaining some useful accommodation in primates and will be further facilitated by modern technology. Capsular opacification is one of the essential problems to be overcome. The technique shown here may provide a breakthrough for possible clinical application to refilling of the lens capsule.

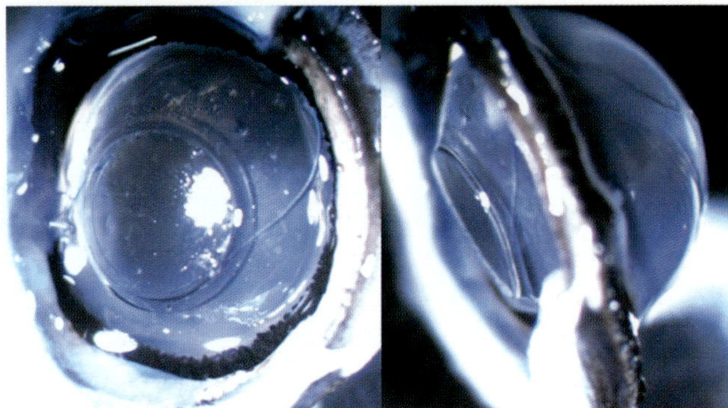

Fig. 7: A well-refilled pig cadaver capsule. The anterior capsule-supported IOL was firmily fixed, and there was no leakage of the material injected

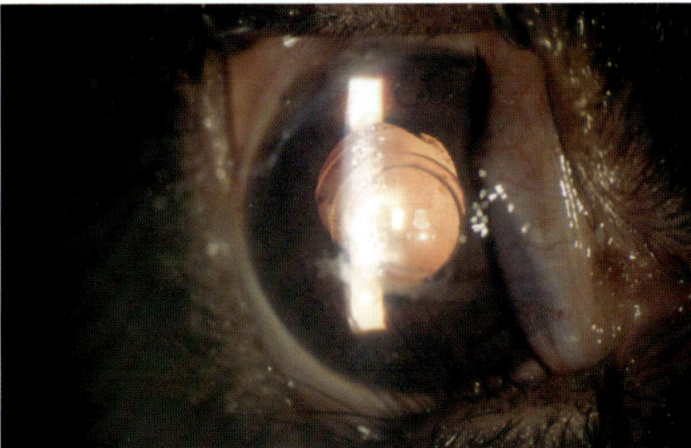

Fig. 8: A refilled rabbit crystalline lens. Three weeks after surgery. Note that the IOL was firmly and securely fixed. There was no leakage of the injected silicone compound. Posterior synechia

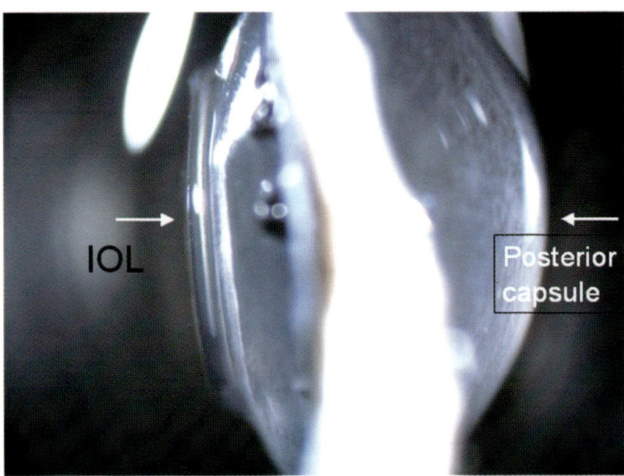

Fig. 9: An enucleated rabbit lens refilled

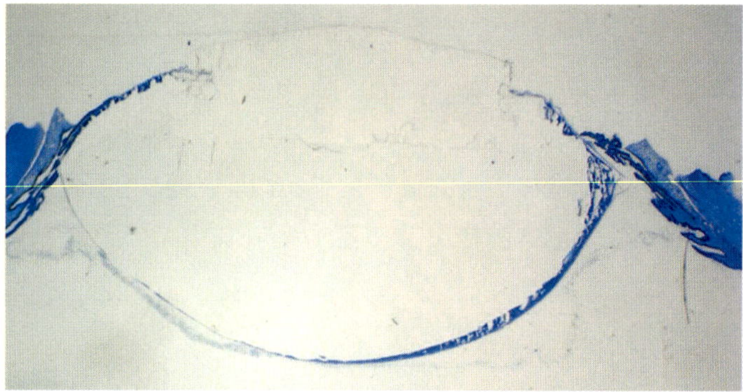

Fig. 10: Histopathological findings of an enucleated rabbit lens refilled. Three weeks after surgery

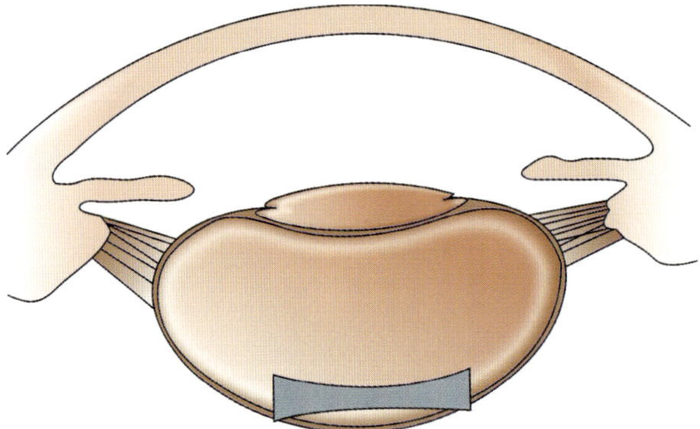

Fig. 11: Dual optic refilling concept I. The concave posterior IOL with a minus power and sharp edges is pressed on the posterior capsule, so that LEC migration might be prevented

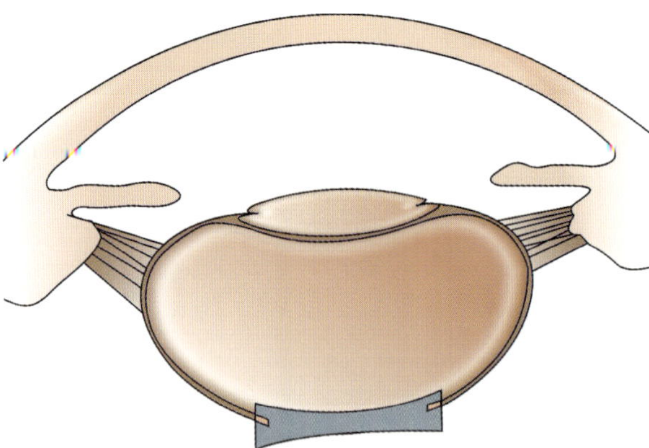

Fig. 12: Dual optic refilling concept II. The concave posterior IOL optic is captured by the posterior CCC. The posterior visual axis is expected to remain PCO-free

24

New Options for Sutureless IOL Implantation in Aphakic Eyes with Lacking Capsule

Peter W Rieck (Germany)

Introduction

Absence of capsular or zonular structures in aphakic eyes might occur in cases of primary or secondary luxation of the crystalline lens, i.e. in patients with Marfan syndrome or after trauma, in patients after former intracapsular cataract extraction or after explantation of an in-the-bag subluxated capsule/intraocular lens (IOL).

Secondary IOL implantation is the standard of care for treating aphakia when spectacle or contact lens correction is not viable. There is controversy about the relative efficacy and safety of the different IOL implantation approaches, as well as their indications. Up to now, options included implantation of an anterior chamber (AC) IOL or suture-fixating an IOL in the ciliary sulcus which was usually accomplished by scleral fixation.

The design of modern open-loop AC angle-supported IOLs has been refined, but most of these developments have recently been achieved for phakic AC IOLs in refractive surgery including the AcrySof SA3M13 (Alcon, USA), the Kelman Duet Implant (Tekia, USA), the Vivarte-IOL (Ioltech, France) and the ICARE (Corneal, France). However, the two latter IOLs have been taken off the market very recently, showing that AC IOL still deals with severe side effects. The two former are presently not aimed for implantation in aphakic eyes. Thus, for correction of aphakia, standard AC IOLs still appear less desirable due to a greater potential for corneal decompensation, long-term inflammation and secondary glaucoma. In consequence, AC-IOL implantation should be avoided in patients with glaucoma, diabetes, cornea guttata or low endothelial cell count, peripheral anterior synechiae, or known or suspected cystoid macular edema. Furthermore, the main disadvantage of angle-supported AC IOLs lies in their dependence on the internal dimensions and anatomy of the anterior chamber. This might soon be overcome with the advent of high-frequency ultrasound biometry instruments such as the Visante OCT (Carl Zeiss, Germany) and the Artemis (Ultralink, Canada) to better adapt AC-IOLs sizes to the specific dimensions of the anterior chamber.

As an alternative to AC IOL, ciliary sulcus fixation of standard posterior chamber (PC) IOls to the sclera by means of sutures has been widely used in these cases for a long period of time. However, the technique is relatively complex and reveals a large range of possible complications (macular edema, IOL tilt / decentration, suture erosion, choroidal hemorrhage and late endophthalmitis). The use of a foldable PC IOL may reduce postoperative astigmatism due to small incision surgery but does not reduce the risk of the above mentioned complications. Recent surgical and technological advances, including the technique of burying the suture knot in sclera, use of an ab externo suturing approach in the normotonic eye, and the use of intraoperative endoscopy, have improved the accuracy of the transsclerally sutured PC IOL technique but it remains a rather laborious approach.

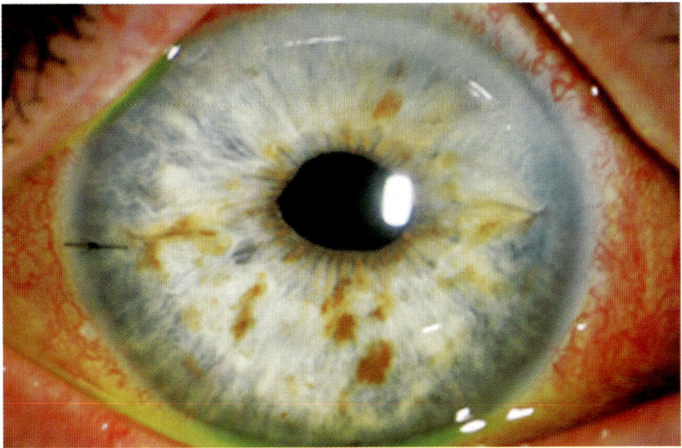

Fig. 1: Postoperative appearance of an inversely implanted, retropupillary fixated iris claw lens. Anterior segment overview. Note the contraction of iris tissue in the mid periphery which corresponds to the site of the enclavations

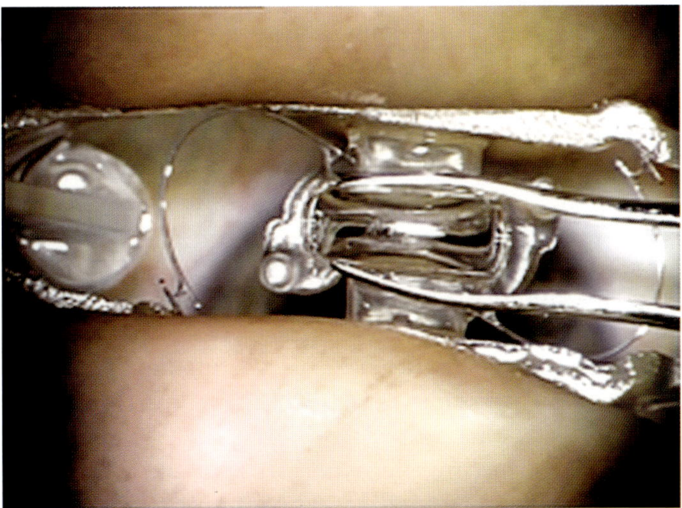

Fig. 2: The Binderflex IOL has been folded in its cartridge and is picked up with a folding forceps

Schein et al have shown that peripheral iris fixation is the safest way to support a PC IOL in aphakic eyes without capsular support. In a large randomized trial (176 patients) of IOL fixation techniques during penetrating keratoplasty, the authors found that the risk of macular edema was significantly less in the iris fixation group compared to AC IOL implantation or PC IOL scleral fixation. Iris suture fixation, however, is a techniqually demanding procedure when no open-sky situation exists as this is the case during penetrating keratoplasty. A refined technique for small-incision peripheral iris fixation of a standard foldable acrylic PC IOL has recently been proposed.

A literature analysis related to IOL implantation in the absence of capsular support by Wagoner et al in 2003 yielded 217 citations for the years 1980 to 2002. The literature supports the safe and effective use of open-loop anterior chamber, scleral-sutured posterior chamber, and iris-sutured posterior chamber IOLs for the correction of aphakia in eyes without adequate capsular support. At that time, no evidence was deteced to demonstrate the superiority of one lens type or fixation site. However, up to now, a precise distinction of complication rates remains difficult since only few quantitative data are available from these studies.

In the following part of this chapter, the progress in this field to avoid the complication-prone use of sutures is described.

New Developments of Sutureless Anterior Chamber IOL

An interesting alternative, combining sutureless iris fixation with anterior chamber implantation of an IOL that does not affect the angle region is the "revival" of the Worst iris claw lens. Originally designed by J Worst in 1978 as an IOL to correct aphakia after cataract extraction, this lens has gained rising popularity in a concave version as a phakic IOL to correct high myopia. Named Artisan® (Ophtec, Netherlands) or Verisyse® (AMO, USA), respectively, different refractive models to correct myopia, hypermetropia, and astigmatism have been developed in the mean time. A foldable version (Artiflex®, Veriflex®) for small incision refractive surgery has been released only recently. An aphakic model of this lens made of PMMA is also available and has successfully been employed to correct aphakia in patients with various ocular pathologies. A recent study, however, has shown a higher rate of endothelial cell loss (10.9%) 36 months postoperatively. The cell loss occurred predominantly during the first year (7.78%). This complication may result from the marked anterior-posterior mobility of the IOL that follows the movements of the often loosened iris diaphragm in aphakic eyes.

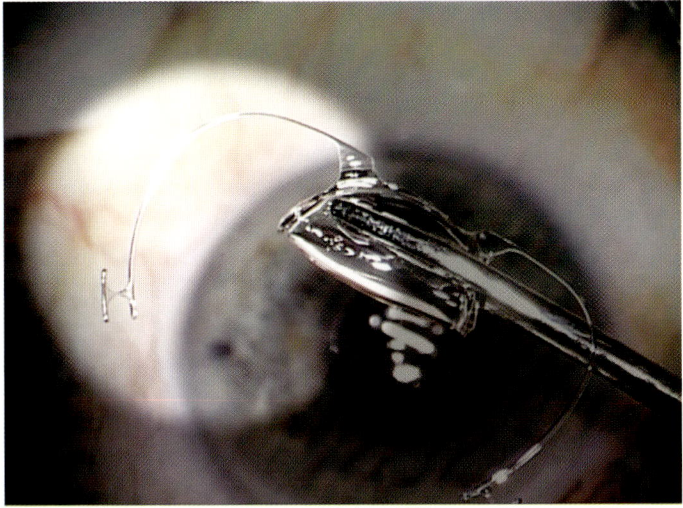

Fig. 3: The folded Binderflex showing the long haptics and the anchors

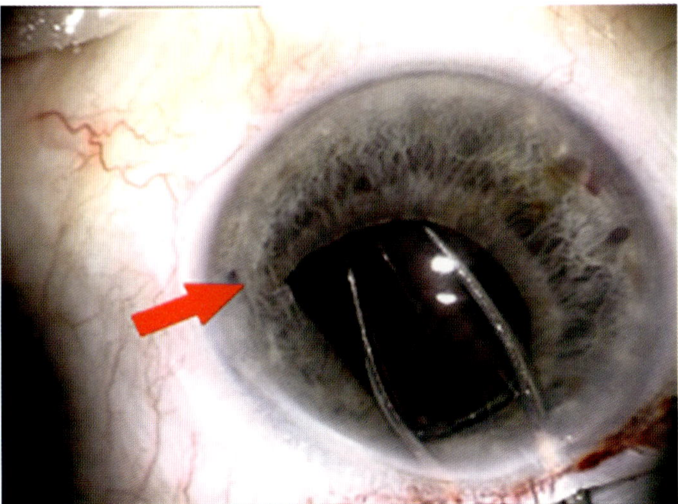

Fig. 4: Implantation of the Binderflex IOL through a scleral tunnel. The IOL is inserted behind the iris plane with the anchor of the leading haptic being hooked on the pupil (red arrow)

In order to stabilize an AC-IOL in aphakic eyes, J Reiter (Landshut, Germany) has developed a sulcus-fixated, but sutureless AC lens with long haptics, each of which is twisted into one of two opposing peripheral iridectomies and thus securely placed in the ciliary sulcus. This IOL, the MP 614 (Human Optics, Germany) made of PMMA has an optic diameter of 6 mm and a total diameter of 14 mm. The configuration of the haptics was designed in a way to follow the curvature of the sulcus in order to enlarge the contact area of the haptics with the sulcus. The haptics are fixed at an angle of 5° backwards from the optic plane. According to Dr Reiter, the implantation is easy to perform for the experienced surgeon. In a preliminary series of 17 eyes, he noted a stabilized iris diaphragm after implantation with no irido- or pseudophakodonesis. In a postoperative follow-up period up to one year for seven of the eyes operated on, he was unable to detect any endothelial cell loss. Attempts are currently under way to develop a foldable version of this lens.

New Developments of Sutureless Posterior Chamber IOL

In order to avoid AC IOL associated problems as mentioned above it appears advantageous to achieve a retropupillary fixation of the iris claw lens. Amar was the first to propose a fixation at the posterior iris as an alternative method to the conventional anterior fixation. However, due to the danger of possible pigment dispersion via rubbing of the anterior IOL surface at the posterior pigmented layer of the iris, the idea was rapidly abandoned and adapted years later by Mohr et al, who implanted the IOL in the inverted position with the convex side up, thus leaving a distance between the IOL surface and the pigmented posterior iris. The enclavation procedure of iris tissue into the "claw"-like haptics is even easier with the retropupillary fixation, due to the facilitated "feeding" of iris tissue into the claw of the firmly fixed IOL. Our experience with at present 32 posterior chamber implantations of an inversed iris claw lens in aphakic eyes without capsular support is excellent. The technique can be handled very easily with a short learning curve. In comparison to the AC implantation, the posterior approach has the advantage of less endothelial cell loss. Furthermore, the more anatomical position of the lens is achieved with much less surgical trauma compared to scleral suture fixated PC IOLs.

A disadvantage might still be the higher mobility of the lens due to iridodonesis in these aphakic eyes, above all after vitrectomy, and thus the danger of late loosening of the IOL as well as the occurrence of possible reflections of the incoming light. In addition, due to the inversed optic there is an increase in optical abberations although patients complaints have not been noticed up to now, probably due to the small pupils in this cohort of mostly elderly patients and an often compromised macular situation due to previous surgeries.

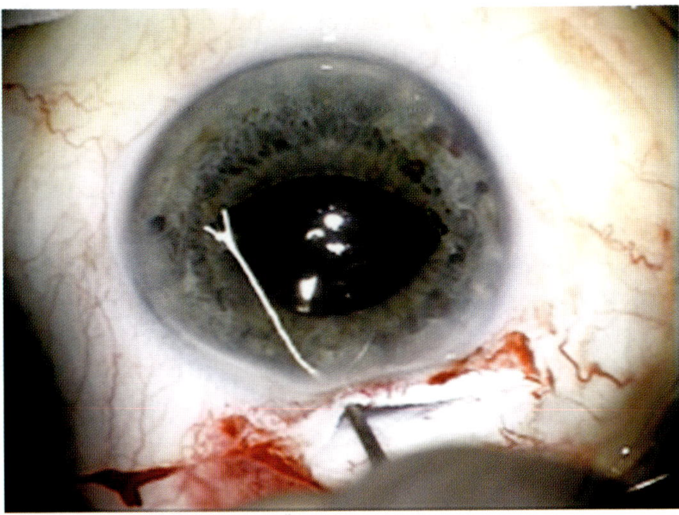

Fig. 5: With the second haptic hung onto the iris, the lens is rotated towards 3 and 9 o'clock position with a rotating device and a Y-hook

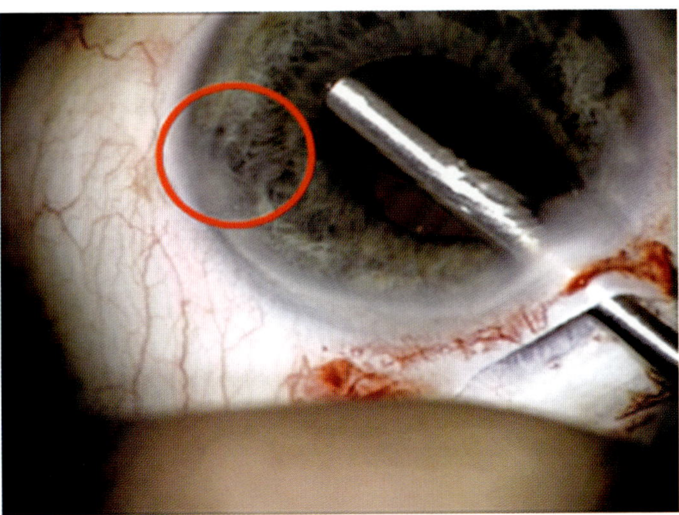

Fig. 6: A haptic forceps is introduced through the tunnel or paracenteses to grasp and position an anchor through an iridotomy (red circle)

In order to combine the advantages of a sutureless implanted PC IOL like the inversed iris claw lens with the stability and optical performance of a standard sutured PC IOL, we developed a technique for a sutureless iris-fixated ciliary sulcus implantation of a new PC IOL designed especially for such cases.

This PC IOL, named "Binder"-IOL after its designer H Binder (Olbertshausen, Germany), has an optic diameter of 6 mm and an overall diameter of 15 mm. The long, C-shaped haptics are only 0.14 mm thick and therefore very flexible. Angulation of the haptics is 12° from the optic plane and they thus provide reciprocal support in the ciliary sulcus. At the end of both haptics, a T-shaped, so-called anchor is mounted at 45° from the optic plane. These anchors are designed to pass through and button in peripheral iridotomies. This design of the haptics stabilize the IOL in every spatial axis. The prototype of this IOL was made of PMMA. In between, a foldable version made of hydrophilic acryl is available that can be prefolded in the delivered cartridge and then picked up with a folding forceps. The IOL is produced by Morcher AG, Germany and distributed by Iolution, Germany.

The key to the stability of this lens is its special design. The haptics have three main functional areas: the long C-haptics, which lodge in the sulcus; the neck of the anchors, which extend through iridotomies, and the head of the anchors, which lie on the surface of the iris.

Implantation of the Binderflex lens involves placing two paracenteses at about 3 and 9 o'clock, a little wider as is done in phaco surgery. A scleral tunnel is prepared in case of an IOL explantation, e.g. after subluxation. A clear corneal incision is made in cases without extractions.

Viscoelastic is injected at 3 and 9 o'clock. Next, two iridotomies are made in dry modus with the vitrectomy machine, using the smallest diameter.

The Binderflex is pre-folded in a cartridge, which allows the surgeon to easily take it with his forceps, with the lens already in position.

The lens is inserted through the tunnel or clear corneal incision, watching that the anchor of the leading haptic does not get caught. Once inside, the first anchor is allowed to hang onto the inner circumference of the iris, and letting go with the forceps, allowed the lens to unfold within the eye. Then the second haptic is hung onto the iris, and the lens is rotated towards 3 and 9 o'clock. Once positioned, a haptic forceps is put through the scleral/clear corneal tunnel or paracenteses to grasp and position the haptic-ends (anchors) through the iridotomies. This step is pivotal to a successful operation, and affords a certain learning curve for the right-handed surgeon since one of the haptics has to be inserted with the left hand. The properly positioned end-anchors can be made visible by means of gonioscopy.

We have implanted this IOL in 22 aphakic eyes with excellent results. After both anchors are securely placed in the iridotomies, the optic of the IOL is

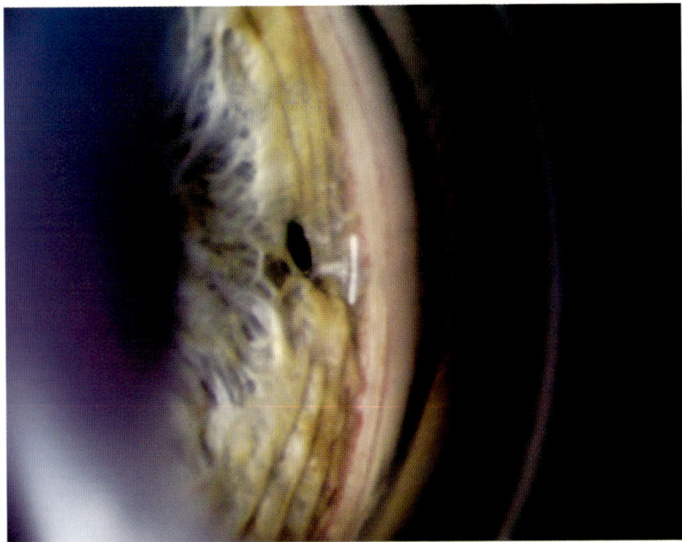

Fig. 7: Gonioscopic view of one of the anchors securely positioned in an iridotomy

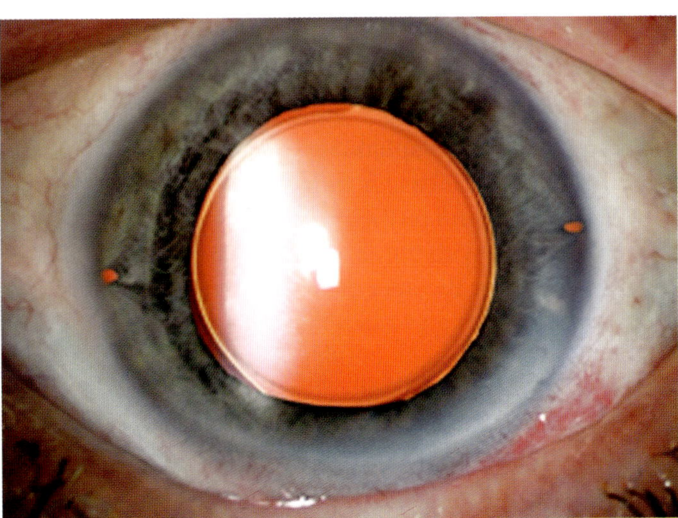

Fig. 8: Postoperatve position of the Binder-IOL after implantation. The lens is perfectly centered and stable

always exactly centered and precisely positioned in the iris plane. The learning curve is somewhat longer compared to the enclavation technique of an iris claw lens. However, the procedure is rapidly adapted with repeated surgery. The Binderflex has the advantage of offering stability in every special dimension with negligible side effects. We had very few complications after these surgeries. A slight early, reversible hyperemia of the iris vessels around the haptic-end anchor disappeared within several weeks. Later-onset, slightly enlarged iridotomies that began three to six months postoperatively also occurred. If the iridotomies had been performed too centrally, an ovalisation of the pupil might occur. The side effects by no means affected the stability of the lens. However, a prerequisite for safe implantation of the anchors is good visibility of the peripheral iris.

The Binder intraocular lens thus combines the advantages of a sutureless technique for aphakic eyes with the stable position and well-known optical properties of a standard PC IOL implanted in the capsular bag or sulcus after cataract extraction.

Furthermore, the Binder IOL can replace the still widely used but laborious and complication-prone scleral or iris suturing techniques of standard posterior chamber intraocular lenses.

Summary

Secondary IOL implantation in aphakic eyes without capsular support remains challenging. Each individual case is different, and the chosen IOL as well as fixation technique will depend on the preoperative pathology of the eye and the experience of the surgeon with the above mentioned methods. We believe that sutureless implantation of the specific lenses mentioned above represents a significant improvement for a visual rehabilitation of these patients in a rapid and atraumatic manner.

25

Laser Cataract Surgery

Kumar J Doctor, Shilpa Kodkany, P Kaushik (India)

Introduction

Cataract surgery is the most common intraocular surgery performed today world wide and ultrasound phacoemulsification is the preferred technique among cataract surgeons. Reduced phaco energy and heat, smaller incisions, improved visual outcomes and efficiency—these are the goals driving advances in cataract phacoemulsification technology. The most negative factor in ultrasound phacoemulsification is the increase in water temperature, which causes an inflammatory response and potential injury to the incision and to the intracameral structures like corneal endothelium, iris, and posterior capsule. To solve these problems, different types of lasers have been developed. Current studies favor the infrared wavelength, particularly the erbium:YAG (Er:YAG) laser (wavelength 2940 nm) and the neodymium:YAG (Nd:YAG) laser (wavelength 1064 nm).

How does Laser Phaco Work?

Both the Er:YAG laser and the Nd:YAG laser use the acoustic effect to fragment cataracts. The energy required by laser surgery is reported to be much lower than that generated by ultrasound, and this could be a significant advantage of the new technology. The principal difference between these 2 lasers is the level of water absorption, i.e. the absorption with the Er:YAG laser is very high and with the Nd:YAG, very low. This determines the manner in which they function. The Er:YAG laser beam can be focused directly on the cataract, and the high tissue water level shields the adjacent tissues from injury. The Nd:YAG laser beam is not totally absorbed at the desired point, and may damage adjacent structures. Hence Er:YAG laser is more popularly used and many multicentric clinical trials have been conducted to study the safety and efficacy of this procedure of **laser phakoemulsification.**

The Er:YAG laser was initially investigated for cataract surgery by Peyman and Katoh and Tsubota in the 1980s

WORDWIDE UNIQUE LASER CATARACT SURGERY SYSTEM

- Laser - phaco - MICS
- No heat at hand piece tip, no corneal burns possible
- Microincision cataract surgery (1.4 mm/1.2 mm in preparation)

Technique of Er: YAG Laser Phaco

The laser procedure is performed using a bimanual technique. The Phacolaser is connected to an optical fiber made of zirconium fluoride and a nontoxic biocompatible quartz tip and the fluidics system from the Sovereign®

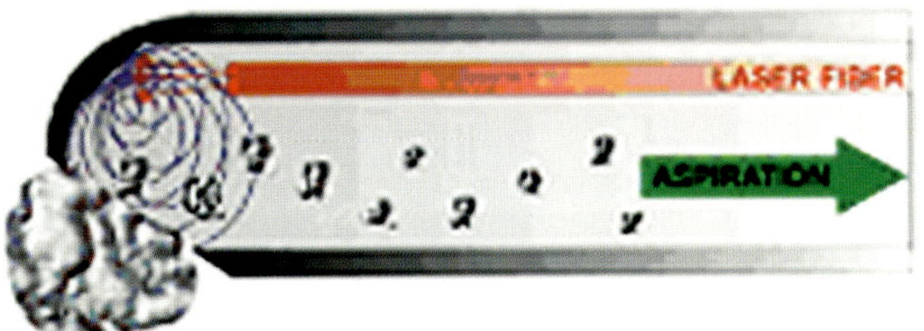

Fig. 1: Laser cataract surgery system

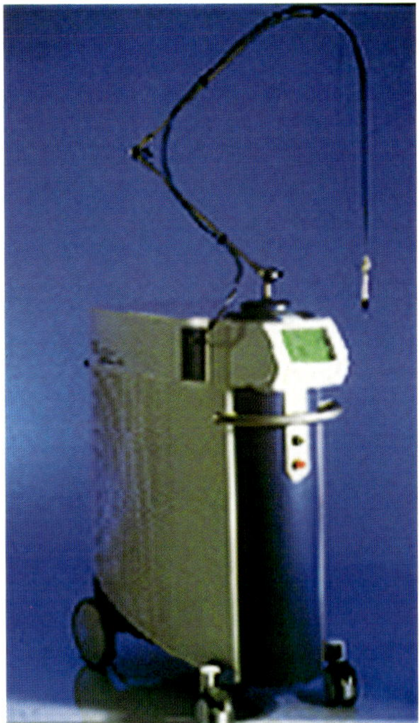

Fig. 2: The Er: YAG laser

phacoemulsification system (AMO). The procedure begins with creation of a 1.2 mm incision in the temporal cornea and a 1.0 mm corneal incision at the 2 o'clock position. The phaco needle is inserted into the first incision with the optical fiber and connected to the aspiration system. The chopper with an irrigation system, which is specifically designed for this surgery, is introduced through the smaller incision. The laser needle has an external diameter of 0.9 mm and an internal diameter of 0.7 mm. A modified needle opening facilitates aspiration of the cortex fragments; there is no need to change the probe to an irrigation/aspiration (I/A) tip, as usually occurs during ultrasound. The 200 μm diameter optical fiber is placed inside the chopper 0.5 mm from the needle opening (which differs from procedures to date) to facilitate suctioning of the cataract fragments and improve the efficacy of the emulsification.

The Er:YAG laser (wavelength 2940 nm), provides maximal water absorption. Erbium radiation is absorbed at all fluencies better than other types of radiation. It has a short penetration depth, 1.0 μm, which produces a small volume of ablated tissue, improving efficacy and minimizing the thermal effects. In addition, the Er:YAG laser has a lower ablation threshold and a greater photovaporization rate than other infrared systems such as the Nd:YAG laser. The Er:YAG laser ablates lens material directly, which may be more effective than disrupting lens material indirectly as with the Nd:YAG laser, which uses a target or photofragmentation chamber.

Advantages of Er: YAG Phaco over Ultrasound Phaco

Erbium laser phacoemulsification is a surgical method that makes the emulsification of softer nuclei under clinical conditions possible with a low rate of complications. For higher nucleus hardnesses, technical and surgical parameters have to be optimized. Advantages of erbium laser phacoemulsification compared to ultrasonic phacoemulsification are less energy transmission into the eye, no heating of anterior chamber, impossibility of corneal burns and easier access in eyes that are deep into the orbit.

Disadvantages of Er: YAG Phaco

The difficulties incurred with the laser surgical procedure depend on cataract hardness and result in longer surgical times, especially with cataract densities of 3+ and 4+. At these levels, the intraocular irrigation time, including phacoemulsification and I/A is longer in patients who had laser surgery than in those who had an ultrasound procedure. The greater hydrodynamic trauma results in greater endothelial cell loss, the development of corneal edema, and the delay in visual recovery.

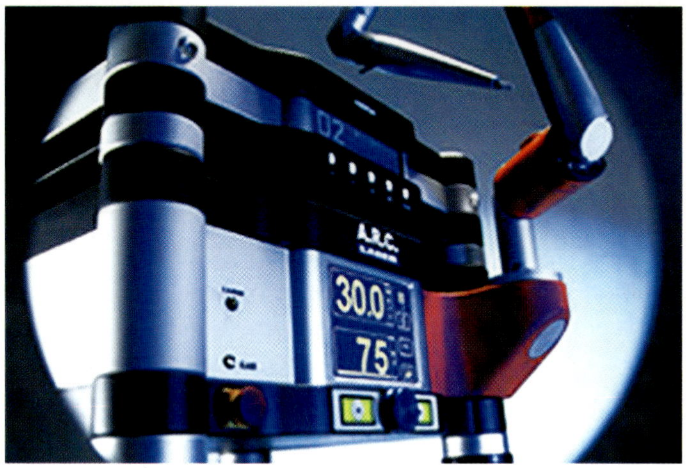

Fig. 3: Venturi fludices – a touch screen control panel

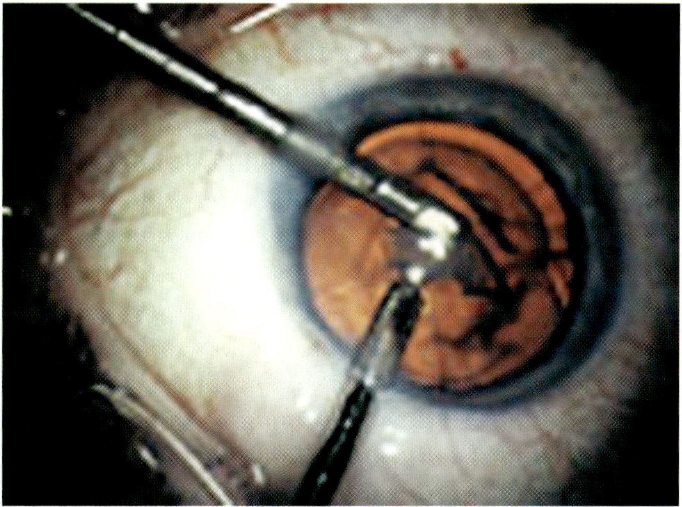

Fig. 4: Ultrasound handpiece port for cataracts

Complications include subclinical cystoid macular edema (CME) diagnosed by fluorescein angiography, irreversible corneal edema, rupture of posterior capsule rupture, elevated IOP level.

Nd:YAG Laser Phacoemulsification

ARC LASER CORPORATION DODICK PHOTOLYSIS

The Dodick Photolysis system, introduced in June 2000, uses Q-switched Nd:YAG laser energy instead of standard ultrasound waves to break up the cataract. The Nd:YAG laser (1,064 nm) systems employ plasma formation and shock wave generation to produce photolysis of lens material. The shock wave results from the impact of laser radiation on a titanium plate. How does it work: First, the surgeon creates a 1.4 mm incision. Surgeons generally use a groove and crack technique with the laser, sculpting in a bimanual fashion and cracking as soon as possible. Alternatively, a prechopping technique may be used as taught by Jack Dodick, MD. He also creates a separate 0.9 mm incision for the infusion probe. He then inserts the laser aspiration probe through the first incision. The probe delivers laser energy via a quartz fiber onto a titanium target at the end of the probe. When the laser energy hits the titanium target, it creates shockwaves—the effect is like a 'mini earthquake.' It generates laser shock waves at 200 to 400 nanoseconds by striking a titanium target at the end of the aspirating hand piece. The system includes ***Venturi fluidics, a touch-screen control panel*** and an ***ultrasound hand piece*** port for cataracts that are too dense for laser phaco.

A significant disadvantage of the system is that it doesn't work well on dense nuclei. The total time that the tip is in the eye varies with the grade of nucleus, from 2.15 minutes for 1+ nuclear sclerosis to 9.8 minutes for 3+ nuclear sclerosis.

FDA-APPROVED

The only FDA-approved laser system is the Dodick Photolysis, Q-switched Nd:YAG system (A.R.C. Laser Corp.).

Nonetheless, laser is safe and efficacious. It provides cold phaco and small incisions, among other advantages. The addition of ultrasound capabilities to laser machines allows surgeons to switch back and forth between modalities for denser cataracts.

Conclusion

Laser phakoemulsification with either Er: YAG or Nd:YAG do help in reducing the energy levels in the eye, they work well while dealing with soft cataracts but for hard cataracts their efficacy and safety are still questionable.

26

Glued IOL

Amar Agarwal, A Dhivya, Soosan Jacob,
Athiya Agarwal, Chandresh Baid, Ashok Garg (India)

Introduction

We devised a new surgical technique for implantation of a posterior chamber intraocular lens (IOL) in eyes with deficient or absent posterior capsule with the use of biological glue. We used a quick acting surgical fibrin sealant derived from human blood plasma, with both hemostatic and adhesive properties.

Scleral Fixated IOL

Intraocular lens implantation (IOL) in eyes that lack posterior capsular support has been accomplished in the past, by means of iris fixated IOL, anterior chamber intraocular lens and transscleral IOL fixation through the ciliary sulcus or pars plana. Surgical expertise, prolonged surgical time, suture induced inflammation, suture degradation, and delayed IOL subluxation or dislocation due to broken suture are some of the limitations in sutured scleral fixated intraocular lenses (SFIOL). It is also difficult and time consuming requiring minute and perfect adjustment of suture length and tension to ensure good centration of SFIOL.

Fibrin Glue

Fibrin glue has been used previously in various medical specialities as a hemostatic agent to arrest bleeding, seal tissues and as an adjunct to wound healing. The fibrin kit we used was ReliSeal™ (Reliseal, Reliance Life Sciences, India). It is available in a sealed pack, which contains freeze dried human fibrinogen (20 mg/0.5 ml), freeze dried human thrombin(250 IU/0.5 ml), aprotinin solution (1500 kiu in 0.5 ml), one ampoule of sterile water, four 21 G needles, two 20 G blunt application needles and an applicator with two mixing chambers and one plunger guide.

Surgical Technique

After inserting the infusion cannula or anterior chamber maintainer, localized peritomy is done. Two partial thickness limbal based scleral flaps about 4 mm × 4 mm are created exactly 180 degrees diagonally apart and about 1.5 mm from the limbus. This is followed by vitrectomy via pars plana or anterior route to remove all vitreous traction. Two straight sclerotomies with a 22 G needle are made about 1.5 mm from the limbus under the existing scleral flaps. The sclerotomies are positioned such a way that the superior one lies close to the upper edge of the flap and the inferior one close to the lower edge of the flap. A scleral tunnel incision is then prepared about 2 mm from the limbus for introducing the IOL. While the IOL is being introduced with the left hand of the surgeon using a McPherson forceps, an end gripping 25 G micro rhexis forceps (Micro Surgical Technology, USA) is passed through the inferior sclerotomy.

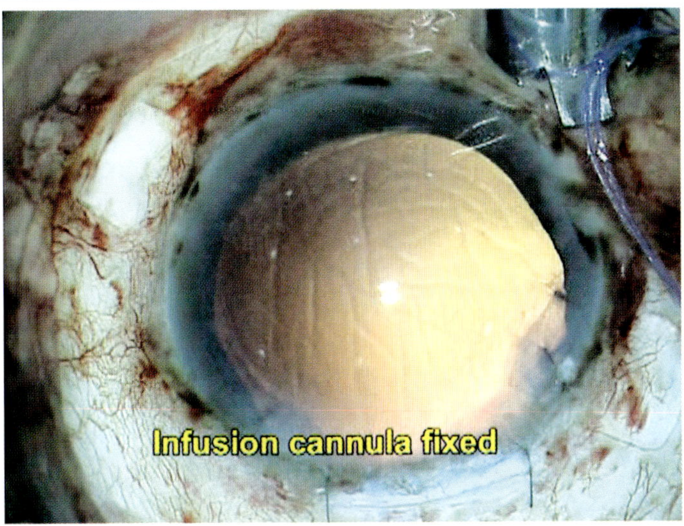

Fig. 1: Scleral flaps prepared 180 degrees diagonally apart. Note the infusion cannula fixed in and eye without any capsule

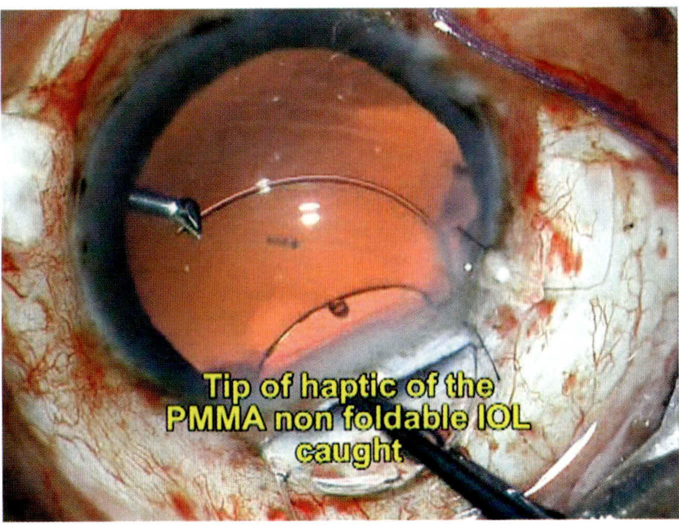

Fig. 2: Tip of the haptic grabbed by the 25 gauge microrhexis forceps (MST, USA) and then that haptic is externalized under the scleral flap

The tip of the leading haptic is then grasped with the microrhexis forceps, pulled through the inferior sclerotomy following the curve of the haptic and is externalized under the inferior scleral flap. Similarly, the trailing haptic is also externalized through the superior sclerotomy under the scleral flap. Then, the reconstituted fibrin glue thus prepared is injected through the cannula of the double syringe delivery system under the superior and inferior scleral flaps. Local pressure is given over the flaps for about 10 to 20 seconds for the formation of fibrin polypeptides. The anterior chamber maintainer or the infusion cannula is removed. Conjunctiva is also closed with the same fibrin glue.

In case of those patients who had a luxated IOL, similar lamellar scleral flaps as described earlier were made and the luxated IOL haptic was then grasped with the 25 gauge rhexis forceps and exteriorized and glued under the scleral flaps. The haptic of the IOL if protruding beyond the scleral flap can be tucked in a tunnel created in the sclera. Our follow-up anterior segment OCT showed postoperative perfect scleral flap adhesion as early as day 1 and continues to remain well maintained at one week and one month.

Discussion

This fibrin glue assisted sutureless PC IOL implantation technique as described by us would be useful in a myriad of clinical situations where scleral fixated IOLs are indicated, such as, luxated IOL, dislocated IOL, zonulopathy or secondary IOL implantation. In dislocated posterior chamber PMMA IOL, the same IOL can be repositioned thereby reducing the need for further manipulation. Externalisation of the greater part of the haptics along its curvature stabilises the axial positioning of the IOL and thereby prevents any IOL tilt. In the 12 eyes of our 12 patients, no complications like postoperative inflammation, hyphema, decenteration, glaucoma or corneal edema were seen after a regular follow-up till now. We expect less incidence of UGH syndrome in fibrin glue assisted IOL implantation as compared to sutured scleral fixated IOL. This is because, in the former the IOL is well stabilized and stuck onto the scleral bed and thereby, has decreased intraocular mobility whereas in the latter, there is increased possibilty of IOL movement or persistent rub over the ciliary body. Visually significant complications due to late subluxation which has been known to occur in sutured scleral fixated IOL may also be prevented as sutures are totally avoided in this technique. Moreover, the frequent complications of secondary IOL implantation like secondary glaucoma, cystoid macular edema or bullous keratopathy were not seen in any of our patients. Another important advantage of this technique is the prevention of suture related complications like suture erosion, suture knot exposure or dislocation of IOL after suture disintegration or broken suture. Chances of scleral melt and haptic exposure is not increased by this technique except possibly, in high risk patients like rheumatoid arthritis.

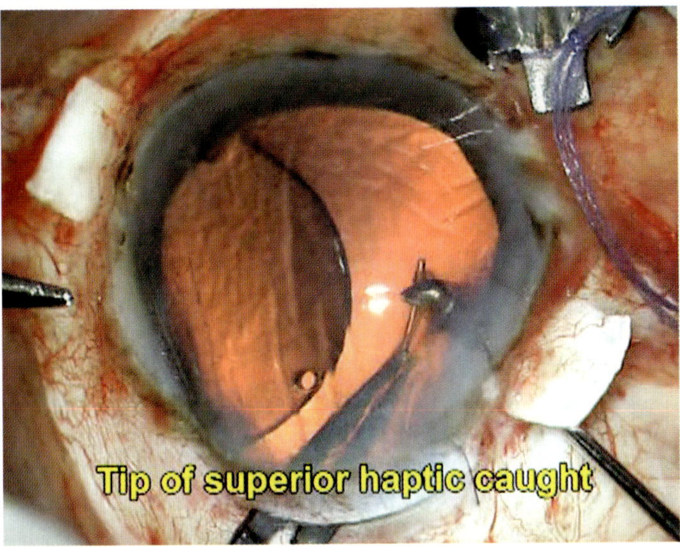

Fig. 3: Superior haptic grabbed by the 25 gauge microrhexis forceps (MST, USA) and then externalized under the scleral flap

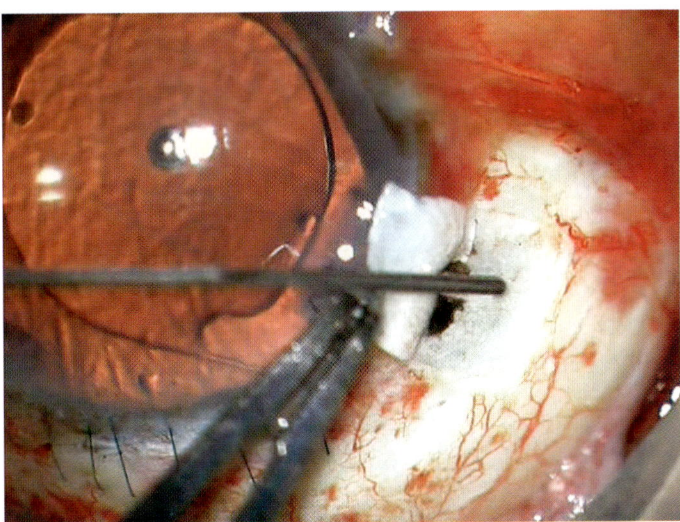

Fig. 4: Fibrin glue applied. Note the haptic which is externalized

The other advantage of this technique is the rapidity and ease of surgery. Since all the steps of tying the difficult to handle 10-0 prolene suture to the IOL haptic eyelets, the time required to ensure good centration before tying down the knots as well as time for suturing scleral flaps and closing conjunctiva are done away with, the total surgical time is significantly reduced. It is also easier and does not require much surgical expertise to use the 25 gauge forceps to grasp and exteriorize the haptic. Fibrin glue takes only 20 seconds to act in the scleral bed and it helps in adhesion as well as hemostasis. Fibrin glue has been shown to provide airtight closure and by the time the fibrin starts degrading, surgical adhesions would have already occurred in the scleral bed. This is well shown in the commercially available fibrin glue that we used is virus inactivated and is checked for viral antigen with polymerase chain reaction, hence the chances of transmission of infection is very low. But with tissue derivatives, there is always a theoretical possibility of transmission of viral infections, therefore it is mandatory to get informed consent from the patient before the procedure. Though the use of fibrin glue in ophthalmology is considered off-label, it has been successfully used in the eye since long. Its various uses in the eye include repair of lacerated canaliculi to seal full thickness macular holes, to seal cataract incisions, corneal perforations, and traumatic lens capsule perforations, It has also been used for temporary closure of scleral flaps after trabeculectomy in eyes with hypotony, conjunctival fistula closure conjunctival autografts, and amniotic membrane transplantation.

Gabor et al have shown sutureless scleral IOL fixation by placing the IOL haptic in a scleral tunnel. Our technique differed from other sutureless methods by use of the fibrin glue which enhances the rate of adhesion with hemostasis. We also used scleral flaps as in conventional sutured SFIOLs and this makes the learning curve very simple. There is also no danger of intra-ocular infection gaining entry through the tunnel as the fibrin glue hermetically seals the flaps leaving behind no possible entry route for microbes. There was no glue induced intraocular inflammation in any of our patients and all 12 eyes had clear media on the postoperative visits. Scleral indentation performed in the operated eyes showed no change in the axial positioning of the IOL. After one month of follow-up, we found no IOL decentration or any other complications in any of the operated 12 eyes.

Summary

Fibrin glue assisted sutureless PC IOL implantation is appropriate for eyes with deficient or absent posterior capsule and this can be performed easily with the available IOL designs, instruments and with less surgical time. However, a longer duration followup might be necessary to judge the long-term functional and anatomical results of the procedure.

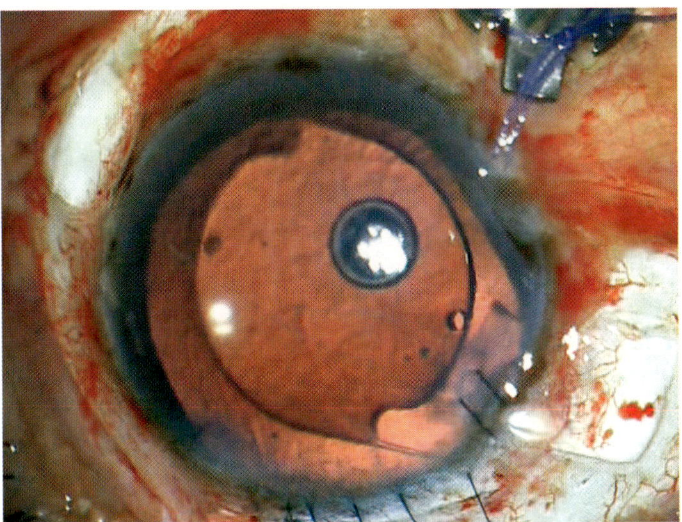

Fig. 5: PC IOL well positioned and centered

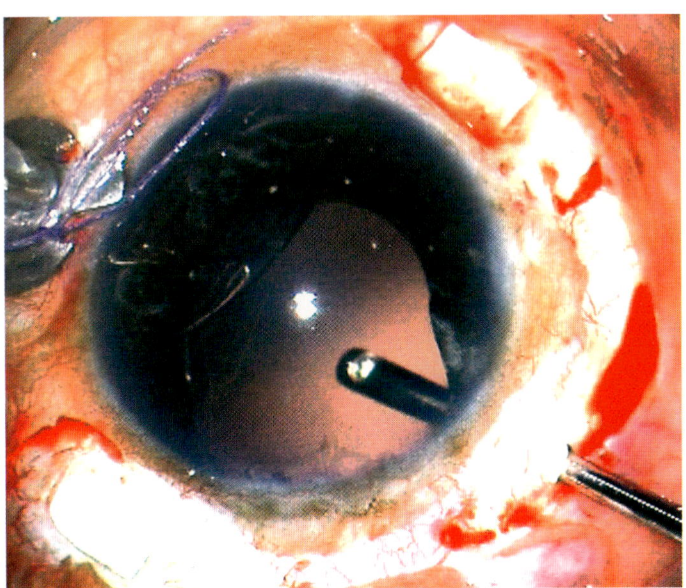

Fig. 6A: Subluxated IOL. Note the infusion cannula fixed and scleral flaps prepared. Vitrectomy being done

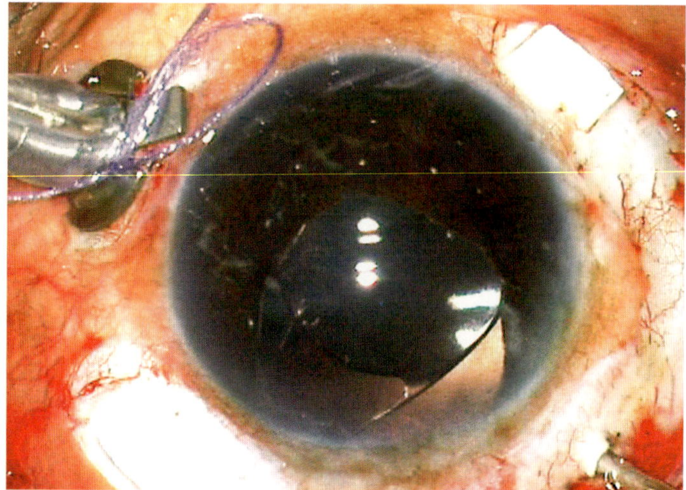

Fig. 6B: Haptics externalized under the scleral flaps and IOL well centered

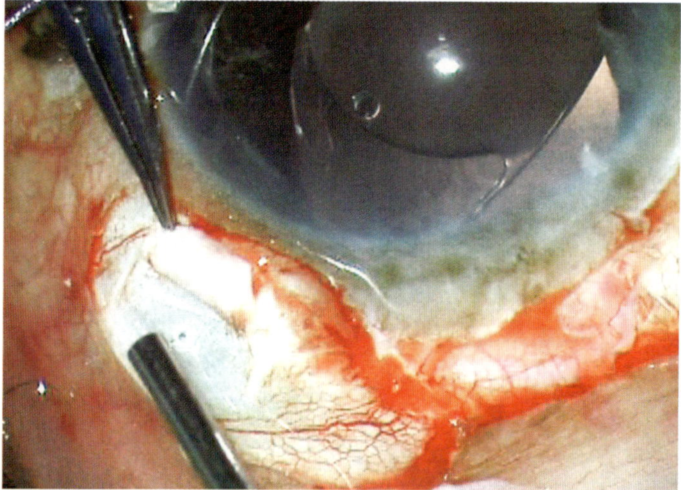

Fig. 6C: Fibrin glue applied and scleral flaps seal the haptic of the IOL

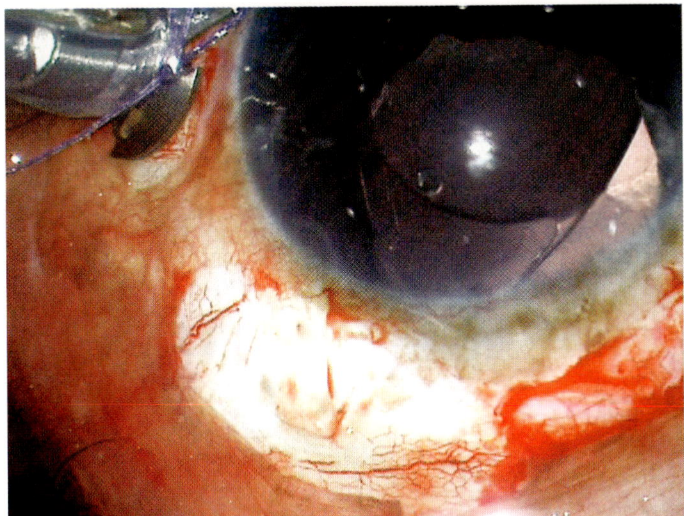

Fig. 6D: IOL haptic now glued by the fibrin glue

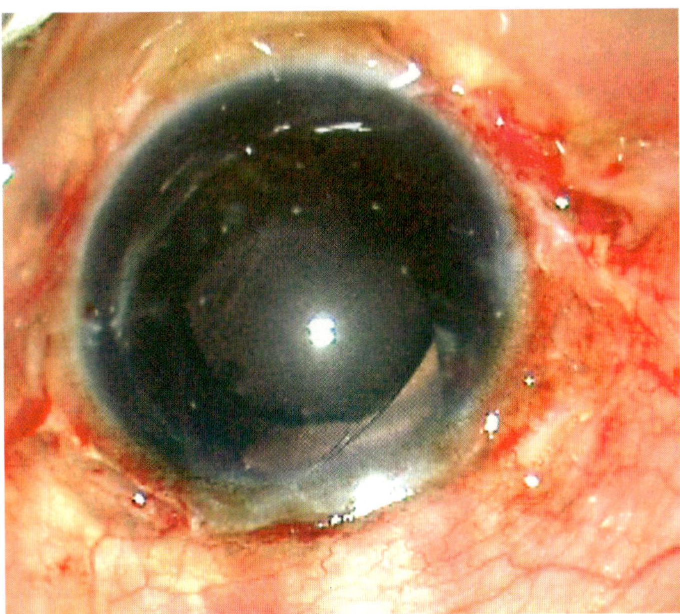

Fig. 6E: Fibrin glue seals the conjunctiva

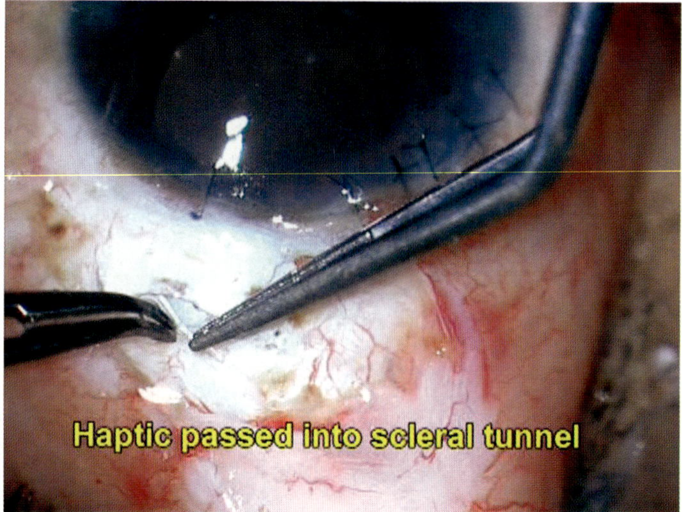

Fig. 7: IOL haptic tucked through a scleral tunnel

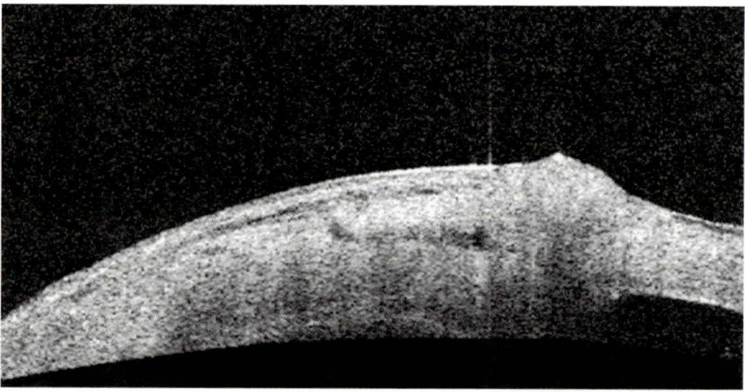

Fig. 8A: Anterior segment OCT of scleral flap

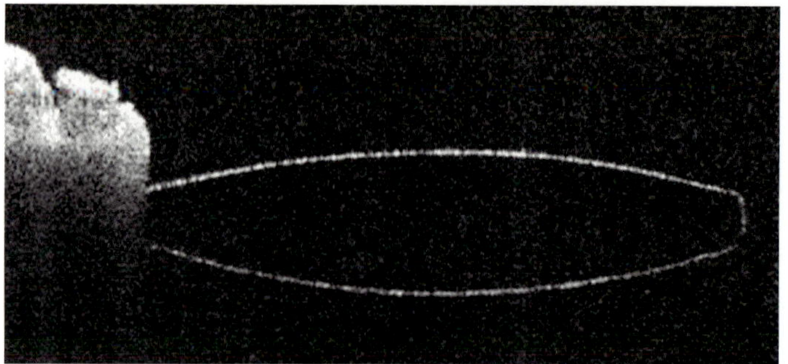

Fig. 8B: Anterior segment OCT of the IOL. Note IOL well centered

27

PCO Prevention and Management in MICS

Frederic Hehn (France)

Introduction

None can prevent posterior capsule opacification (PCO), which results from the proliferation of the lens epithelial cells (LEC) that remain in the lens bag, especially in the equatorial region. Depending on the length of the follow-up, the PCO occurs and has been reported in up to 80% of eyes having a cataract extraction with an IOL Implantation.

Albert Galand developed in 1996 the concept of a systematic posterior continuous curvilinear capsulorhexis (PCCC), but there is some risks of retinal detachment, and the learning curve of this technique is hard. Marie-josé Tassignon developed the concept of 'the bag in the lens ' to avoid the PCO, but the stability of the lens and the realization of this difficult technique are in concern. The square edge IOL design provides a lower rate of PCO, but does not eradicate it.

With MICS (Microincision cataract surgery), bimanual technique consisting in separate irrigation and aspiration; it allows microincision of 1.5 mm width for entirely procedure from corneal incision until IOL implantation. But in regard of PCO the problem is the same that it was in conventional 3.2 incision cataract surgery.

The well known preventing factors of a PCO are: no IOL decentration, a 360° IOL overlapping of capsulorhexis, an ablation of visco-elastic behind the optic, a reduction of the retro-optical space, no folds on posterior capsule the speed of the capsular bend formation, the adhesion between the optic and posterior capsule by fibronectin, IOL materials, and of course Square Edge IOL design. But only a total cleaning of anterior and equatorial LEC could be efficient to avoid the PCO.

The LEC gives always anterior or posterior capsular bag opacification in the shape of fibrosis or pearls and sometimes shrinkage with IOL displacement.

The problem of PCO is not only the cost and the morbidity of Nd:yag capsulotomy, but the real challenge is to keep a soft capsular bag. With a soft capsular bag, LEC free, it will be possible to restore accommodation in pseudophakic eyes with the "phacoersatz" and avoid to practice anterior vitrectomy and PCCC in children's cataract surgery.

There are only two ways to avoid PCO, Block LEC migration, or kill the LEC.

Block LEC Migration

There are two possibilities to block cell migration ; the first is to block them by IOL shape " the square edge", the second is to block LEC in equatorial region with a capsular ring.

SQUARE EDGE

What are we speaking about ? We are speaking about cell. The LEC become 'fibroblast like' from 10 μm diameter << IOL' optic diameter (500 μ or more).

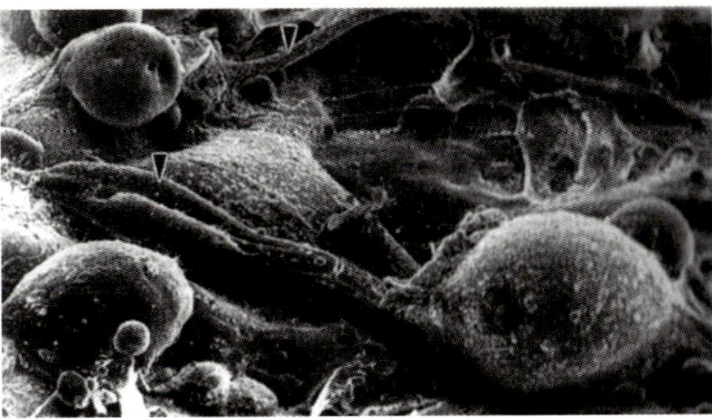

Fig. 1: "Fibroblast like": At time of pearls and fibrosis game is over

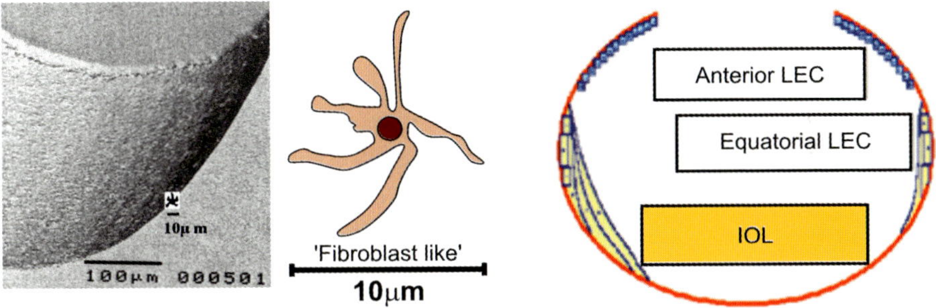

Figs 2 and 3: Escobar-Gomez a SEM of the SA30AL at the scale of 100 μm. (On this figure a virtual 'fibroblast like' wide of 10 μm has been drawn by the author)

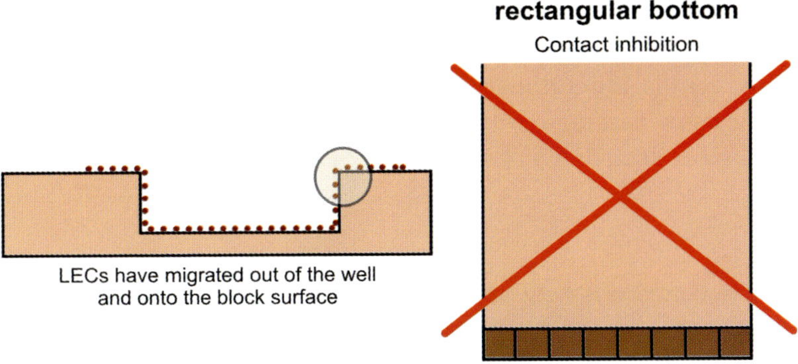

Figs 4 and 5: Failure of discontinuous bend to prevent LEC migration *in vitro* Bhermi GS, Spalton DJ

'Fibroblasts like' have got *'arms and legs and hands and feet'* and they try to conquer the retro-optical space. Be sure that 'Fibroblast like' are not afraid of a SE IOL design and that they can pass it round. Obviously the square edge shape concept does not exist at the cellular scale ; because the fibroblast like cells are not at all cubic, and they have got three-dimensional coordinates. Secondly, the IOL itself at the cellular scale of 10 µm is not smooth at all and it is not perfectly polished but rough and porous.

At the scale of 10 µm the IOL optic material, seems to be porous and rough, and the SE sharp of the IOL becomes a very academic point of view. That the reason why some authors demonstrate a failure of discontinuous bend to prevent LEC migration *in vitro*.

But is there nothing right at all about a SE IOL design effect ? Some studies show there is a SE effect on the PCO regardless of the type of IOL material Other studies show that the difference in terms of PCO rate is due to the IOL material, and not statistically due to the SE effect. Obviously both factors, SE IOL design and type of IOL's material, influence the PCO rate .We now know that, of course, there is a SE effect but it is not a contact cellular inhibition, but it is a mechanical tension effect. Boyce, Bhermi and Spalton have shown, by a mathematical model, that in fact a SE IOL design exerts twice more pressure than a round edge at the point P . This 'P' point is the contact between the corner of the edge and the posterior capsule. This high pressure blocks the LEC migration.

Capsular Rings: CBR and CTR Respective Actions Against PCO

Many other systems failed to completely clean the capsular bag without any risk for the zonula, the endothelium or the posterior capsule. Only a ring is able to go to the equatorial region, to try to mechanically block the LEC, or to block it by a disposable drug delivery system like 5FU and so on...

CBR

There are two methods with rings ; the first is to block LEC in equatorial region by a CBR : capsular bending ring which is large enough 700 µm, that the study of NISHI, but with this technique, because the CBR is large it avoid the collapse and adhesion between anterior and posterior capsule (which increase the risk of LEC migration)

Nishi O, Nishi K Study

HEMA IOL HM60 STORZ + 13 mm CTR PMMA square edge not polished 0.7 mm width and 0.2 mm thickness One eye IOL + CTR Second eye only IOL 2 years follow up.

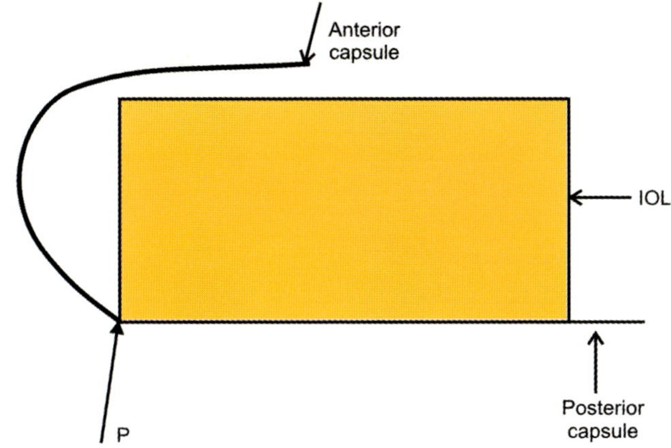

Fig. 6: A square edge exerts twice more pressure on posterior capsule than a round edge

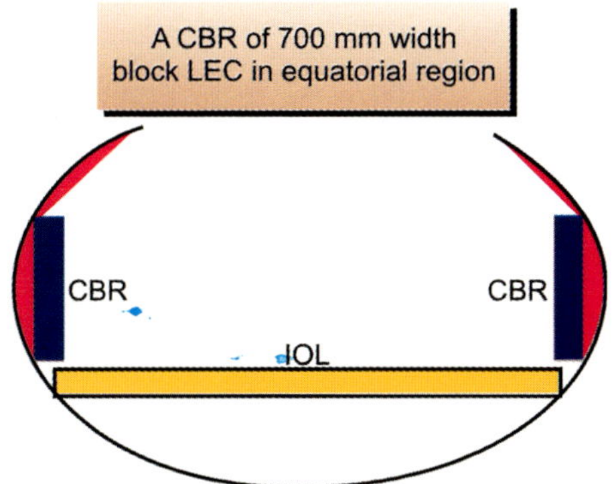

Fig. 7: Capsular bending ring inside the capsular bag

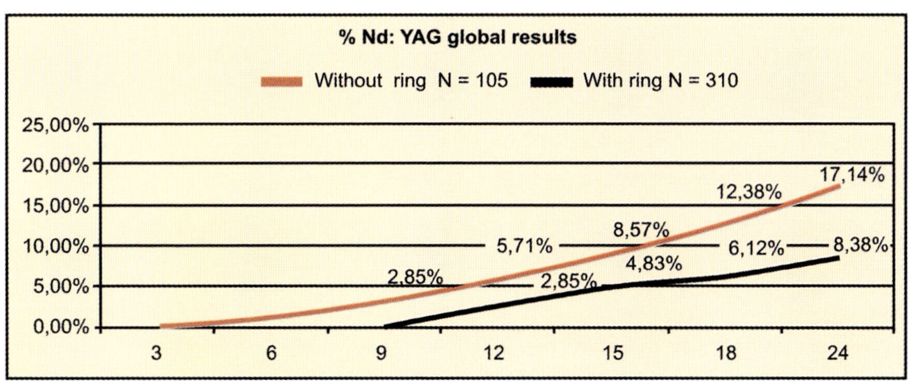

Fig. 8: Global mean results % Nd:YAG for PCO 24 months follow-up

84 eyes of 42 patients EPCO computer image analysis

Rate of Nd:yag capsulotomy	5%	ring	20%	without
Folds post cap	0%	ring	25 %	without

CTR

HEHN F: Clinical trial

At the contrary we explore the way of classical CTR which increases the speed of the adhesion between anterior and post capsule. We have analyzed 415 eyes with 24 months follow up. Two groups of patients with (n = 310) and without (n = 105) a CTR, during the months after a cataract surgery and we have compared the rate of Nd yag capsulotomy and EPCO grading for evaluate the PCO. We have got 3 groups of 3 kinds of IOL's materials. Hydrophilic acrylic (Stabibag Ioltech), silicone (Clariflex AMO) and hydrophobic acrylic(SA60AT Alcon). The CTR was simply a choice from the same laboratory than the IOL: Tensiobag Ioltech, Reform Alcon, Injectoring AMO.

TABLE 1: Rate % of Nd:yag for PCO at 24 months follow up

Hydrophobic	without CTR	n=41	12,19%(5)	with CTR	n= 96	5,20%(5)	p<0.01
Hydrophilic	without CTR	n=33	21, 21%(7)	with CTR	n=106	10,37%(11)	p<0.001
Silicone	without CTR	n=31	19,35%(6)	with CTR	n=108	9,25%(10)	p<0.01

EPCO Results

Globally EPCO score index is less with CTR : 0.254 than without : 0.396 p< 0.01

TABLE 2: At one year follow-up in 23 eyes EPCO score is less with CTR than without

Hydrophobic	without CTR N = 3	0,229	With CTR	N = 5	0,107	p<0,01
Hydrophilic	without CTR N = 2	0,523	With CTR	N = 4	0,360	p<0,01
Silicone	without CTR N = 4	0,459	With CTR	N = 5	0,317	p<0,01

When the ring is inside the bag, it exerts a tangential tension of the posterior capsule all around 360°. Therefore a CTR increases the pressure at the 'P' point and then the SE tension effect of IOL, to mechanically block the LEC migration. That is the most fundamental effect of a CTR against the PCO but it is not the only one.

Previous research, by Rupert **Menapace** suggested that capsular tension rings prevent the PCO through more than one mechanism. First, the ring causes posterior capsule stretching, which reduces the IOL capsule distance. The well

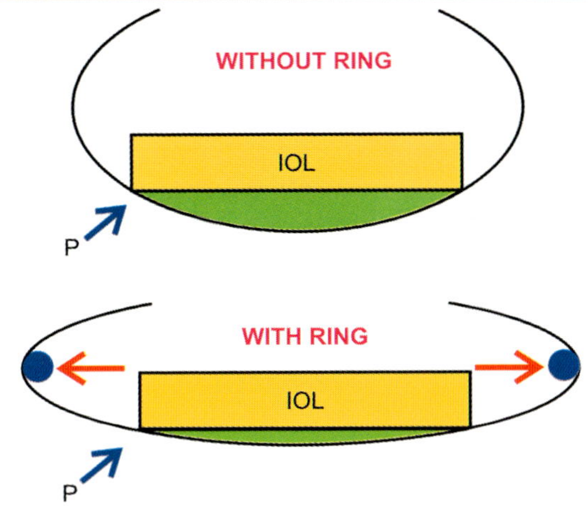

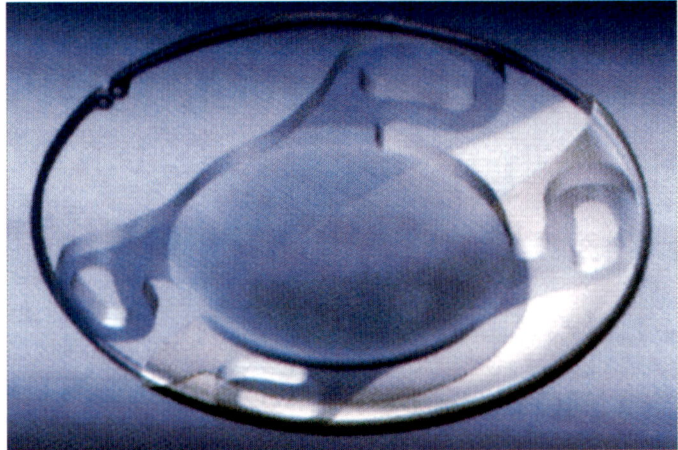

Figs 9 and 10: Effect of a capsular tension ring inside the bag

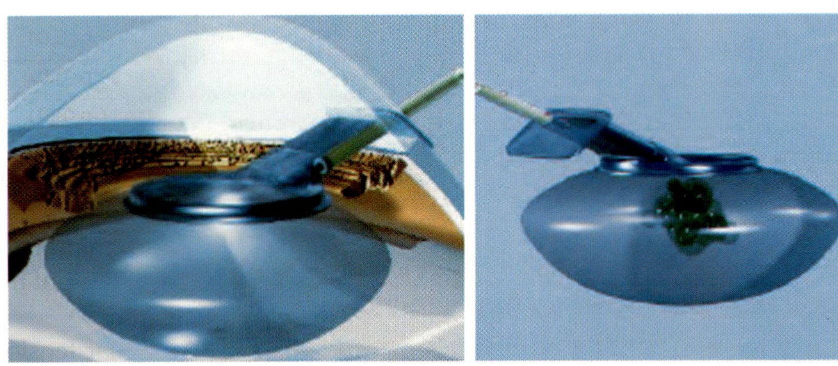

Fig. 11

tension of the capsular bag reduces the retro-optical space: the CTR increases the 'no space no cell ' theory. The immediate well tension of the bag with the ring (before the natural retraction of the capsular bag), increases the speed of the capsular bend formation, before the LEC get enough time to conquer the retro-optical space: the CTR increases the CBI (Capsular bending index), which is fundamental, to avoid the LEC migration. The instantaneous tension of the bag by the ring facilitates the capsular adhesion between the posterior capsule and the IOL optic by fibronectin, laminin or collagen type IV, which are present on capsular or on LEC surface, and so on, are free to absorb the IOL surface after the break of the blood aqueous barrier: the CTR increases the 'sandwich' theory.

I expect so that a CTR would probably increase the LEC destruction by a direct cell compression. Other well known properties of the ring can be combined to reduce the PCO rate, like the better long terms centration for all lens with a CTR. CTR facilitates the equatorial LEC removal by an IOL rotation inside the capsular bag without any risk for the zonula, it facilitates the retro-optical viscoelastic ablation too, according to the 'no space no cell' theory, it facilitates the anterior capsular bag cleaning to prevent capsular shrinkage. Eventually, a CTR decreases capsular fold of posterior capsule and then it avoids the LEC migration along the folds.

Ten specific CTR preventing PCO factors :

1 The CTR increases the pressure at the 'p' point and then the SE IOL design tension effect.
2. The CTR reduces the retro-optical space too, according to the 'no space, no cell' theory.
3. The CTR increases the speed of the capsular bend formation.
4. The CRT facilitates the adhesion between the capsule and the IOL according to the 'sandwich' theory.
5. The CTR probably makes some equatorial LEC destruction by direct cell compression.
6. The CTR prevents IOL decentration, deformation and tilting with soft IOL.
7. The CTR facilitates the equatorial LEC removal by an IOL rotation inside the capsular bag.
8. The CTR facilitates the retro-optical viscoelastic ablation too, according to the 'no space no cell' theory.
9. The CTR facilitates the anterior capsular bag cleaning to prevent capsular shrinkage.
10 The CTR decreases the capsular folds of posterior capsule.

Kill the LEC

1. **Perfect capsule™:** This system, which is able to kill the LEC by hypo-osmolarity. But is there some risk for endothelium if the suction leaks ?

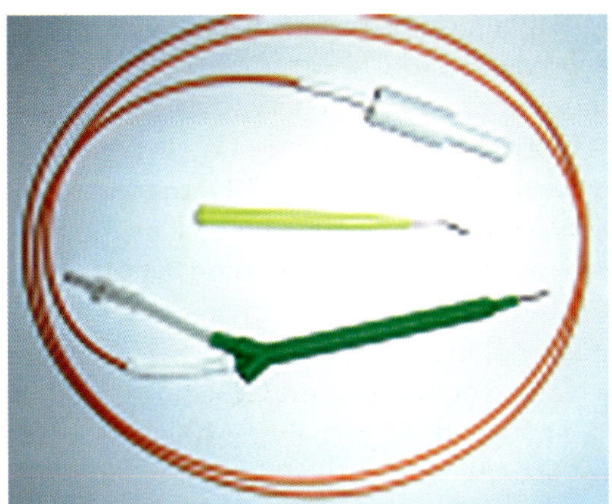

Fig. 12

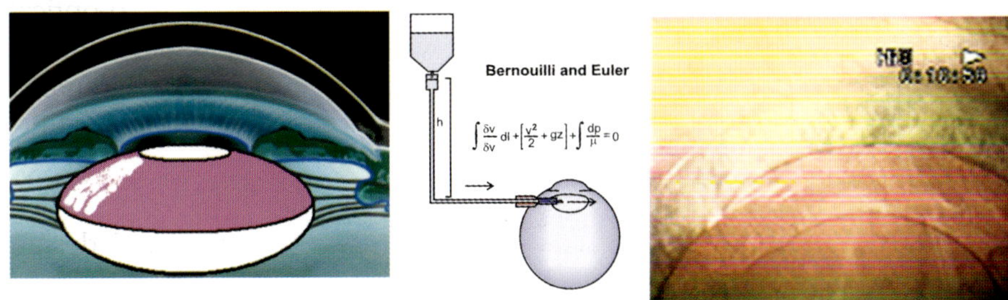

Fig. 13

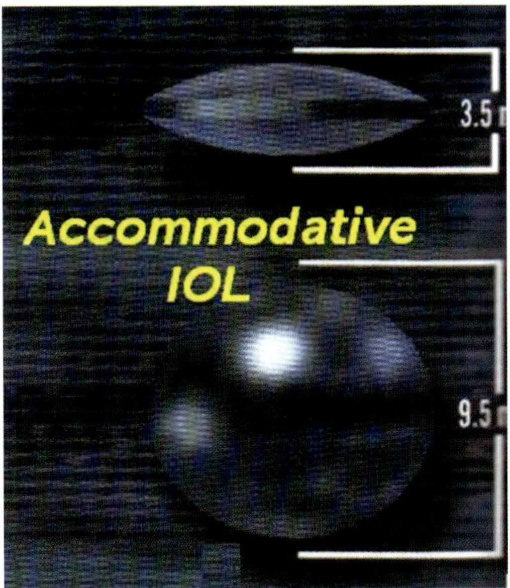

Fig. 14: Phacoersatz

Actually perfect capsule device is not available for MICS because it needs a 3.2 mm width cornea incision.

2. **Aqualase®:** An hot hydrojet, able to hydrolyse the nucleus of the crystalline. Is there any possibilities to hydrolyse the LEC in equatorial region? Actually aqualase is compatible with bimanual technique, but not with MICS because the needle of aqualase handpiece needs of 3.2 incision, the next generation of aqualase certainly will be compatible with MICS.
3. **Phaco-laser** (the Dodick photolysis) is compatible with MICS, recently at ARVO 2004 meeting, it has been shown the possibility of direct LEC destruction by Nd yag laser on anterior capsule.
4. **CBJ: Cleanbagjet®** is a new phaco handpiece, which produce a micro hydrojet able to clean the LEC even in equatorial region, developed by IOL tech laboratories, first clinical results are expected at ASCRS 2005 congress.

Conclusion

With MICS or not, PCO remains the really final frontier in cataract surgery. Until we will not be able to take off or kill entirely the equatorial LEC, PCO occurs irreversibly from month to month after cataract surgery. The more IOL becomes softer smaller and thinner CTR will take a greater place especially against PCO. Without PCO it will be possible to treat accommodation in pseudophakic eye and perform cataract surgery as easily in children than in adult without anterior vitrectomy nor PCCC.

Index

E

F

G

H

I

K

L

M

N

O

P

S

T

V

W

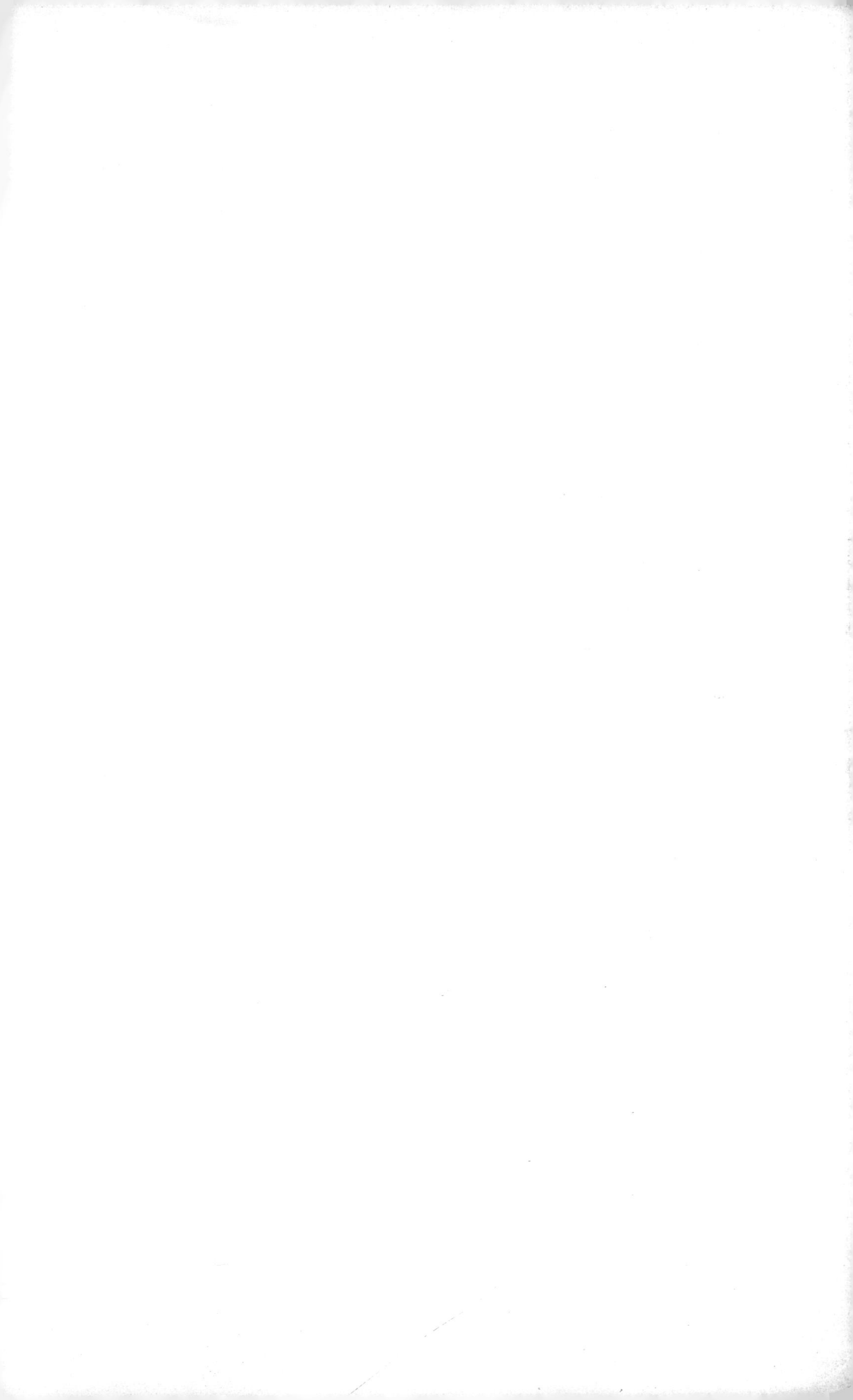